PEDIATRIC ONCOLOGY

Nai-Kong V. Cheung
Susan L. Cohn
(Eds.)

Neuroblastoma

With 51 Figures and 48 Tables

Springer

Library of Congress
Control Number 2004113134
ISBN-10 3-540-40841-X
Springer Berlin Heidelberg New York
ISBN-13 978-3-540-40841-3
Springer Berlin Heidelberg New York
ISSN 1613-5318

Nai-Kong V. Cheung, MD, PhD
(e-mail: cheungn@mskcc.org)
Department of Pediatrics, Memorial Sloan-Kettering Cancer Center, 1275 York Avenue, New York, NY 10021, USA

Susan L. Cohn, MD
(e-mail: scohn@northwestern.edu)
Department of Pediatrics and the Comprehensive Robert H. Lurie Cancer Center, Northwestern University, Feinberg School of Medicine, Children's Memorial Hospital
2300 Children's Plaza, Chicago, IL 60614, USA

Springer is a part of Springer Science+Business Media

springeronline.com

Printed in Germany

Medical Editor: Dr. Julia Heidelmann, Heidelberg, Germany
Desk Editor: Meike Stoeck, Heidelberg, Germany
Cover design: Erich Kirchner, Heidelberg, Germany
Layout: Bernd Wieland, Heidelberg, Germany
Production: Pro Edit GmbH, Heidelberg, Germany
Reproduction and typesetting: AM-productions GmbH, Wiesloch, Germany

21/3151 – 5 4 3 2 1 0
Printed on acid-free paper

Preface

The rapid advances in our understanding of the biology and treatment of neuroblastoma make it difficult to keep up to date. The clinical facets of neuroblastoma are endlessly fascinating. Its "natural history" overtly displays the difference between cancer and a truly extraordinary non-malignant proliferative disease. An interesting and potentially promising research emphasis is to unravel the difference between the "good" and "bad" forms of the disease. Our interest in neuroblastoma was kindled by clinical observations going back many decades. For example, is it likely that neuroblastoma "metastasizes" from one adrenal to the other and to the posterior mediastinum, or that malignant secondary deposits in these three unlikely sites will disappear spontaneously? Our early observations of this phenomenon were made in the days when there were no effective treatments for neuroblastoma so it was easier willy-nilly to observe the natural history.

We have seen disease wax and wane over time, such as skin lesions which became increasingly mature with each new "crop"; thus, the last one seen at 36 months was diagnosed as a neurofibroma. The results coming from the screening programs underline these concepts. They have shown that many more infants actually harbor occult neuroblastoma than are diagnosed clinically (in the nonscreened cohort population). This establishes that most such foci would have regressed spontaneously had they not been detected through screening. Observations such as these suggest that 4S neuroblastoma could teach us more about what clonal growth implies than clonal growth teaches us about neuroblastoma.

Obviously neuroblastoma can be a relentless, malignant disease, and these children need far better therapies than we now can muster. But the future may not lie so much in new classes of compounds or even drug adjuvants. It lies, instead, in the final understanding of what makes neuroblastoma mature into ganglioneuroma or, even more importantly, what prompts it to disappear spontaneously. Success will be measured when widespread disease in children with high-risk neuroblastoma is made to vanish through molecular genetic manipulations. Then cure will have achieved its true and very special meaning: disappearance of a life-threatening malignant disease without incurring the side effects of currently available avenues of treatment.

Audrey E. Evans
Professor of Pediatrics, Emeritus at the University of Pennsylvania, Senior Physician, Children's Hospital of Philadelphia, Philadelphia, Pennsylvania

Giulio J. D'Angio
Professor of Radiation Oncology, Radiology and Pediatrics, Emeritus at the University of Pennsylvania, Philadelphia, Pennsylvania

Contents

13 Management of Neurologic Complications

Kim Kramer, Michael R. Pranzatelli

14 Immunology and Immunotherapy

Nai-Kong V. Cheung, Paul M. Sondel

15 Differentiation and Retinoids

Carol J. Thiele, C. Patrick Reynolds

16 Angiogenesis
Darrell J. Yamashiro, Susan L. Cohn

17 Experimental Therapeutics and Preclinical Models
Jennifer K. Peterson, Peter J. Houghton

18 Late Effects of Treatment
Caroline Laverdière, James Gurney, Charles A. Sklar

19 Perspectives and Future Directions
Nai-Kong V. Cheung, Susan L. Cohn

Contributors

Sara J. Abramson, MD
(e-mail: abramsos@mskcc.org)
Department of Radiology,
Memorial Sloan-Kettering Cancer Center,
1275 York Avenue, New York, NY 10021, USA

Inge M. Ambros, MD
(e-mail: inge.ambros@ccri.univie.ac.at)
Children's Cancer Research Institute,
St. Anna Kinderspital, Kinderspitalgasse 6,
1090 Vienna, Austria

Peter F. Ambros, PhD
(e-mail: peter.ambros@ccri.univie.ac.at)
Children's Cancer Research Institute,
St. Anna Kinderspital, Kinderspitalgasse 6,
1090 Vienna, Austria

Frank Berthold, MD
(e-mail: Frank.Berthold@medizin.uni-koeln.de)
Children's Hospital, Department of Pediatric
Oncology and Hematology, University of Cologne,
Joseph-Stelzmann-Strasse 9, 50924 Cologne,
Germany

Garrett M. Brodeur, MD
(e-mail: brodeur@email.chop.edu)
Division of Oncology, The Children's Hospital
of Philadelphia and the University of Pennsylvania,
Abramson Pediatric Research Center 902,
Philadelphia, PA 19104, USA

Irene Y. Cheung, ScD
(e-mail: cheungi@mskcc.org)
Department of Pediatrics, Memorial Sloan-Kettering
Cancer Center, 1275 York Avenue, New York,
NY 10021, USA

Nai-Kong V. Cheung, MD, PhD
(e-mail: cheungn@mskcc.org)
Department of Pediatrics, Memorial Sloan-Kettering
Cancer Center, 1275 York Avenue, New York,
NY 10021, USA

Susan L. Cohn, MD
(e-mail: scohn@northwestern.edu)
Department of Pediatrics and the Comprehensive
Robert H. Lurie Cancer Center, Northwestern
University, Feinberg School of Medicine,
Children's Memorial Hospital,
2300 Children's Plaza, Chicago, IL 60614, USA

William L. Gerald, MD
(e-mail: geraldw@mskcc.org)
Department of Pathology, Memorial Sloan-Kettering
Cancer Center, 275 York Avenue, New York,
NY 10021, USA

Stephan A. Grupp, MD, PhD
(e-mail: grupp@email.chop.edu)
Director, Stem Cell Biology, Division of Oncology,
Children's Hospital of Philadelphia
and University of Pennsylvania,
3615 Civic Center Blvd., ARC 902, Philadelphia,
PA 19104, USA

Epidemiology

Andrew F. Olshan

Contents

This chapter reviews the epidemiology of neuroblastoma including the descriptive epidemiology and the evidence for an association with environmental exposures such as parental occupation, medication use during pregnancy, parental smoking and alcohol consumption, pregnancy history, and other exposures.

1.1 Descriptive Epidemiology

In the United States neuroblastoma accounts for 7.2% of all cancers among children younger than 15 years of age (SEER 2003). It is the most common extracranial solid tumor of childhood. Approximately 650 children are diagnosed with neuroblastoma in the United States each year (Goodman et al. 1999).

Based upon 1424 incident cases identified by the Surveillance, Epidemiology, and End Results Program of the U.S. National Cancer Institute (NCI) for 1975–2000, the total incidence of neuroblastoma was 10.2 per million children under age 15 years (age-adjusted to the 2000 U.S. standard million population; SEER 2003). The rates were 10.3 per million for males and 10.1 for females. Rates by race and ethnicity were 10.8 for whites, 8.4 for black children, and 7.5 for children of other racial/ethnic groups. The incidence rates by age category were 19.6 per million for ages 1–4 years, 2.9 for ages 5–9 years, and 0.7 for 10–14 years. Neuroblastoma is the most common malignancy among infants (61.3 per million). The incidence rate among infants was slightly higher among males (62.8) than females (59.8).

Based upon international registry data, the incidence of neuroblastoma is highest among Caucasians

Table 1.1. Neuroblastoma survival by gender, race, age, and stage

	5-year relative survival rate (%)[a]
Male	64
Female	65
White	65
Black	60
<1 year old at diagnosis	86
1–4 years at diagnosis	54
5–9 years at diagnosis	44
10–14 years at diagnosis	61
Local and regional stages (all ages)	85
Local and regional stages (<1 year old)	95
Local and regional stages (≥1 year old)	80
Distant metastatic stage (all ages)	48
Distant metastatic stage (<1 year old)	77
Distant metastatic stage (≥1 year old)	34

[a] Based on SEER (www.seer.cancer.gov) registry data 1985–2000

from North American, Europe, Australia, and Israeli Jews (Stiller and Parkin 1992). Lower rates were found for registries in southern and eastern Asia, including India and China, and in Latin America. Overall, the incidence appeared to be higher for regions or ethnic groups with a higher standard of living (Stiller and Parkin 1992). A previous study by SEER data found no total increase in incidence over time but reported a 3.4% average annual percentage (APC) increase for infants diagnosed between 1973 and 1992 (Gurney et al. 1996). The average annual increase was twice as high for infant boys as for infant girls. Other studies in the United States and elsewhere have noted increases in the incidence of neuroblastoma (Olshan and Bunin 2000). Improvements in diagnostic procedures, prenatal diagnosis, and possibly screening in some countries contributed to some of the increase during the 1970s through the early 1990s; however, analysis of the most recent SEER data (1973–2000) showed no significant increase in incidence overall (annual percentage change=0.3%) or among infants (APC=0.7%). There is some variability in 5-year relative survival rates based on age and stage (Table 1.1). Based upon SEER data for the years 1985–2000 the 5-year relative survival rate for neuroblastoma was 65%. No overall differences were found by race or gender. Survival was highest among infants and those with local or regional disease. Poorer survival was found for older children and those with distant metastases disease.

1.2 Risk Factors

The odds ratio provides an estimate of the relative risk, the risk among those with the exposure relative to the risk among those without the exposure. The odds ratio is estimated using exposure data collected in a case-control study, an efficient study design for a rare disease such as neuroblastoma. Odds ratios above the null value of 1.0 (indicating no case-control differences in the prevalence of a given exposure or factor) suggest a positive association, whereas odds ratios below 1.0 suggest that the factor may be associated with decreased risk. The assessment of the statistical associations should also include consideration of study design and analysis issues, such as the role of chance, confounding variables, and selection and exposure misclassification bias. Except where specifically indicated, the majority of epidemiologic studies have not examined any potential heterogeneity in risk among neuroblastoma subgroups defined by stage, age, or molecular markers.

1.2.1 Pregnancy and Childhood Factors

Several epidemiologic studies have investigated the role of reproductive history and birth characteristics in the etiology of neuroblastoma (See Review by Olshan and Bunin 2000). Conflicting results have been found for risk of neuroblastoma and maternal history of prior miscarriage, history of one or more induced abortions (Hamrick et al. 2001; Buck et al. 2001), repeat Cesarean birth and history of vaginal infection during pregnancy and sexually transmitted infection (Michalek et al. 1996; Hamrick et al. 2001). Studies also conflict with regard to the relationship between preterm birth (<37 weeks gestation) and low birth weight (<2500 g). One study reported that neuroblastoma patients were less likely than controls to have been born preterm (Johnson and Spitz 1985); however, a trend toward increasing risk with lower birth weight was observed among term births. Two recent studies have reported positive associations: one with very preterm birth (<33 weeks odds ratio=1.9; Hamrick et al. 2001); and preterm birth among patients with stage-3 or stage-4 neuroblastoma (odds ratio=3.4; Schuz et al. 2001). Low birth weight and very low birth weight (<1500 g) have been found to increase risk in two studies (Johnson and Spitz 1985; Hamrick et al. 2001). Two studies have reported no differences in birth weight or gestational age, and no associations with birth order, maternal age, or parity have been reported (Hamrick et al. 2001).

A German study reported that a history of tonsillectomy and/or appendectomy increased the risk threefold for stage-3 or stage-4 neuroblastoma patients (Schuz et al. 2001). Breastfeeding for more than 6 months was shown to decrease the risk of neuroblastoma by 40% in one study (Daniels et al. 2002).

A recent review indicated that some studies have found a significant excess of birth defects among children with neuroblastoma compared directly with controls or using expected rates (Foulkes et al. 1997). Associations with defects, including neurofibromatosis type 1, Beckwith-Wiedemann syndrome, Hirschsprung's disease, musculoskeletal and cardiovascular malformations, Turner's syndrome, and neurodevelopmental abnormalities, have been reported. Some of these associations were not consistent across studies, and over- or under-ascertainment could bias the comparisons. Molecular studies of familial neuroblastoma cases have not provided evidence of linkage with the genes thought to be responsible for Hirschsprung's disease or neurofibromatosis (Maris et al. 1997).

1.2.2 Medication Use

Case series reports from Israel, Australia, and Japan identified a possible relationship with maternal use of hormones for bleeding, history of miscarriage, and ovulation induction (see review by Olshan and Bunin 2000). Four case-control studies have examined hormone use before or during pregnancy. Positive associations (odds ratio>2.0) have been reported with maternal use of sex hormones 3 months prior to or during pregnancy and among women with a history of miscarriage or stillbirth. Indications for hormone usage included contraception, vaginal bleeding, and previous miscarriage. The largest case-control study (504 cases) found no overall association with infertility, infertility treatment, and other hormone use, although an elevated risk (odds ratio=4.4) was found for Clomid use among male offspring, consistent with a previous finding (Olshan et al. 1999a). Other maternal medications used during pregnancy that have been found in some studies to increase the risk of neuroblastoma include a group termed "neurally active" drugs (amphetamines, antidepressants, antipsychotics, muscle relaxants, prescription pain medications, and tranquilizers), antinauseants, diuretics, analgesics, and antibiotics (odds ratio=2.8; Kramer et al. 1987).

A recent report suggested that maternal multivitamin use during pregnancy was associated with a 30–40% reduction in the risk of neuroblastoma (Olshan et al. 2002). The analysis was unable to isolate any specific vitamin that might be responsible for the association. The finding requires replication in epidemiologic studies and possible investigation in laboratory experiments.

1.2.3 Lifestyle Exposures

Although a possible increased risk exists for mother's smoking during pregnancy, other studies have failed to confirm this finding (Olshan and Bunin 2000; Yang et al. 2000). No association with paternal smoking has been found. A possible association between fetal alcohol syndrome and neuroblastoma has been reported (Kinney et al. 1980). Case-control studies have not reported a difference in the proportion of case and control mothers who reported alcohol consumption during pregnancy; however, daily drinking or drinking three or more drinks on one occasion was associated with a nine- and sixfold elevated risk, respectively (Kramer et al. 1987). Other studies have not found an association with the amount or frequency of alcohol consumption.

1.2.4 Parental Occupation and Environmental Exposures

Parental occupation, specifically paternal occupation, has been found to increase the risk of neuroblastoma in offspring in several studies (Olshan and Bunin 2000; Olshan et al. 1999b; DeRoos et al. 2001a–c). Two of the studies found an association with fathers employed in electronics-related occupations including electricians, electric and electronics workers, electrical equipment assembly, linemen, utility employees, welders, and electric equipment salesmen and repairmen. The risk estimates were relatively large (>2.0) but imprecise. Other paternal occupations and industries that had an increased risk included food product packers and warehouse men, farmers and agricultural workers, rubber processing, painting, chemistry occupations, tire manufacturing, rubber/plastics/synthetics industry, service occupations, packaging and materials handling, and processing occupations.

Bunin et al. (1990) reported an increased risk (odds ratio=2.2) for maternal occupations including stock girls, textile and food product packers, plastic product packers, electrical products assembly, and metal product fabrication workers. Parental occupational exposures reported to be associated with risk included dusts, aromatic and aliphatic hydrocarbons, electromagnetic fields, metal fumes and dusts, benzene, asbestos, and pesticides/herbicides. The studies did not include direct measurement of occupational exposures but indirectly inferred the potential exposures using job title and industry.

All the parental occupation studies thus far have a number of limitations including the lack of a complete occupational history in studies using birth certificates, broad occupational groupings, crude exposure assessment, and small sample sizes. Nonetheless, the current epidemiologic evidence suggests that the risk of several occupations (e.g., electronics-related jobs) warrants further evaluation.

Two studies have reported associations with self-reported use of home and garden pesticides (Daniels et al. 2001; Schuz et al. 2001). One study reported a twofold increased risk for garden pesticides among children with stage-3 or stage-4 disease (Schuz et al. 2001). Another study did not find any differences in risk among subgroups defined by MYCN tumor status or stage (Daniels et al. 2001). There have been reports of "clusters" of neuroblastoma cases in communities in the United States. Environmental factors, such as proximity to hazardous waste sites, have been suggested as possibly related to the etiology of these clusters, but firm evidence to confirm the causality of these speculative associations has been consistently lacking.

1.3 Conclusions

Several epidemiologic studies have been conducted to evaluate potential risk factors for neuroblastoma. No causal factor(s) has been isolated. Few of the reported associations have been replicated in multiple studies. Moreover, the studies have suffered from methodologic limitations such as small sample size (most studies had fewer than 200 cases), incomplete exposure data collection, and inadequate control groups.

Despite these limitations, the previous studies have provided leads that warrant evaluation in future studies. Certain pregnancy and birth factors, parental occupation, and medications deserve more careful investigation. Besides addressing the methodologic concerns outlined above, future studies should take advantage of the developments in molecular epidemiology and identification of specific genetic variation in the human genome. The sharp distinction between favorable (local reginal-4S) and high-risk (stage 4 and MCYN-amplified stage 3) groups, as well as apparent biologic heterogeneity of neuroblastoma, should be incorporated directly in future epidemiologic studies. Biologic subgroups that represent different etiologic pathways for neuroblastoma can refine our ability to detect risk factors operating in those pathways. Finally, the incorporation of genetic susceptibility factors, such as common polymorphisms for genes involved in carcinogen metabolism and DNA repair, may help elucidate gene-environment interactions that have otherwise gone undetected with only the exposure data.

References

Buck GM, Michalek AM, Chen CJ, Nasca PC, Baptiste MS (2001) Perinatal factors and risk of neuroblastoma. Paediatr Perinat Epidemiol 15:47–53

Bunin GR, Ward E, Kramer S, Rhee CA, Meadows (1990) Neuroblastoma and parental occupation. Am J Epidemiol 131:776–780

Daniels JL, Olshan AF, Teschke K, Hertz-Picciotto I, Savitz DA, Blatt J, Bondy ML, Neglia JP, Pollock BH, Cohn SL, Look AT, Seeger RC, Castleberry RP (2001) Residential pesticide exposure and the risk of neuroblastoma. Epidemiology 12:20–27

Daniels JL, Olshan AF, Pollock, BH, Shah NR, Stram DO (2002) Breastfeeding and the occurrence of neuroblastoma. Cancer Causes Control 13:401–405

De Roos AJ, Olshan AF, Poole C, Teschke K (2001a) An application of hierarchical regression in the investigation of multiple paternal occupational exposures and childhood cancer. Am J Industr Med 39:477–486

De Roos AJ, Olshan AF, Teschke K, Poole C, Savitz DA, Blatt J, Bondy ML, Pollock BH (2001b) Parental occupational exposures to chemicals and the incidence of neuroblastoma in offspring. Am J Epidemiol 154:106–114

De Roos AJ, Teschke K, Savitz DA, Poole C, Grufferman S, Pollock BH, Olshan AF (2001c) Parental occupational exposures to fields and radiation in the electromagnetic spectrum and the incidence of neuroblastoma in offspring. Epidemiology 12:508–517

Foulkes WD, Buu PN, Filiatrault D, Leclerc J-M, Narod SA (1997) Excess of congenital abnormalities in French-Canadian children with neuroblastoma: a case series study from Montreal. Med Pediatr Oncol 29:272–297

Goodman MT, Gurney JG, Smith MA, Olshan AF (1999) Sympathetic nervous system tumors, chap IV. In: Ries, LAG, Smith MA, Gurney JG, Linet M, Tamra T, Young JL, Bunin GR (eds) Cancer incidence and survival among children and adolescents: United States SEER Program 1975–1995, National Cancer Institute, SEER Program. NIH Publ no 00–4649. Bethesda, MD

Gurney JG, Davis S, Severson RK, Fang JY, Ross JA, Robison LL (1996) Trends in cancer incidence among children in the US. Cancer 78:532–541

Hamrick SEG, Olshan AF, Neglia JP, Pollock BH (2001) Association of pregnancy history and birth characteristics with neuroblastoma. A report from the Children's Cancer Group and Pediatric Oncology Group. Paediatr Perinat Epidemiol 15:328–337

Johnson CC, Spitz MR (1985) Neuroblastoma: a case-control analysis of birth characterisitics. J Natl Cancer Inst 74: 789–192

Kinney H, Faix R, Brazy J (1980) The fetal alcohol syndrome and neuroblastoma. Pediatrics 66:130–132

Kramer S, Ward E, Meadows AT, Malone KE (1987) Medical and drug risk factors associated with neuroblastoma: a case-control study. J Natl Cancer Inst 78:797–804

Maris JM, Kyemba SM, Rebbeck TR, White PS, Sulman EP, Kensen SJ, Allen C, Biegel JA, Brodeur GM (1997) Molecular genetic analysis of familial neuroblastoma. Eur J Cancer 33:1923–1928

Michalek AM, Buck GM, Nasca PC, Freedman AN, Baptiste MS, Mahoney MC (1996) Gravid health status, medication use, and risk of neuroblastoma. Am J Epidemiol 143:996–1001

Olshan AF, Bunin GR (2000) Epidemiology of neuroblastoma. In: Brodeur GM, Sawada T, Tsuchida Y, Voute PA (eds) Neuroblastoma. Elsevier, Amsterdam, pp 33–39

Olshan AF, Smith J, Cook MN, Grufferman S, Pollock BH, Stram DO, Seeger RC, Look AT, Cohn SL, Castleberry RP, Bondy ML (1999a) Hormone and fertility drug use and the risk of neuroblastoma: a report from the Children's Cancer Group and the Pediatric Oncology Group. Am J Epidemiol 150: 930–938

Olshan AF, DeRoos AJ, Teschke K, Neglia JP, Stram DO, Pollock BH, Castleberry RP (1999b) Neuroblastoma and parental occupation. Cancer Causes Control 10:539–549

Olshan F, Smith JC, Bondy ML, Neglia JP, Pollock BH (2002) Maternal vitamin use and reduced risk of neuroblastoma. Epidemiology 13:575–580

Schuz J, Kaletsch U, Meinert R, Kaatsch P, Spix C, Michaelis J (2001) Risk factors for neuroblastoma at different stages of disease. Results from a population-based case-control study in Germany. J Clin Epidemiol 54:702–709

SEER (2003) Surveillance, Epidemiology, and End Results (SEER) Program (www.seer.cancer.gov) SEER*Stat Database: Incidence – SEER 9 Regs, Nov 2002 Sub (1973–2000), National Cancer Institute, DCCPS, Surveillance Research Program, Cancer Statistics Branch, released April 2003, based on the November 2002 submission

Stiller CA, Parkin DM (1992) International variations in the incidence of neuroblastoma. Int J Cancer 52:538–543

Yang Q, Olshan AF, Bondy ML, Shah NR, Pollock BH, Seeger RC, Look AT, Cohn SL (2000) Parental smoking and alcohol consumption and risk of neuroblastoma. Cancer Epidemiol Biomark Prevent 9:967–972

Screening for Neuroblastoma

William G. Woods

Contents

2.1 Introduction

Pediatricians are by training the most prevention oriented of all the primary care physicians. Immunizations for various potentially life-threatening infectious diseases and early screening for inborn errors of metabolism are two shining examples of childhood disease prevention. Prior to 1970, no one had attempted to reduce the morbidity, or more importantly, the mortality, of any childhood cancer through preclinical detection, specifically by mass screening for this disease. Over the past 30 years there has been much effort put into better understanding the role of preclinical detection of neuroblastoma, and potentially lowering mortality from this most challenging of childhood solid tumors. This chapter addresses various aspects of screening for neuroblastoma in children.

2.2 The Rationale for Neuroblastoma Screening

Neuroblastoma has an incidence of about 10 per million children 0–14 per year throughout the developed world (Young et al. 1986; Bernstein et al. 1992). In North America neuroblastoma will develop in approximately one in 7000 children before the age of 5 years, and over 700 cases are expected to be diagnosed annually. The incidence of neuroblastoma is about twice that of phenylketonuria, almost tenfold higher than that of galactosemia, and slightly less common than neonatal hypothyroidism (Woods and Tuchman 1987), all diseases which are mandated by most neonatal screening programs throughout the U.S.

Neuroblastoma is a fascinating neoplasm because of several clinical and biologic characteristics. The tumor is unique biochemically because it possesses metabolic pathways for catecholamine synthesis and metabolism. Homovanillic acid (HVA), the main metabolite of dopamine, and vanillylmandelic acid (VMA), the main metabolite of adrenalin and noradrenalin, are sensitive and convenient markers of neuroblastoma since they are excreted in excessive amounts in a patient's urine (Hinterberger and Bartholomew 1969). Homovanillic acid and VMA have routinely been measured in patients with neuroblastoma for the past 30 years, and have been found to be invaluable aids in both neuroblastoma diagnosis and follow-up.

The treatment and outcome of neuroblastoma are highly age- and stage dependent. Children who are diagnosed with early-stage localized disease or under 1 year of age, irrespective of stage, can often be treated with limited therapy and have excellent survival (Bernstein et al. 1992; Matthay et al. 1989). In contrast, children over the age of 1 year who present with advanced-stage disease have a very poor survival despite aggressive chemotherapeutic treatment regimens, including bone marrow transplantation (Bernstein et al. 1992; Matthay et al. 1989). While some authors have hypothesized that neuroblastoma presents as at least two discreet clinical pathologic entities (Woods et al. 1992; Brodeur and Nakagawara 1992), others believe that malignant progression is a natural transition from benign-acting neuroblastoma in an infant to advanced-stage disease in a child. We presently know that favorable prognosis is strongly associated with specific tumor cellular characteristics (see Chaps. 4, 5, and 8) But in the 1980s, in the absence of this molecular genetic information, it was hypothesized that this natural transition may be interrupted by early detection to eradicate preclinical neuroblastomas.

2.3 Early Pioneering Studies Investigating Neuroblastoma Screening in Japan

The identification of elevated urinary catecholamines in infants with neuroblastoma was first made in 1957 (Mason et al. 1957). Over the next 15 years, methods for measuring the main urinary metabolic byproducts of dopamine and epinephrine, HVA, and VMA were refined. Twenty-four-hour collections were the rule, and elevated urinary catecholamines became extremely important in aiding in the diagnosis of children with "small round cell tumors" and subsequent follow-up of catecholamine-secreting neuroblastomas (Tuchman et al. 1987). A urinary VMA "spot test" based on the reaction of phenolic acids with diazotized p-nitroaniline became commonplace in pediatric oncology practice (LaBrosse 1968). In the early 1970s, Sawada and colleagues from the Kyoto Prefectural University of Medicine began pilot studies which led to implementing a mass screening program for 6-month-old children in eight cities and prefectures in Japan using the VMA spot test on random urine samples (Sawada et al. 1984). The annual incidence of neuroblastoma in Japan, 8 per million children, was similar to that reported in the U.S. at the time. Originally, 282,000 infants were screened by Sawada et al., representing 50–75% of all births in the areas studied (Sawada et al. 1984). Because of a positive test or logistic problems with the initial sample, almost 11,000 infants (3.8%) were retested. Among 264 infants (1 in 1000) who required clinical evaluation for neuroblastoma at a medical center because they had three consecutive positive urinary tests, 16 cases of neuroblastoma were subsequently identified, giving an incidence by screening of 1 in 17,600 infants. As opposed to the high expected incidence of metastatic disease at diagnosis, 5 patients were found with Evans stage-I tumor, 4 with stage II, 2 with stage III, 5 with stage IV-S, and none with stage IV. The 16 patients were treated with surgery and limited chemotherapy, 15 of whom were alive more than 5 years after diagnosis. The only death occurred 1 month after surgery in a patient with stage-II disease. Of the original screened cohort, an additional 6 children were found to have neuroblastoma 14–29 months after their urinary spot tests gave negative results. Hence, the false-negative rate of the Kyoto screening program was 6 of 22, or 27%, similar to what one would have expected using a VMA spot test (Sawada et al. 1984).

This encouraging early trial was reconfirmed by Sawada in longer-term follow-up of the screened population (Sawada 1986). Subsequently, many other screening trials were initiated in Japan, increasingly using quantitative assays for measuring both VMA and HVA. In an important trial from Sapporo City, Nishi, Takeda and colleagues demonstrated markedly improved survival in children in that city offered screening compared with neighboring rural areas in Hokkaido Prefecture, in which no screening was available (Nishi et al. 1987). Several childhood cancer experts throughout Europe and North America called for the institution of neuroblastoma screening programs on their continents. Many other Japanese investigators began trials in their own prefectures, and by 1986, screening for neuroblastoma was mandated by law in Japan.

A more careful analysis of the Japanese neuroblastoma screening studies revealed many methodologic limitations (Tuchman et al. 1990). Firstly, there was no utilization of a population-based cohort of infants: studies were generally performed in prefectures which did not have the ability to guarantee ascertainment of all neuroblastoma cases occurring in that region, either detected by screening, or missed and subsequently clinically found. Secondly, the data were all based on survival rather than mortality. To the untrained observer, one would surmise that mortality is the reverse of survival (or "one minus survival"). In fact, mortality represents the number of deaths in a given population, and is not affected by the incidence of a disease in that given population. This difference from "survival" becomes most important in evaluating neuroblastoma screening trials. For example, as the Japanese increasingly used more sensitive and specific quantitative assays for measuring VMA and HVA in their trials, there were increasing data suggesting a rise in neuroblastoma incidence (Yamamoto et al. 2002). As can be seen graphically in Fig. 2.1, if one has an incidence in a disease of 1X, with a survival of 50%, of 100 children, 50% will die. If one artificially raises the incidence to 2X, or 200 individuals in this case, and one maintains the same mortality (50 deaths), there is an artificial increase in the survival to 75% (150 of 200). Hence, looking at survival only, when the actual relevant end point is death rate, can greatly mislead an investigator. In addition, the early Japanese studies utilized no control groups other than historical controls; therefore, potential declines in neuroblastoma mortality could

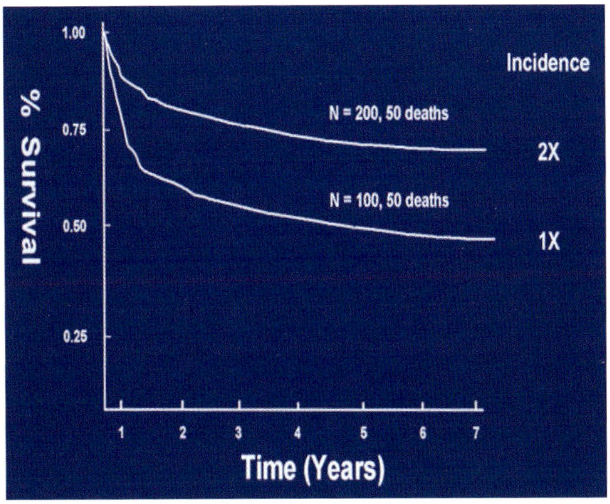

Figure 2.1
Effect of incidence on survival

have been attributed to improvements in therapy, rather than preclinical detection. Finally, without the utilization of a population-based cohort trial, several other classic methodologic issues, such as lead time or length bias, could produce falsely optimistic results.

2.4 Initial North American and European Neuroblastoma Screening Trials

In the context of the potentially exciting results coming out of Japan mixed with the realities of those studies' limitations, several groups throughout Europe and North America began early pilot studies looking at the potential effectiveness of neuroblastoma screening. Small exploratory studies were initiated in Quebec (Scriver et al. 1987), Minnesota (Tuchman et al. 1989), northern England (Craft et al. 1989), Germany (Schilling et al. 1991), France (Mathieu et al. 1996), Austria (Kerbl et al. 1997), and elsewhere (Bergeron et al. 1998). Newcastle hosted the first International Symposium on Neuroblastoma Screening in 1988, where investigators had the opportunity to share logistical challenges and early results. Several important methodologic aspects of

Table 2.1. Principles to be considered for a cancer screening program (Adapted from Prorok and Connor 1986)

1. The disease should be a "common" serious health problem, with substantial morbidity and mortality
2. The target population should be clearly defined and have a reasonable disease prevalence
3. The target population should be accessible, with reasonable compliance to screening expected
4. The screening test should be acceptable in its performance (sensitivity, specificity) and acceptable to those screened
5. Effective treatment should exist for the disease to be detected by screening
6. There should be a reasonable expectation that patients with positive screening will comply with recommended work-up, diagnosis, therapy, and follow-up
7. Sufficient resources should be available to perform the screening
8. Develop policies for early recall of patients testing positive and follow-up of those testing negative
9. Quality control procedures to maintain sensitivity and specificity of the screening test should be in place0

neuroblastoma were revealed. These aspects deserve some comment, given that they represent challenges of any population-based screening approaches for any diseases:

- Sample collection. In a series of important studies, Tuchman and colleagues from Minnesota demonstrated that measuring spot urines to determine HVA and VMA were as valid as 24-hour sample collections, thus obviating long collections for children in whom neuroblastoma was suspected clinically (Tuchman et al. 1985). In Japan, urine was squeezed out of diapers into plastic soy sauce bottles which held 5–10 ml of urine. North American and European investigators began collecting urine on diapers blotted against a 10×10 cm piece of filter paper which, when dried, could be mailed by regular mail to the screening laboratory for accurate determination of VMA and HVA, with urinary creatinine as the internal standard.
- Assays. Multiple laboratory assays for measuring catecholamines were debated, from the totally qualitative VMA spot test and the semi-quantitative thin layer chromatographic approach, through high performance liquid chromatography (HPLC), ELISA immuno-assays, and ultimately gas chromatography/mass spectroscopy (GC-MS) as the gold standard.
- Compliance. No adequate population-based screening trial can be done without a high compliance rate among the participants. Early studies in Minnesota (Tuchman et al. 1989), Texas (Ater et al. 1998), and Austria (Kerbl et al. 1997) found compliance rates of returning filter papers by parents of 6 month olds to be as low as 9 percent, pointing out the need for a massive public health infrastructure to support adequate compliance, even for something as simple as collecting urine from a diaper. Because of such issues, investigators in Minnesota joined forces with those in Quebec, combining clinical trials expertise (Bernstein et al. 1992), an infrastructure already in place for collecting urine in a large majority of 3-week olds, as part of a urinary metabolic screening program for various inborn errors of metabolism (Scriver et al. 1987); and a rapid GC-MS assay for VMA and HVA determination (Tuchman et al. 1983).
- Sample sizes. It became rapidly clear that to adequately study neuroblastoma screening, one might need a trial studying up to a million children or more to get meaningful results (Esteve et al. 1995). This sobering reality led to major modifications in many trials, some of which were abandoned due to the cost, and others that waited years for adequate funding before they proceeded.
- Case and control ascertainment. In-place state and country-wide tumor registries collecting incidence and mortality data with greater than 90–95% ascertainment are an important requirement for an adequate prevention study.

Table 2.1, from Prorok and Connor (1986), lists principles to be considered for a cancer screening program. One could argue that any childhood disease is not a "common" serious health problem with substantial morbidity and mortality, to warrant the expense of a screening program; however, based on past precedent and the fact that children represent the future of the world, should screening of any childhood disease lower mortality, implementation would be seriously considered.

2.5 Follow-up Studies from Japan and Europe

Since 1986, when screening for neuroblastoma in Japan was mandated by law, compliance with the Japanese screening program has been much greater than 80% nationwide (Sawada and Takeda 2000). Although highly successful in recruiting parents to participate in this program, such widespread mass screening also led to less ability to measure the efficacy of this approach, for example, by comparing mortality from neuroblastoma in a population offered screening versus that not offered screening; however, subsequent attempts to document screening efficacy were performed in Japan on relatively small populations. Investigators in general found no diminution in the incidence of late-stage disease, an early marker of potential screening success, in the incidence of the disease with unfavorable biologic features, or in mortality (Yamamoto et al. 2002; Bessho et al. 1991; Yamamoto et la. 1995; Kaneko et al. 1990; Suita et al. 1998).

During the 1990s, as noted above, several smaller studies were also performed in Europe, usually without controls, with preliminary results suggesting that screening increased the incidence of the disease (Mathieu et al. 1996; Bergeron et al. 1998). Ultimately, only two prospective population-based controlled trials examining the role of neuroblastoma screening in reducing mortality from this disease were implemented that had adequate funding to guarantee a high screening compliance rate; uniform neuroblastoma evaluation, staging, treatment, and follow-up; and optimum ascertainment procedures for determining incidence and mortality. These were the Quebec Neuroblastoma Screening Project (Woods et al. 1996, 2002) and the German Project on Neuroblastoma Screening (Schilling et al. 1998, 2002). Both of these studies deserve special mention, noting similarities and differences.

2.6 Definitive Controlled Trials from Quebec and Germany

2.6.1 Studies, Designs, and Logistics

The greatest strength of both the Quebec and German trials was that they were prospective, population-based controlled studies in which neuroblastoma mortality was the definitive end point, rather than survival (vide supra). Both studies had considered a randomized trial approach, but "randomized controlled trials in population-based intervention studies are not always feasible" (Woods et al. 1999) as pointed out by the Quebec researchers. To clarify, the North American group had to decide what they were actually studying by introducing a new screening procedure in an infant population. Were they going to evaluate the screening test itself (urine sampling of 6-month-old babies by parents at home), or were they going to study the entire public health intervention which included introducing a new screening test? They decided that the latter question was much more relevant to improving scientific knowledge, and that to achieve a reasonable compliance rate multiple population-based education methods would be necessary, as noted below. If these measures led to a "halo effect," with an increased incidence in the non-screened population, the study results would have been viewed with skepticism. There were also practical matters including the fact that there were no other infant urinary screening programs in place in North America with a high compliance rate. Hence, control populations were picked throughout North America where no public health interventions were performed, and where had such been attempted they would have required millions of dollars in resources to be successful. These areas included the states of Minnesota and Florida, the Greater Delaware Valley, and the Province of Ontario (Woods et al. 1996). German investigators faced a similar problem. They im-

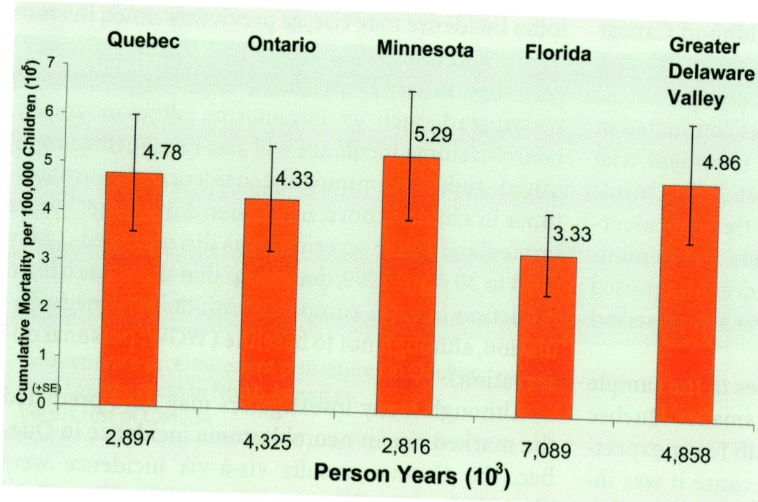

Figure 2.2

Cumulative mortality due to neuroblastoma among children younger than 8 years of age

al. 2002). Despite no deaths in the screened detected children in the Quebec trial, in 1 child with stage 2-B neuroblastoma that was detected by screening at 6 months and who was treated with doxorubicin and cyclophosphamide, a secondary leukemia with an abnormality in chromosome 11q23 subsequently developed. That child underwent bone marrow transplantation and is alive but has severe graft-vs-host disease. An additional child whose disease was detected by screening is in a persistent vegetative state as a result of complications of surgery for severe gastrointestinal obstruction and necrosis. The gastrointestinal problems were attributed to adhesions that resulted from the surgery to remove the neuroblastoma 7 years previously (Woods et al. 2002).

As an intermediate end point, both studies examined the incidence of advanced-stage neuroblastoma (INSS 3–4) in children over 1 year of age. Both showed, if anything, an increase in that incidence in the screened groups (Table 2.2). These results suggested that the screening procedure or the public health interventions instituted as part of the screening projects actually raised the incidence of advanced-stage disease in older infants, perhaps through clinical detection of cases that may have spontaneously regressed, the "halo effect." In the Quebec trial, there was a significant increased incidence in neuroblastoma over 1 year of age (Woods et al. 1996). In the German trial, even the incidence of advanced-stage disease over the age of 2 years was not lowered by the screening procedure (Schilling et al. 2002).

Finally, and most importantly, cumulative mortality in the study populations in both the Quebec and German trials was not reduced compared with appropriate controls. Mortality was higher in the Quebec screened cohort than in the German, but included a 9-year analysis (Woods et al. 2002). Only preliminary mortality results were presented for the German trial, examining cumulative figures between 1 and 5 years of age (Schilling et al. 2002); however, in examining standardized mortality ratios (SMR) of neuroblastoma comparing study versus control groups, neither showed any reduction, with an SMR of 1.4 in Quebec and 1.1 in Germany (Table 2.2). In fact, in the Quebec trial, examining the rate of death due to neuroblastoma compared with the rest of Canada, as compiled by Statistics Canada, the overall SMR for Quebec was 1.39, with 95 % confidence intervals of 0.85–2.30. Figure 2.2 displays cumulative deaths in the Quebec population versus the four control populations whose deaths were ascertained by study investigators.

2.7 Biologic, Psychologic, Economic, and Clinical Aspects of Neuroblastoma Screening

2.7.1 Biologic Aspects

Had neuroblastoma screening actually been associated with a reduction in mortality, one should have seen children with unfavorable biology detected preclinically with subsequent good outcomes. In general, this was not the case. Even in early Japanese trials, virtually all children with neuroblastomas detected by screening demonstrated favorable biologic features, including histology, triploid DNA content, and lack of MYCN amplification (Kaneko et al. 1990). In only one international trial, that conducted in Austria, were any substantial number of patients found through screening with unfavorable biology (Kerbl et al. 1997): results from this study are a bit controversial because of various methodologic issues. Preliminary results from the Quebec trial documented that, similar to the Japanese uncontrolled studies, virtually all children detected clinically had favorable biologic features (Brodeur et al. 1998, 2001); however, the vast majority of children who died after being missed by screening had unfavorable biologic features; for example, amplified MYCN oncogene identified in 11 of 19 patients studied (Woods et al. 2002). The German project is expected to publish biologic results in the future.

In summary, the current data overwhelmingly suggest that patients with favorable biology neuroblastoma are able to be successfully detected preclinically; however, those with poor biologic characteristics are missed by screening at 3 weeks, 6 months, and 1 year of age. This suggests that such tumors are either in general not present at these ages, or small enough not to be excreting catecholamines in excess of normal urinary amounts, with subsequent other cellular events leading to a great expansion of the cancer, often with metastatic spread, and clinical detection at an advanced stage.

2.7.2 Psychologic Aspects

Unfortunately, very few studies have examined the potential psychological implications of screening infants for neuroblastoma (Bell et al. 1994). Investigators in the Quebec trial tried unsuccessfully to obtain funding for what they believed to be an important secondary aim of their trial. Austrian investigators fortunately were able to conduct interviews on parents of children who underwent neuroblastoma screening with negative results (Dobrovoljski et al. 2003). They found that a large portion of parents of infants who were referred to cancer centers because of elevated catecholamines and were found not to have neuroblastomas remained very concerned about their children, even years later. Hence, the screening procedure was felt to be very psychologically stressing with long-term consequences. The Quebec screening trial was geared toward a very high specificity, and in the end, less than 1 in 10,000 normal children were evaluated at medical centers for neuroblastoma and found not to have the cancer. The number and percent of such children who falsely tested positive was a log higher in the German study, and remains high in Japan today.

2.7.3 Economic Aspects

Very little has been written on the potential cost-effectiveness of neuroblastoma screening. Because screening has been found to be ineffective, one could argue that such studies would by necessity be negative. The Quebec investigators, however, did prospectively examine cost-effectiveness and the data have yet to be published; however, preliminary results lead to a very important and provocative conclusion: over $8 million USD were spent on the Quebec trial in funds provided through the peer-review grant mechanism of the National Cancer Institute. In addition, significant resources were provided by the Quebec Institute of Genetic Medicine for neuroblastoma screening, including costs associated with setting up the infrastructure for metabolic screening that enabled this study to be done as economically as possible. The German Trial cost more than $20 million USD; hence, at first glance these were highly expensive "negative" studies. But over 4 million children are born in the U.S. every year, compared with 100,000 in Quebec. To put in place an effective infrastructure to screen a large portion of American newborns would have cost easily hundreds of millions of dollars. As importantly, such an infrastructure would have cost tens of millions of dollars to maintain on an annual basis. As noted above, major pediatric voices clamored for institution of neuroblastoma screening in the U.S. before definitive trials proving or disproving its efficacy were performed. Not only did the Quebec and German trials show that neuroblastoma screening was ineffective, but ultimately they saved the American, Canadian, German, and other health care system billions of dollars over a generation. The economic value of well-done research cannot be overestimated, even if results obtained are negative.

2.7.4 Clinical Implications

With the determination that a substantial number of preclinically detected neuroblastomas undergo spontaneous regression, it is highly likely that a substantial amount of favorable-biology neuroblastoma detected clinically would also spontaneously regress; hence, the results of the neuroblastoma screening studies may have practical implications for the care of infants with clinically detected disease. Yamamoto and colleagues have now defined criteria for observing patients with neuroblastomas detected by screening without incurring any untoward risk. The criteria include the identification of small masses on radiographic examinations but no invasion of the intraspinal canal or infiltration around the great vessels; relatively moderate catecholamines secretions; and parental consent (Yamamoto et al. 1998). Their initial results reveal that a substantial proportion of observed tumors regress, and even those infants that need subsequent treatment do well. It is therefore likely that a similar proportion of infants in whom neuroblastoma is detected clinically at less than 6 months of age can also be observed for potential regression of the tumor, rather than undergo major surgery.

2.8 Conclusions

The idea that one could detect childhood cancer preclinically by screening has been and remains an appealing prospect. In well-performed trials in the only childhood cancer in which proper studies could be performed at the end of the twentieth century, neuroblastoma screening for elevated urinary catecholamines led to a marked increase in the incidence of the disease with no reduction in its mortality; hence, in 2004 using the markers studied, neuroblastoma screening has been and should be abandoned throughout the world: in Japan, screening was finally halted in March of 2004 (Tsubono et al. 2004). In the future, there may be better opportunities as more selective markers for poor-biology neuroblastoma are discovered that can be utilized as screening tools. In the meantime, one needs to remember that even collecting urine from a wet diaper may have horrendous long-term consequences, as evidenced by the outcome of some infants screened in the Quebec, German, and Japanese trials. Physicians should always practice the "golden rule" of medicine: *primum non nocere.*

References

Ater JL, Gardner KL, Foxhall LE et al. (1998) Neuroblastoma screening in the United States: results of the Texas Outreach Program for neuroblastoma screening. Cancer 82:1593–1602

Bell S, Parker L, Cole M et al. (1994) Screening infants for neuroblastoma: the parents' perspective in false-positive cases. Pediatr Hematol Oncol 11:157–163

Bergeron C, Tafese T, Kerbl R et al. (1998) European experience with screening for neuroblastoma before the age of 12 months. Med Pediatr Oncol 31:442–449

Bernstein M, Leclerc J, Bunin G et al. (1992) A population-based study of neuroblastoma incidence, survival, and mortality in North America. J Clin Oncol 10:323–329

Bessho F, Hashizume K, Nakajo T, Kamoshita S (1991) Mass screening in Japan increased the detection of infants with neuroblastoma without a decrease in cases in older children. J Pediatr 119:237–241

Brodeur G, Ambros P, Favrot M (1998) Biological aspects of neuroblastoma screening. Med Pediatr Oncol 31:394–400

Brodeur GM, Look AT, Shimada H et al. (2001) Biological aspects of neuroblastomas identified by mass screening in Quebec. Med Pediatr Oncol 36:157–159

Brodeur GM, Nakagawara A (1992) Molecular basis of clinical heterogeneity in neuroblastoma. Am J Pediatr Hematol-Oncol 14:111–116
Carlsen NLT (1986) Epidemiological investigations on neuroblastomas in Denmark, 1943–1980. Br J Cancer 54:977–988
Craft AW, Dale G, McGill A et al. (1989) Biochemical screening for neuroblastoma in infants: a feasibility study. Med Pediatr Oncol 17:373–378
D'Angio G, Evans A, Koop C (1971) Special pattern of widespread neuroblastoma with a favourable prognosis. Lancet 1:1046–1049
Dobrovoljski G, Kerbl R, Strobl C et al. (2003) False-positive results in neuroblastoma screening: the parents' view. J Pediatr Hem Oncol 25:14–18
Esteve J, Parker L, Roy P et al. (1995) Is neuroblastoma screening evaluation needed and feasible? Br J Cancer 71:1125–1131
Hinterberger H, Bartholomew RJ (1969) Catecholamines and their acidic metabolites in urine and tumor tissue in neuroblastoma, ganglioneuroma and pheochromocytoma. Clin Chim Acta 26:291–294
Kaneko Y, Kanda N, Maseki N et al. (1990) Current urinary mass screening for catecholamine metabolites at 6 months of age may be detecting only a small portion of high risk neuroblastomas: a chromosome and N-myc amplification study. J Clin Oncol 8:2005–2013
Kerbl R, Urban C, Ladenstein R et al. (1997) Neuroblastoma screening in infants postponed after the sixth month of age: a trial to reduce "overdiagnosis" and to detect cases with unfavourable" biological features. Med Pediatr Oncol 29: 1–10
LaBrosse EH (1968) Biochemical diagnosis of neuroblastoma; use of the urine spot test. Proc Am Assoc Cancer Res 9:39
Mason GA, Hart-Mercer J, Miller ES et al. (1957) Adrenaline-secreting neuroblastoma in an infant. Lancet 2:322–325
Mathieu P, Frappaz D, Chauvin F et al. (1996) A 5-year (1990–1994) neuroblastoma screening feasibility study in France. Methodology and preliminary observations. Early Hum Dev 46:177–196
Matthay KK, Sather HN, Seeger RC et al. (1989) Excellent outcome of stage II neuroblastoma is independent of residual disease and radiation therapy. J Clin Oncol 7:236–244
Matthay KK, Villablanca JG, Seeger RC et al. (1999) Treatment of high-risk neuroblastoma with intensive chemotherapy, radiotherapy, autologous bone marrow transplantation, and 13-cis-retinoic acid. N Engl J Med 341:1165–1173
Nishi M, Miyake H, Takeda T et al. (1987) Effects of the mass screening of neuroblastoma in Sapporo City. Cancer 60: 433–436
Prorok P, Connor R (1986) Screening for the early detection of cancer. Cancer Invest 4:225–238
Ross JA, Severson RK, Pollock BH et al. (1996) Childhood cancer in the United States: a geographical analysis of cases from the pediatric cooperative clinical trials groups. Cancer 77:201–207
Sawada T (1986) Outcome of 25 Neuroblastomas revealed by screening in Japan. Lancet 1:377
Sawada T, Nakata T, Takasugi N et al. (1984) Mass screening for neuroblastoma in infants in Japan. Lancet 2:271–273
Sawada T, Takeda T (2000) Screening for neuroblastoma in infancy in Japan. In: Brodeur GM, Sawada T, Tsuchida Y, Voûte PA (eds) Neuroblastoma. Elsevier, Amsterdam, pp 245–264
Sawada T, Todo S, Fujita K et al. (1982) Mass screening of neuroblastoma in infancy. Am J Dis Child 136:710–712
Schilling F, Oberrauch W, Schanz F et al. (1991) Evaluation of a rapid and reliable method for mass screening for neuroblastoma in infants. Prog Clin Biol Res 366:579–583
Schilling F, Spix C, Berthold F et al. (1998) German neuroblastoma screening study at 12 months of age: statistical aspects and preliminary results. Med Pediatr Oncol 31:435–441
Schilling F, Spix, C, Berthold F et al. (2002) Neuroblastoma screening at one year of age. N Engl J Med 346:1047–1053
Scriver C, Gregory D, Bernstein M et al. (1987) Feasibility of chemical screening of urine for neuroblastoma case finding in infancy in Quebec. Can Med Assoc J 136:952–956
Suita S, Tajiri T, Akazawa K et al. (1998) Mass screening for neuroblastoma at 6 months of age: difficult to justify. J Pediatr Surg 33:1674–1678
Tsubono Y, Hisamichi S (2004) A halt to neuroblastoma screening in Japan. N Engl J Med 350:2010
Tuchman M, Crippin PJ, Krivit W (1983) Capillary gas chromatographic determination of urinary homovanillic acid and vanillylmandelic acid. Clin Chem 29:828–831
Tuchman M, Robison LL, Maynard RC et al. (1985) Assessment of the diurnal variations in urinary homovanillic acid and vanillylmandelic acid excretion for the diagnosis and follow up of patients with neuroblastoma. Clin Biochem 18:176–179
Tuchman M, Ramnaraine ML, Woods WG et al. (1987) Three years of experience with random urinary homovanillic and vanillymandelic acid levels in the diagnosis of neuroblastoma. Pediatrics 79:203–205
Tuchman M, Fisher E, Heisel M, Woods WG (1989) Feasibility study for neonatal neuroblastoma screening in the United States. Med Pediatr Oncol 17:258–264
Tuchman M, Lemieux B, Woods WG (1990) Editorial: screening for neuroblastoma in infants: investigate or implement? Pediatrics 86:791–793
Woods WG, Tuchman M (1987) Neuroblastoma: the case for screening infants in North America. Pediatrics 79:869–873
Woods WG, Lemieux B, Tuchman M (1992) Neuroblastoma represents distinct clinical–biologic entities: a review and perspective from the Quebec Neuroblastoma Screening Project. Pediatrics 89:114–118
Woods WG, Tuchman M, Robison L et al. (1996) A population-based study of the usefulness of screening for neuroblastoma. Lancet 348:1682–1672

Woods WG, Bernstein M, Lemieux B (1999) Commentary: randomized controlled trials in population-based intervention studies are not always feasible. Med Pediatr Oncol 33:360–361

Woods WG, Gao R, Shuster J et al. (2002) Screening of infants and mortality due to neuroblastoma. N Engl J Med 346: 1041–1046

Yamamoto K, Hayashi Y, Hanada R et al. (1995) Mass screening and age-specific incidence of neuroblastoma in Saitama Prefecture, Japan. J Clin Oncol 13:2033–2038

Yamamoto K, Hanada R, Kikuchi A et al. (1998) Spontaneous regression of localized neuroblastoma detected by mass screening. J Clin Oncol 16:1265–1269

Yamamoto K, Ohta S, Ito E et al. (2002) Marginal decrease in mortality and marked increase in incidence as a result of neuroblastoma screening at 6 months of age: Cohort study in seven prefectures in Japan. J Clin Oncol 20:1209–1214

Young JL, Ries LG, Silverberg E et al. (1986) Cancer incidence, survival and mortality for children under 15 years of age. Cancer 58:598–602

Genetics

John M. Maris, Garrett M. Brodeur

Contents

3.1 Introduction

Multiple somatically acquired genetic alterations have been described in neuroblastoma, but the genetic events that initiate tumorigenesis remain largely unknown. Like most other human cancers, a small subset of neuroblastoma cases have an apparent heritable genetic etiology. Familial neuroblastoma was first described in 1945 (Dodge and Brenner 1945), and multiple pedigrees have been reported in the literature since that time (Knudson and Strong 1972; Kushner et al. 1986; Maris and Brodeur 2001). In addition, there have been several patients with neuroblastoma and associated constitutional abnormalities and/or other conditions reported, suggesting the underlying genetic defect predisposed to the development of neuroblastoma.

This chapter reviews the genetics of neuroblastoma, emphasizing germline aberrations that predispose to the development of this neoplasm. Somatic genetic events associated with neuroblastoma pathogenesis and with clinical phenotype are reviewed in Chaps. 4 and 5.

3.2 Associated Genetic Conditions

It is likely that any neuroblastoma predisposition gene will have an essential role in the normal development of neural crest-derived tissues. Interestingly, the coincident occurrence of neuroblastoma in patients with global disorders of neural crest-derived cells (i.e., "neurocristopathies"), such as Hirschsprung disease (HD) and/or congenital central hypoventilation syndrome (CCHS, Ondine's curse),

Table 3.1. Candidate regions for neuroblastoma predisposition gene

Regions with evidence for genetic linkage	Regions of allelic deletion	Regions of chromosomal gain	Regions containing genes mutated in HD, CCHS, and/or NF1
4p16	1p36.2-.3	1q21–32	1p36.1 (*ECE1*)
16p12–13	3p21-pter	2p24 (*MYCN*)	2q22 (*ZFHX1B*)
	4p16	7q	4p12 (PHOX2B)
	9p21–24	17q23–25	5p12 (*GDNF*)
	11q14–23		10q11 (*RET*)
	14q32		11p13 (*BDNF*)
	16p12–13		13q22 (*EDNRB*)
	18q21		17q11.2 (NF1)
	19q13		20q13 (EDN3)

has been described (Verloes et al. 1993). In addition, there have been reports of the coexistence of neuroblastoma and neurofibromatosis type 1, including the coincidence of these disorders in familial neuroblastoma (Maris et al. 1997, 2002). Indeed, homozygous inactivation of the NF1 gene in primary neuroblastomas has also been described (Origone et al. 2003; Martinsson et al. 1997). These data suggest that the genes implicated in the genesis of Hirschsprung disease (*RET, EDNRB, EDN3, GDNF, ECE1*, and *ZFHX1B*), central hypoventilation (*RET, GDNF, EDN3, BDNF*, and *PHOX2B*) and/or NF1 may be causally involved in the initiation or progression of human neuroblastoma, especially in the context of a neurocristopathy (Table 3.1). A recent study reported a germline mutation in *PHOX2B* in a patient with neuroblastoma (Amiel et al. 2003), although previous reports have found no evidence for linkage at the 4p12 *PHOX2B* locus (Maris et al. 2002). GDNF and related molecules, neurturin (*NRTN*), artemin (*ARTN*), and persephin (*PSPN*), signal through a unique multicomponent receptor system consisting of RET tyrosine kinase and glycosyl-phosphatidylinositol-anchored coreceptor (*GFRalpha1–4*) (Sariola and Saarma 2003; Takahashi 2001); however, other than *RET* and *GDNF*, mutations in the genes encoding these ligands and coreceptors have not yet been implicated in the pathogenesis of HD or CCHS.

3.3 Constitutional Chromosomal Abnormalities

Discovery of cancer predisposition genes has been facilitated by the identification of rare patients with constitutional genomic DNA aberrations. Although neuroblastoma patients with de novo karyotypic abnormalities are rare, detailed analyses of these cases have been informative. Satge and colleagues recently reviewed 51 cases of constitutional karyotypic aberrations in neuroblastoma patients and confirmed recurrent constitutional deletions at chromosomal regions 1p36, 2p23, 3q, 11q14–23, and 15q (Satge et al. 2003). High-resolution genetic mapping of some of these deletions has aided in determining the location of putative neuroblastoma suppressor genes at chromosomes 1p36 and 11q14–23 (White et al. 2001; Mosse et al. 2003). The three children with constitutional 1p36 interstitial deletions all had profound neurocognitive deficits and were diagnosed with neuroblastoma during infancy. The constitutional deletions overlap the location of a putative 1p36 tumor suppressor gene (see Chaps. 4 and 5), suggesting that germline absence of a gene within this region may predispose to the development of neuroblastoma. Constitutional balanced translocations have been identified rarely in neuroblastoma patients, and no common region is apparent. Whole chromosome gains or losses are also rare in neuroblastoma patients. Interestingly, there appears to be an excess incidence of neuroblastoma in patients with 45,X (Turner) syndrome and perhaps trisomy 13, whereas trisomy 21 (Down syndrome) appears to be associated with a decreased risk for developing neuroblastoma (Satge et al. 2003; Blatt et al. 1997; Satge et al. 1998).

3.4 Hereditary Neuroblastoma

Neuroblastoma, like retinoblastoma and Wilms' tumor, is an embryonal malignancy that is notable for both a sporadic and hereditary form of the disease. Knudson and Strong provided the first genetic hypothesis of neuroblastoma tumorigenesis in 1972. In a comparison of 29 cases of hereditary neuroblastoma (from 13 families) to 504 unselected cases, they showed that 56% of familial cases were diagnosed at less than 1 year of age compared with 26% of the nonfamilial cases. In addition, 23% of the familial cases had multiple primary tumors documented, compared with 5% of the nonfamilial cases. Analysis of the pedigree structures was consistent with an autosomal-dominant mode of inheritance with incomplete penetrance that they calculated to be 0.63 (63% chance carriers will be affected). These data strongly suggested that the genetics of neuroblastoma initiation are similar to retinoblastoma, and subsequent studies indicated that, like *RB1*, a hereditary neuroblastoma predisposition gene should be a tumor suppressor. Nevertheless, for many of the reasons listed below, the genetic etiology of neuroblastoma has remained elusive over three decades since Knudson and Strong's original observations.

Despite the unequivocal data supporting a genetic hypothesis for the initiation of neuroblastoma tumorigenesis, it is relatively uncommon to obtain a positive family history of the disease for an individual neuroblastoma patient. Shojaei-Brosseau and colleagues recently used an epidemiological approach to show that only 5 of 426 consecutive neuroblastoma patients (1.2%) at a single institution had documentation of at least one first- or second-degree relative with neuroblastoma (Shojaei-Brosseau et al. 2004). This translates to a relatively high standardized incidence ratio (SIR) of 11.4 (95% confidence interval of 3.7–26.5) for the development of neuroblastoma among index-case relatives, but the risk to siblings was estimated at only 0.2%. Patients who present with multiple primary tumors or congenital neuroblastoma are more likely to harbor a germline mutation in a predisposition gene, but in many cases these may be de novo mutations. Taken together, these data suggest that heritable neuroblastoma is a rare phenomenon, and the pediatric oncologist should reassure parents of any newly diagnosed patient that the risk to siblings (particularly in the absence of high-risk features such as multifocal primary tumors) is very low.

The vast majority of reported neuroblastoma pedigrees are small, and large, multiplex, or three-generation families have been identified only rarely. Analyses of the published pedigrees in the past three decades strongly support the original conclusion of an autosomal-dominant mode of inheritance with incomplete penetrance. Although some families show multiple-affected individuals with few unaffected individuals between generations (obligate carriers), other families show multiple-affected individuals in the same generation (i.e., cousins) with no disease detected in intervening relatives (Maris et al. 2002; Perri et al. 2002; Lemire et al. 1998). Therefore, it is very difficult to determine precisely the penetrance of a mutant hereditary neuroblastoma gene segregating within a family, and this interfamilial heterogeneity may suggest that there is more than one heritable predisposition gene with different likelihoods of initiating neuroblastoma tumorigenesis.

Similar to patients with sporadic neuroblastoma, the clinical course in familial cases is also extremely variable (intrafamilial heterogeneity), with often striking contrast in the ages at presentation, disease stage, biological features of the tumor, and disease outcome. In addition, there are several reports of asymptomatic obligate carriers with elevated urinary catecholamines or in whom clinically occult tumors have been detected (Maris et al. 1997); therefore, reduced penetrance secondary to clinically occult or spontaneously regressing tumors, on the one hand, and the lethality of the condition prior to reproductive age, on the other, may both contribute to the

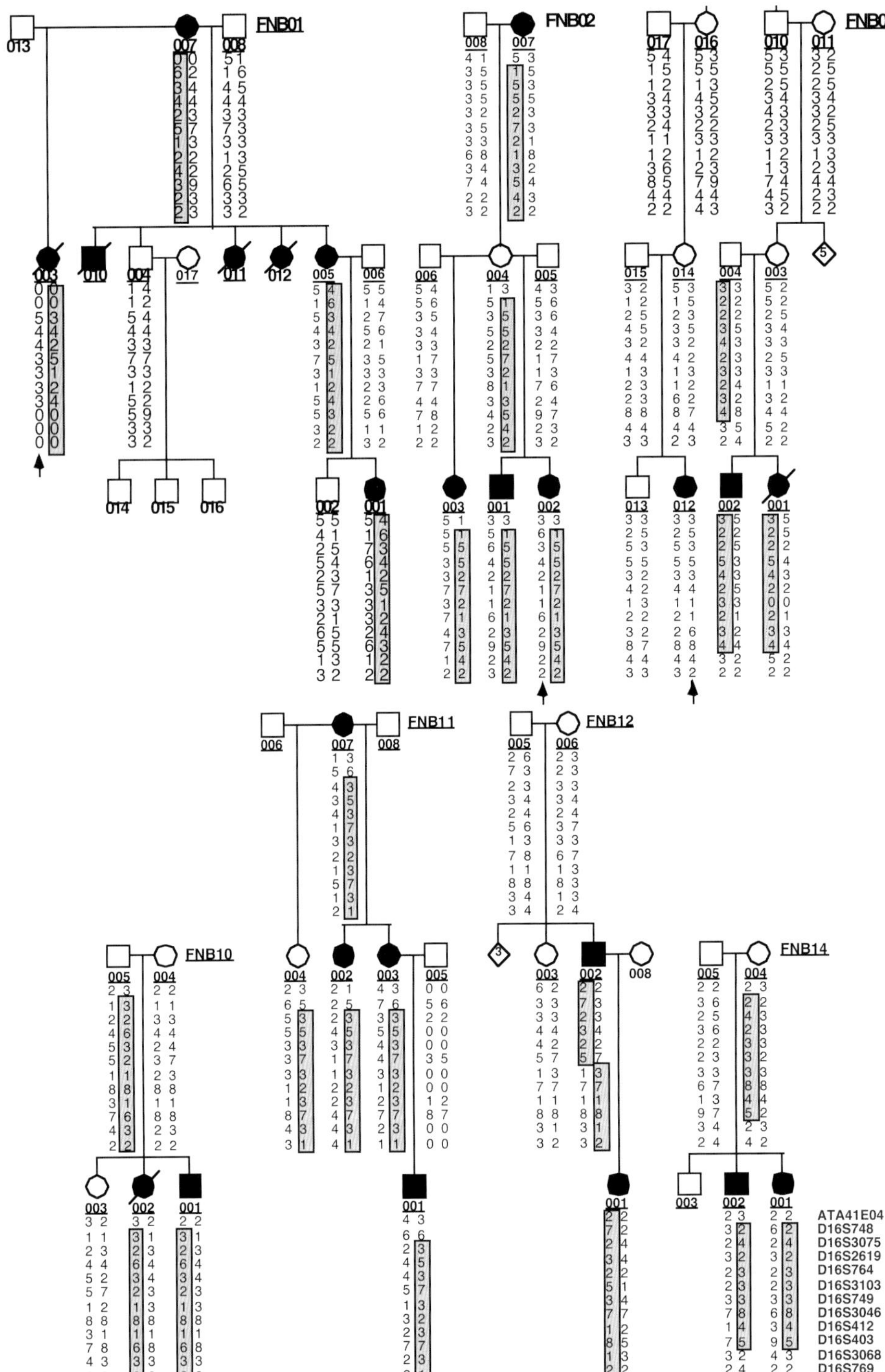
FNB01
FNB02
FNB03
FNB11
FNB12
FNB10
FNB14
ATA41E04
D16S748
D16S3075
D16S2619
D16S764
D16S3103
D16S749
D16S3046
D16S412
D16S403
D16S3068
D16S769

◀ Figure 3.1

The pedigrees from seven neuroblastoma families with evidence for linkage to chromosome bands 16p12–13. *Filled symbols* indicate individual affected with neuroblastoma, ganglioneuroblastoma, or ganglioneuroma. Genotyping data are arranged into probable haplotypes based on minimization of recombination events for 16p polymorphic markers listed at *bottom right* and are displayed for each individual with an available DNA sample. *Gray box* indicates common haplotype segregating with disease in each family and shows genetic homogeneity at 16p. *Arrowheads* indicate haplotype lost when LOH was detected in corresponding tumor specimen

rarity of familial neuroblastoma. These facts have also contributed to the difficulty in approaching this disease with classic genetic approaches in order to isolate genes that predispose to the development of neuroblastoma when mutated in the germline.

3.5 Genetic Studies of Familial Neuroblastoma

There are two published studies that used classic genetic linkage methods to localize hereditary neuroblastoma predisposition genes. In a genome-wide search for linkage in seven pedigrees with at least two first-degree relatives affected with neuroblastoma, convincing evidence was discovered that a hereditary neuroblastoma predisposition gene (*HNB1*) is located on the distal short arm of chromosome 16 (16p12–13; Fig. 3.1) (Maris et al. 2002). Subsequent identification of a three-generation family with seven individuals affected with neuroblastoma appeared to confirm linkage to 16p with a cumulative LOD score of 3.7 (Maris et al. 2003). Loss of heterozygosity has been observed in 13% of sporadic neuroblastomas, suggesting that somatic inactivation of a 16p tumor suppressor gene might contribute to neuroblastoma initiation or progression in at least a subset of nonfamilial cases (Furuta et al. 2000). The genomic region likely to harbor *HNB1* remains relatively large and the positional cloning of this gene is ongoing.

Perri and colleagues studied two families in which ≥ third-degree relatives (cousins) were affected with neuroblastoma. They showed no evidence for linkage to 16p (Perri et al. 2002), in agreement with the original 16p linkage report in which two families consisting of cousins with neuroblastoma also showed no evidence of linkage to 16p (Maris et al. 2002). However, using a candidate-locus approach, they did show evidence for linkage to the distal short arm of chromosome 4p that overlapped a common region of hemizygous deletion observed in some primary neuroblastomas (Perri et al. 2002). Of note, the seven families linked to 16p showed strong evidence refuting linkage to 4p (J.M. Maris, unpublished data). Taken together, these observations support the hypothesis that at least two hereditary neuroblastoma predisposition genes exist, and that the penetrance of the two predisposition genes is different. The literature also strongly suggests that each of the major candidate loci and/or genes listed in Table 3.1 have been excluded as harboring a hereditary neuroblastoma predisposition gene through candidate-locus and/or genome-wide analyses (Maris et al. 1996, 2002; Tonini et al. 2001).

3.6 Conclusions

The rare neuroblastoma patients with a family history of the disease, associated genetic disorder, and/or constitutional chromosomal abnormality offer unique insights into the molecular pathogenesis of this enigmatic tumor. The identification of at least two putative familial neuroblastoma predisposition loci supports the assumption that neuroblastoma is a complex disease genetically, with multiple pathways to tumor initiation. Although identification of hereditary neuroblastoma predisposition genes would be of immediate benefit to those rare families that show evidence for predisposition to the disease, it is likely that the larger impact will be drawn from the insights these discoveries will provide for neuroblastoma tumorigenesis in general.

Acknowledgements. This work was supported in part by National Institutes of Health grants CA78545 and CA87847 (J.M.M.), and by NIH grants CA39771 and CA94194, and by the Audrey E. Evans Endowed Chair (G.M.B.).

et al. 1996). Loss of the whole chromosome 11 appears to be strongly associated with low stage tumors, whereas unbalanced deletion of 11q is predominantly observed in high-stage tumors without amplified *MYCN* (Guo et al. 1999, 2000; Maris et al. 2001b). Deletion events affecting 11q are predominantly large and terminal. A single region of 2.1 cM within 11q23.3, flanked by markers *D11S1340* and *D11S1299*, was deleted in all tumors with 11q LOH (Guo et al. 1999). Constitutional rearrangements of 11q have been observed in some neuroblastoma patients, including a deletion of 11q23-qter, balanced translocations involving 11q21 and 11q22, and an inversion of 11q21-q23 (Bown et al. 1993; Hecht et al. 1982; Koiffmann et al. 1995). The role of these constitutional changes is not clear, but it has been speculated that disruption of one or more 11q genes may predispose to the development of neuroblastoma.

4.4.2.1 Chromosome 11 Deletion and 17q Gain

Fluorescence in situ hybridization (FISH) analyses have demonstrated that, after 1p, chromosome arm 11q is the second most common partner for 17q translocations (van Roy et al. 1994). Such translocations, resulting in concurrent loss of distal 11q and gain of 17q, account for approximately half of the 11q deletion cases (Vandesompele et al. 2001); thus, LOH studies assessing the prognostic value of chromosome losses must take into account the 17q status of each individual tumor.

4.4.3 LOH of Additional Chromosomes

Genome-wide surveys at randomly selected loci have revealed several chromosomal regions with LOH including. 9p21 (Marshall et al. 1997), 14q32 (Hoshi et al. 2000; Thompson et al. 2001), and others (Westermann and Schwab 2002). Although numerous investigators have speculated that TSGs may reside in these sites, to date, in spite of laborious efforts, not one neuroblastoma TSG has been identified.

4.4.4 LOH and Tumor Suppressor Genes: an Evasive Connection or Flawed Hypothesis?

There are several possible explanations for the failure to identify a neuroblastoma TSG. Firstly, the two-hit model, in its original form, may not be applicable to neuroblastoma. In addition, the current logic of utilizing LOH studies to determine the SRO and then surveying the chromosomally intact homologue for genes in this region and for mutations may be flawed. One possibility is that the loss of a single allele by deletion may be sufficient to produce a biological effect. Evidence for haploinsufficiency is accumulating (Goss et al. 2002; Gruber et al. 2002; Kucherlapati et al. 2002; Spring et al. 2002; Venkatachalam et al. 1998) for a number of genes, including *BLM*, *Fen1*, *TP53*, *ATM*, and others (Table 4.1). It is also possible that deletion of a single allele, such as in 1p, alone or in combination with deletion at another genetic locus, may contribute to tumorigenesis simply by dosage effect, without any mutational or epigenetic change of the remaining allele. Evidence is also emerging that slight gene dosage changes, like segmental duplications, can contribute to human malignant and nonmalignant disorders (Corvi et al. 1995; Gratacos et al. 2001; Savelyeva et al. 2001). Genetic imbalance for 1p36 (at least 2 copies of chromosome 1 present with additional 1p36-deleted chromosome 1 copies) may also be associated with poor prognosis, similar to that seen in patients with tumors with 1p deletion or amplified *MYCN* (Spitz et al. 2002).

Another problem could be genetic heterogeneity for particular LOH regions among neuroblastoma subtypes, and thus, the strategy of analyzing the genes of a consensus region deduced from a larger number of tumors is flawed. One scenario, hypothetical but in principle suggested earlier (Takeda et al. 1994), could be that one biological or clinical group (group 1) of tumors results from the inactivation of one gene, while another clinical group of neuroblastomas (group 2) depends on the inactivation of another gene. Both genes may be in 1p36, but the group-2 gene may be several megabases away from the group-I gene. When LOH data are combined from these two groups, the SRO will be extremely unlikely to harbor the damaged second allele (Fig. 4.4).

Table 4.1. Genes and haploinsufficiency in tumorigenesis

Gene	Function	Reference
AML1/CBFA2	Transcription factor	Barton and Nucifora (2000); Song et al. (1999)
Cdh1	Cell-cell adhesion	Smits et al. (2000)
Dmpl	Cell-cycle control	Inoue et al. (2001)
Lkb1	Kinase with unknown target	Miyoshi et al. (2002)
NF1	Signal transduction	Zhu et al. (2002)
P27^{Kip1}	Cell-cycle control	Fero et al. (1998)
Ptch	Signal transduction	Wetmore et al. (2000)
Pten	Signal transduction	Kwabi-Addo et al. (2001)
Atm	DNA damage response	Spring et al. (2002)
Blm	DNA repair	Goss et al. (2002)
Fenl	DNA repair	Kucherlapati et al. (2002)
p53	Cellular stress response	Ide et al. (2003); Venkatachalam et al. (1998)
H2AX	DNA repair	Celeste et al. (2003)
Nbn	DNA repair	Dumon-Jones et al. (2003)
Anx7	DNA repair	Srivastava et al. (2003)

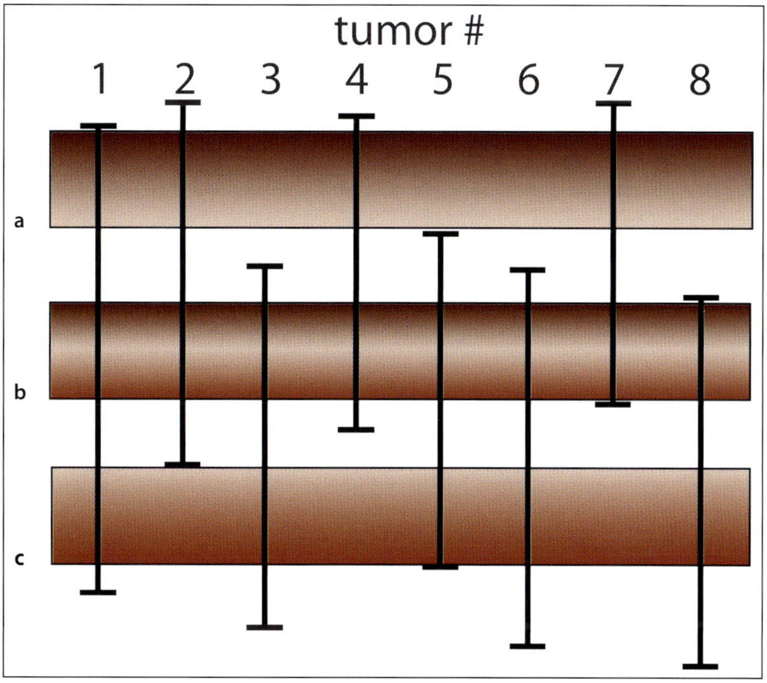

Figure 4.4

Genetic heterogeneity of LOH regions (depicted by *black capped bars*) may explain the failure to find the "neuroblastoma suppressor gene." In case of genetic heterogeneity, there could actually be at least two (*B*, *C*), if not more genes involved, and these might be separated many megabases from each other. Combining these LOH regions into a single consensus region (*A*) would inevitably initiate a gene search in a region that is unlikely to harbor the long-sought NSG

According to this hypothesis, there would actually be two SROs, each harboring a different gene that is damaged only in tumors of the corresponding group. As mentioned above, previous studies have indicated that two, or even more, "neuroblastoma genes" may reside in chromosome 1p (Caron et al. 2001). The existence of two separate 1p regions with relevance to neuroblastoma is also supported by an independent study that indicated two regions of loss, at 1p36 and 1p22 (Mora et al. 2000). Another study concluded that there were three regions of loss at 1p36.1–2, 1p36.3, and 1p32–34, and each was associated with different neuroblastoma groups (Hiyama et al. 2001).

4.5 Comparative Genomic Hybridization

In CGH, differentially labeled tumor DNA and normal DNA are competitively hybridized to normal human metaphase chromosomes (Kallioniemi et al. 1992). This methodology detects quantitative chromosomal changes, such as deletions, duplications or amplifications on the basis of the ratio of the hybridization of the two differently labeled DNAs. The advantage of this approach is that the complete set of quantitative genomic changes can be determined in a single experiment. Limitations are the low level of resolution (several Mb) and the fact that absolute quantitation of the changes is not precise. More recently, array CGH has been performed in an effort to increase the resolution of this technique. This strategy utilizes an array of DNA targets, and both cDNA and BAC arrays have been used (Beheshti et al. 2003; Cowel and Nowak 2003).

Both CGH and array CGH (Cunsolo et al. 2000; Plantaz et al. 2001; Schleiermacher et al. 2003; Stallings et al. 2003; Vettenranta et al. 2001) have largely confirmed previous cytogenetic and LOH studies revealing a high-frequency of 1p loss, 11p loss, 2p gain, and 17q gain (Schleiermacher et al. 2004; Brinkschmidt et al. 1997; Lastowska et al. 1997b, 2002; Plantaz et al. 1997; Vandesompele et al. 1998). The CGH studies have also revealed that about 50% of neuroblastomas have an additional segment of 17q, indicating that gain of 17q is the most frequent genetic alteration in neuroblastoma. Gain of 17q appears more common in advanced-stage tumors, in tumors from children aged over 1 year, and in tumors showing 1p loss, amplified *MYCN*, and diploidy or tetraploidy. In contrast, triploidy with whole chromosome 17 gain is associated more often with neuroblastomas showing favorable clinical and genetic features (Bown et al. 1999). Amplified *MYCN* rarely, if ever, occurs without either 1p deletion or 17q gain or both, implying that *MYCN* amplification is a later event in the sequence of genetic aberrations underlying neuroblastoma progression (Bown et al. 1999). Although several studies appear to suggest 17q gain as a powerful prognostic factor (Abel et al. 1999; Bown et al. 1999, 2001; Caron 1995; Caron et al. 1996; Lastowska et al. 1997a), a recent study could not confirm this association (Spitz et al. 2003).

4.6 Tumor Cell Ploidy

Many neuroblastomas have higher than normal DNA content or hyperploidy. Kaneko and Knudson have suggested that in neuroblastoma, aneuploidy may be a consequence of tetraploidization with subsequent bipolar, tripolar, or tetrapolar divisions (Kaneko and Knudson 2000). Supernumerary centrosomes leading to multipolar divisions have been implicated in both chromosome missegregation and the generation of aneuploid cells in various cancer types, including neuroblastoma (Brinkley 2001). A defect of spindle formation may cause incomplete segregation during mitosis; thus, such a defect in a tetraploid cell undergoing a tripolar division could lead to one near-triploid and one near-pentaploid cell. In fact, in neuroblastoma tumors with more than one tumor cell clone, near-pentaploid tumor cells are often observed together with near-triploid tumor cells.

Recently, Kaneko and Knudson have developed an attractive hypothesis explaining the association between ploidy and neuroblastoma phenotype (Kaneko and Knudson 2000). This hypothesis is based on the assumption that both clinically "favorable" triploid tumors and clinically "unfavorable" diploid tumors arise through the same genetic event, as suggested from observations in familial cases (Knudson and Strong 1972; Kushner et al. 1986). The initiating tumorigenic event may be a mutation in a classical tumor suppressor gene with recessive effect at cellular level (Comings 1973; Knudson and Strong 1972). Tetraploidization and subsequent multipolar division of a diploid cell heterozygous for a mutation in such a gene would give rise to diploid and tetraploid daughter cells with no normal allele and highly malignant phenotype, or triploid daughter cells with at least one normal allele and less malignant phenotype.

4.7 Conclusion

Despite many advances in understanding the genetics and developmental molecular pathways, they have not yet translated into more effective therapy for high-risk neuroblastoma Nevertheless, the fascinating multiplicity of its clinical and biological phenotypes has attracted a growing number of clinical and basic scientists. Their combined efforts will inevitably resolve the intricate pathways that govern both progression and spontaneous regression of this disease. This knowledge should provide the platform for the development of new diagnostic tools and novel therapeutic strategies. Until then, we should be careful and avoid offering simplified suggestions for a rapid clinical translation.

Acknowledgements. Work in the author's laboratory was supported by grants from the Deutsche Krebshilfe, Sander Stiftung, Bundesministerium für Forschung und Technology, and by DKFZ-MOS (Israel) cooperation.

References

Abel F, Ejeskar K, Kogner P et al. (1999) Gain of chromosome arm 17q is associated with unfavourable prognosis in neuroblastoma, but does not involve mutations in the somatostatin receptor 2(SSTR2) gene at 17q24. Br J Cancer 81:1402–1409

Alaminos M, Mora J, Cheung NK et al. (2003) Genome-wide analysis of gene expression associated with *MYCN* in human neuroblastoma. Cancer Res 63:4538–4546

Alt FW, Kellems RE, Bertino JR et al. (1978) Selective multiplication of dihydrofolate reductase genes in methotrexate-resistant variants of cultured murine cells. J Biol Chem 253:1357–1370

Amler LC, Corvi R, Praml C et al. (1995) A reciprocal translocation (1;15) (36.2;q24) in a neuroblastoma cell line is accompanied by DNA duplication and may signal the site of a putative tumor suppressor-gene. Oncogene 10:1095–1101

Amler LC, Bauer A, Corvi R et al. (2000) Identification and characterization of novel genes located at the t(1;15) (p36.2;q24) translocation breakpoint in the neuroblastoma cell line NGP. Genomics 64:195–202

Balaban-Malenbaum G, Gilbert F (1977) Double minute chromosomes and the homogeneously staining regions in chromosomes of a human neuroblastoma cell line. Science 198:739–741

Barton K, Nucifora G (2000) AML1 haploinsufficiency, gene dosage, and the predisposition to acute leukemia. Bioessays 22:214–218

Bauer A, Savelyeva L, Claas A et al (2001) Smallest region of overlapping deletion in 1p36 in human neuroblastoma: a 1 Mbp cosmid and PAC contig. Genes Chromosomes Cancer 31:228–239

Beheshti B, Braude I, Marrano P et al. (2003) Chromosomal localization of DNA amplifications in neuroblastoma tumors using cDNA microarray comparative genomic hybridization. Neoplasia 5:53–62

Berwanger B, Hartmann O, Bergmann E et al. (2002) Loss of a FYN-regulated differentiation and growth arrest pathway in advanced stage neuroblastoma. Cancer Cell 2:377–386

Biedler JL, Spengler BA (1976) A novel chromosome abnormality in human neuroblastoma and antifolate-resistant Chinese hamster cell lives in culture. J Natl Cancer Inst 57:683–695

Biegel JA, White PS, Marshall HN et al. (1993) Constitutional 1p36 deletion in a child with neuroblastoma. Am J Hum Genet 52:176–182

Bishop JM (1981) Enemies within: the genesis of retrovirus oncogenes. Cell 23:5–6

Bishop JM (1982) Retroviruses and cancer genes. Adv Cancer Res 37:1–32

Bishop JM (1987) The molecular genetics of cancer. Science 235:305–311

Bown N, Pearson AD, Reid MM (1993) High incidence of constitutional balanced translocations in neuroblastoma. Cancer Genet Cytogenet 69:166–167

Bown N, Cotterill S, Lastowska M et al. (1999) Gain of chromosome arm 17q and adverse outcome in patients with neuroblastoma. N Engl J Med 340:1954–1961

Bown N, Lastowska M, Cotterill S et al. (2001) 17q gain in neuroblastoma predicts adverse clinical outcome. U.K. Cancer Cytogenetics Group and the U.K. Children's Cancer Study Group. Med Pediatr Oncol 36:14–19

Brinkley BR (2001) Managing the centrosome numbers game: from chaos to stability in cancer cell division. Trends Cell Biol 11:18–21

Brinkschmidt C, Christiansen H, Terpe HJ et al. (1997) Comparative genomic hybridization (CGH) analysis of neuroblastomas: an important methodological approach in paediatric tumour pathology. J Pathol 181:394–400

Martinsson T, Sjoberg RM, Hedborg F et al. (1995) Deletion of chromosome 1p loci and microsatellite instability in neuroblastomas analyzed with short-tandem repeat polymorphisms. Cancer Res 55:5681–5686

Martinsson T, Sjoberg RM, Hallstensson K et al. (1997) Delimitation of a critical tumour suppressor region at distal 1p in neuroblasoma tumours. Eur J Cancer 33:1997–2001

Meddeb M, Danglot G, Chudoba I et al. (1996) Additional copies of a 25 Mb chromosomal region originating from 17q23.1–17qter are present in 90 % of high-grade neuroblastomas. Genes Chromosomes Cancer 17:156–165

Mertens F, Johansson B, Hoglund M et al. (1997) Chromosomal imbalance maps of malignant solid tumors: a cytogenetic survey of 3185 neoplasms. Cancer Res 57:2765–2780

Miller RW, Fraumeni JF Jr, Hill JA (1968) Neuroblastoma: epidemiologic approach to its origin. Am J Dis Child 115: 253–261

Miyoshi H, Nakau M, Ishikawa TO et al. (2002) Gastrointestinal hamartomatous polyposis in Lkb1 heterozygous knockout mice. Cancer Res 62:2261–2266

Mora J, Cheung NK, Kushner BH et al. (2000) Clinical categories of neuroblastoma are associated with different patterns of loss of heterozygosity on chromosome arm 1p. J Mol Diagn 2:37–46

Mora J, Gerald WL, Cheung NK (2003) Evolving significance of prognostic markers associated with new treatment strategies in neuroblastoma. Cancer Lett 197:119–124

Mosse Y, Greshock J, King A et al. (2003) Identification and high-resolution mapping of a constitutional 11q deletion in an infant with multifocal neuroblastoma. Lancet Oncol 4:769–771

Neel BG, Jhanwar SC, Chaganti RS et al. (1982) Two human c-onc genes are located on the long arm of chromosome 8. Proc Natl Acad Sci USA 79:7842–7846

Nowell PC, Hungerford DA (1960a) Chromosome studies on normal and leukemic human leukocytes. J Natl Cancer Inst 25:85–109

Nowell PC, Hungerford DA (1960b) A minute chromosome in human granulocytic leukemia. Science 132:1497–1499

Ohira M, Kageyama H, Mihara M et al. (2000) Identification and characterization of a 500-kb homozygously deleted region at 1p36.2-p36.3 in a neuroblastoma cell line. Oncogene 19:4302–4307

Parada LF, Tabin CJ, Shih C et al. (1982) Human EJ bladder carcinoma oncogene is homologue of Harvey sarcoma virus ras gene. Nature 297:474–478

Perri P, Longo L, Cusano R et al. (2002) Weak linkage at 4p16 to predisposition for human neuroblastoma. Oncogene 21:8356–8360

Plantaz D, Mohapatra G, Matthay KK et al. (1997) Gain of chromosome 17 is the most frequent abnormality detected in neuroblastoma by comparative genomic hybridization. Am J Pathol 150:81–89

Plantaz D, Vandesompele J, van Roy N et al. (2001) Comparative genomic hybridization (CGH) analysis of stage 4 neuroblastoma reveals high frequency of 11q deletion in tumors lacking *MYCN* amplification. Int J Cancer 91:680–686

Sandberg AA, Sakurai M, Holdsworth RN (1972) Chromosomes and causation of human cancer and leukemia. 8. DMS chromosomes in a neuroblastoma. Cancer 29:1671–1679

Santos E, Tronick SR, Aaronson SA et al. (1982) T24 human bladder carcinoma oncogene is an activated form of the normal human homologue of BALB- and Harvey-MSV transforming genes. Nature 298:343–347

Satge D, Moore SW, Stiller CA et al. (2003) Abnormal constitutional karyotypes in patients with neuroblastoma: a report of four new cases and review of 47 others in the literature. Cancer Genet Cytogenet 147:89–98

Savelyeva L, Claas A, Matzner I et al. (2001) Constitutional genomic instability with inversions, duplications, and amplifications in 9p23–24 in BRCA2 mutation carriers. Cancer Res 61:5179–5185

Savelyeva L, Corvi R, Schwab M (1994) Translocation involving 1p and 17q is a recurrent genetic alteration of human neuroblastoma cells. Am J Hum Genet 55:334–340

Schleiermacher G, Peter M, Michon J et al. (1994) Two distinct deleted regions on the short arm of chromosome 1 in neuroblastoma. Genes Chromosomes Cancer 10:275–281

Schleiermacher G, Delattre O, Peter M et al. (1996) Clinical relevance of loss heterozygosity of the short arm of chromosome 1 in neuroblastoma: a single-institution study. Int J Cancer 69:73–78

Schleiermacher G, Janoueix-Lerosey I, Combaret V et al. (2003) Combined 24-color karyotyping and comparative genomic hybridization analysis indicates predominant rearrangements of early replicating chromosome regions in neuroblastoma. Cancer Genet Cytogenet 141:32–42

Schleiermacher G, Raynal V, Janoueix-Lerosey I et al. (2004) Variety and complexity of chromosome 17 translocations in neuroblastoma. Genes Chromosomes Cancer 39:143–150

Schwab M (1998) Amplification of oncogenes in human cancer cells. Bioessays 20:473–479

Schwab M, Alitalo K, Klempnauer KH et al. (1983a) Amplified DNA with limited homology to myc cellular oncogene is shared by human neuroblastoma cell lines and a neuroblastoma tumour. Nature 305:245–248

Schwab M, Alitalo K, Varmus HE et al. (1983b) A cellular oncogene (c-Ki-ras) is amplified, overexpressed, and located within karyotypic abnormalities in mouse adrenocortical tumour cells. Nature 303:497–501

Schwab M, Varmus HE, Bishop JM et al. (1984) Chromosome localization in normal human cells and neuroblastomas of a gene related to c-myc. Nature 308:288–291

Schwab M, Varmus HE, Bishop JM (1985) Human N-myc gene contributes to neoplastic transformation of mammalian cells in culture. Nature 316:160–162

Schwab M, Praml C, Amler LC et al. (1996) Genomic instability in 1p and human malignancies. Genes Chromosomes Cancer 16:211–229

Schwab M, Westermann F, Hero B et al. (2003) Neuroblastoma: biology and molecular and chromosomal pathology. Lancet Oncol 4:472–480

Shaffer LG, Heilstedt HA (2001) Terminal deletion of 1p36. Lancet 358 (Suppl):S9

Shapira SK, McCaskill C, Northrup H et al. (1997) Chromosome 1p36 deletions: the clinical phenotype and molecular characterization of a common newly delineated syndrome. Am J Hum Genet 61:642–650

Smits R, Ruiz P, Diaz-Cano S et al. (2000) E-cadherin and adenomatous polyposis coli mutations are synergistic in intestinal tumor initiation in mice. Gastroenterology 119: 1045–1053

Song WJ, Sullivan MG, Legare RD et al. (1999) Haploinsufficiency of CBFA2 causes familial thrombocytopenia with propensity to develop acute myelogenous leukaemia. Nat Genet 23:166–175

Sotiriou C, Khanna C, Jazaeri AA et al. (2002) Core biopsies can be used to distinguish differences in expression profiling by cDNA microarrays. J Mol Diagn 4:30–36

Sparkes RS, Sparkes MC, Wilson MG et al. (1980) Regional assignment of genes for human esterase D and retinoblastoma to chromosome band 13q14. Science 208:1042–1044

Sparkes RS, Murphree AL, Lingua RW et al. (1983) Gene for hereditary retinoblastoma assigned to human chromosome 13 by linkage to esterase D. Science 219:971–973

Spieker N, Beitsma M, van Sluis P et al. (2001) Three chromosomal rearrangements in neuroblastoma cluster within a 300-kb region on 1p36.1. Genes Chromosomes Cancer 31:172–181

Spitz R, Hero B, Westermann F et al. (2002) Fluorescence in situ hybridization analyses of chromosome band 1p36 in neuroblastoma detect two classes of alterations. Genes Chromosomes Cancer 34:299–305

Spitz R, Hero B, Ernestus K et al. (2003) Gain of distal chromosome arm 17q is not associated with poor prognosis in neuroblastoma. Clin Cancer Res 9:4835–4840

Spring K, Ahangari F, Scott SP et al. (2002) Mice heterozygous for mutation in Atm, the gene involved in ataxia-telangiectasia, have heightened susceptibility to cancer. Nat Genet 32:185–190

Squire J, Gallie BL, Phillips RA (1985) A detailed analysis of chromosomal changes in heritable and non-heritable retinoblastoma. Hum Genet 70:291–301

Srivastava M, Montagna C, Leighton X et al. (2003) Haploinsufficiency of Anx7 tumor suppressor gene and consequent genomic instability promotes tumorigenesis in the Anx7(+/–) mouse. Proc Natl Acad Sci USA 100:14287–14292

Stallings RL, Howard J, Dunlop A et al. (2003) Are gains of chromosomal regions 7q and 11p important abnormalities in neuroblastoma? Cancer Genet Cytogenet 140:133–137

Swanstrom R, Parker RC, Varmus HE et al. (1983) Transduction of a cellular oncogene: the genesis of Rous sarcoma virus. Proc Natl Acad Sci USA 80:2519–2523

Takayama H, Suzuki T, Mugishima et al. (1992) Deletion mapping of chromosomes 14q and 1p in human neuroblastoma. Oncogene 7:1185–1189

Takeda O, Homma C, Maseki N et al. (1994) There may be two tumor suppressor genes on chromosome arm 1p closely associated with biologically distinct subtypes of neuroblastoma. Genes Chromosomes Cancer 10:30–39

Takeda O, Handa M, Uehara T et al. (1996) An increased NM23H1 copy number may be a poor prognostic factor independent of LOH on 1p in neuroblastomas. Br J Cancer 74:1620–1626

Takita J, Hayashi Y, Kohno T et al. (1995) Allelotype of neuroblastoma. Oncogene 11:1829–1834

Thompson PM, Seifried BA, Kyemba SK et al. (2001) Loss of heterozygosity for chromosome 14q in neuroblastoma. Med Pediatr Oncol 36:28–31

Tonini GP, Longo L, Coco S et al. (2003) Familial neuroblastoma: a complex heritable disease. Cancer Lett 197:41–45

Turleau C, de Grouchy J, Chavin-Colin F et al. (1985) Cytogenetic forms of retinoblastoma: their incidence in a survey of 66 patients. Cancer Genet Cytogenet 16:321–334

Van Roy N, Laureys G, Cheng NC et al. (1994) 1;17 translocations and other chromosome 17 rearrangements in human primary neuroblastoma tumors and cell lines. Genes Chromosomes Cancer 10:103–114

Van Roy N, Cheng NC, Laureys G et al. (1995) Molecular cytogenetic analysis of 1;17 translocations in neuroblastoma. Eur J Cancer 31A:530–535

Vandesompele J, van Roy N, van Gele M et al. (1998) Genetic heterogeneity of neuroblastoma studied by comparative genomic hybridization. Genes Chromosomes Cancer 23: 141–152

Vandesompele J, Speleman F, van Roy N et al. (2001) Multicentre analysis of patterns of DNA gains and losses in 204 neuroblastoma tumors: how many genetic subgroups are there? Med Pediatr Oncol 36:5–10

Varmus HE (1982) Form and function of retroviral proviruses. Science 216:812–820

Venkatachalam S, Shi YP, Jones SN et al. (1998) Retention of wild-type p53 in tumors from p53 heterozygous mice: reduction of p53 dosage can promote cancer formation. EMBO J 17:4657–4667

Vettenranta K, Aalto Y, Wikstrom S et al. (2001) Comparative genomic hybridization reveals changes in DNA-copy number in poor-risk neuroblastoma. Cancer Genet Cytogenet 125:125–130

Weith A, Martinsson T, Cziepluch C et al. (1989) Neuroblastoma consensus deletion maps to 1p36.1–2. Genes Chromosomes Cancer 1:159–166

Westermann F, Schwab M (2002) Genetic parameters of neuroblastomas. Cancer Lett 184:127–147 get tissue-derived neurotrophins (Oppenheim 1991). This same death mechanism appears to be conserved in primary neuroblastomas found in infants, leading to the induction of their spontaneous regression (Nakagawara 1998b).

5.2.2 Neurotrophic Factors and Their Receptors

5.2.2.1 Neurotrophins and Their Receptors in Neuroblastoma

The neurotrophin family of growth factors consists of nerve growth factor (NGF), brain-derived neurotrophic factor (BDNF), neurotrophin-3 (NT-3), and neurotrophin-4/5 (NT-4/5; Huang and Reichardt 2003). The corresponding high-affinity neurotrophin receptors with tyrosine kinase activity have been identified as TrkA, TrkB, and TrkC (Snider 1994) (Fig. 5.5 a, b). TrkA is a preferred receptor for NGF, TrkB for BDNF and NT-4/5, and TrkC for NT-3. All of the neurotrophins also bind similarly to a lower-affinity neurotrophin receptor $p75^{NTR}$, a member of the tumor necrosis factor receptor (TNFR)/Fas family (Snider 1994). The targeted disruption of neurotrophins and their receptors has demonstrated that NGF/TrkA signaling supports the survival and differentiation of sympathetic and sensory neurons responsive to temperature and pain, while BDNF/TrkB, NT-4/TrkB, and NT-3/TrkC signaling supports those of sensory neurons responsive to tactile stimuli and motor and sensory neurons responsive to limb movement and position, respectively (Klein 1994). These results suggest that neural development and maintenance of the neural network are spatiotemporally controlled by neurotrophin signaling with or without some redundancy in both peripheral and central nervous systems.

In neuroblastoma, high levels of TrkA are expressed in subsets of tumors with good prognosis, often showing spontaneous regression (Nakagawara et al. 1992, 1993; Suzuki et al. 1993; Kogner et al. 1993). Such tumors usually occur in patients under 1 year of age, and their DNA ploidy is aneuploid. A very limited amount of NGF may be supplied from stromal cells, e.g., Schwannian cells and fibroblasts, which at least partly regulate the differentiation and programmed cell death of neuroblastoma cells (Nakagawara 1998a). On the other hand, TrkA expression is strongly downregulated in tumors with aggressive behavior that usually possess amplification of the *MYCN* oncogene and allelic loss of chromosome 1p36 (Nakagawara et al. 1992, 1993). TrkB is preferentially expressed in aggressive neuroblastomas together with its preferred ligands BDNF and NT-4/5 which stimulate in an autocrine/paracrine manner, conferring an enhanced malignant phenotype to the tumor cells (Nakagawara et al. 1994; Matsumoto et al. 1995). TrkC is expressed in favorable neuroblastomas at variable levels (Yamashiro et al. 1996), but its preferred ligand, NT-3, is nearly undetectable by RT-PCR in primary neuroblastomas (Nakagawara 1998a); thus, in regressing neuroblastomas, tumor cells expressing the TrkA receptor may be dependent on a limited amount of NGF supplied from stromal cell. In the presence of NGF the cells mature, whereas they will die in the absence of this ligand (Nakagawara 1998a,b); however, in clinically aggressive neuroblastomas, the TrkA is downregulated and the downstream signaling cascades are disturbed, and these cells utilize the BDNF or NT-4/TrkB autocrine system for efficient growth. Neurotrophin signaling may also regulate tumor metastasis (Matsumoto et al. 1995), proliferation (Matsumoto et al. 1995), and angiogenesis (Canete et al. 2000). The role of $p75^{NTR}$ in neuroblastoma is unclear. The $p75^{NTR}$ receptor is expressed in both neuroblastoma cell lines (Azar et al. 1990) and primary neuroblastomas (Nakagawara et al. 1993). Interestingly, the expression levels of $p75^{NTR}$ mRNA are significantly higher in favorable neuroblastomas (stages 1, 2 and 4s) as compared with the advanced stage tumors, especially those with *MYCN* amplification (Nakagawara et al. 1993).

5.2.2.2 Neurotrophin Signaling in Neuroblastoma

In a rat pheochromocytoma cell line PC12, differentiation signals by NGF may be mediated through the tyrosine phosphorylation of the Trk receptor and through the subsequent activation of Shc/Grb2/SOS, Ras, Raf, MEK, and ERKs, while survival signals in the same cells may be transduced through the direct

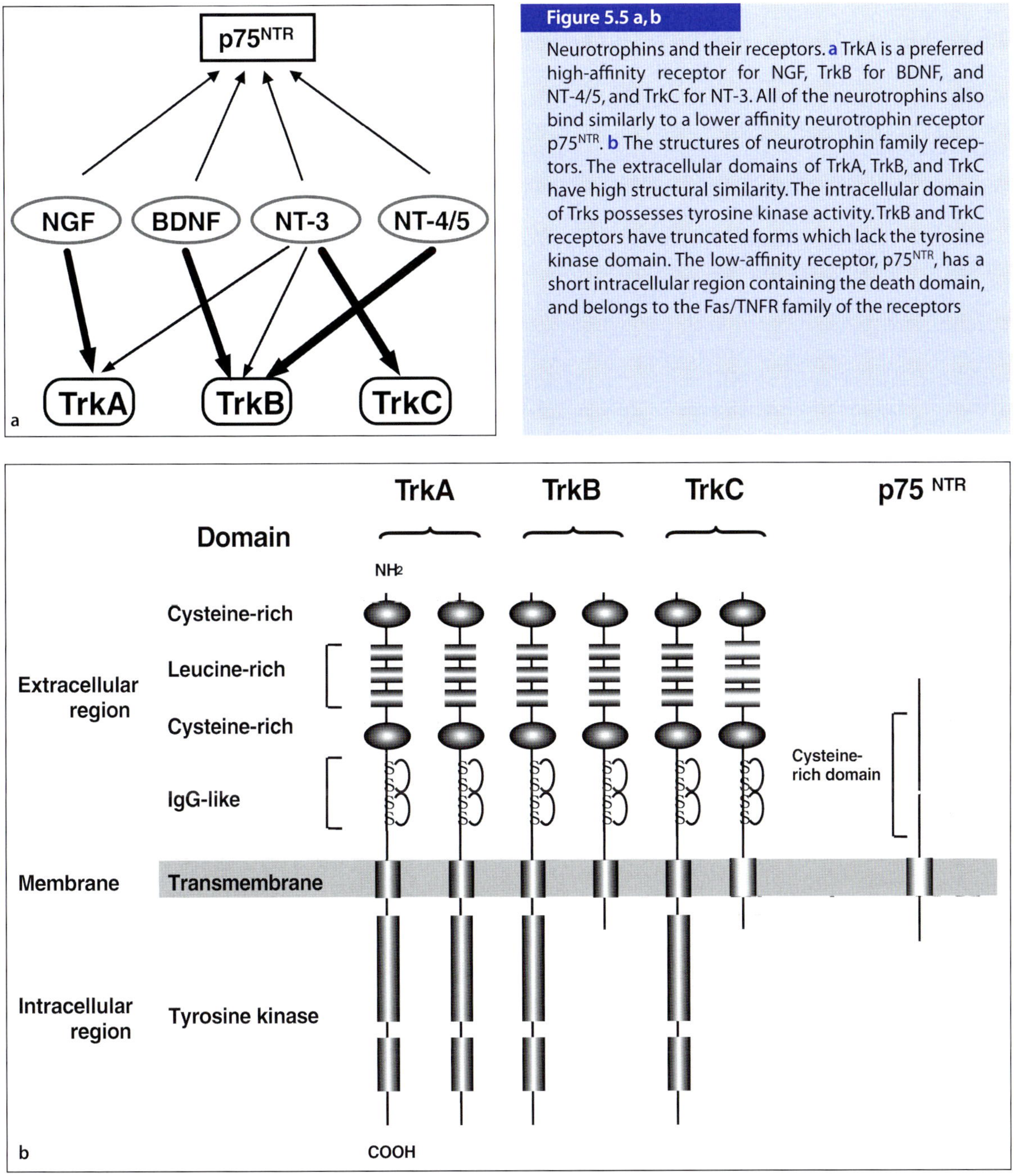

Figure 5.5 a, b

Neurotrophins and their receptors. **a** TrkA is a preferred high-affinity receptor for NGF, TrkB for BDNF, and NT-4/5, and TrkC for NT-3. All of the neurotrophins also bind similarly to a lower affinity neurotrophin receptor $p75^{NTR}$. **b** The structures of neurotrophin family receptors. The extracellular domains of TrkA, TrkB, and TrkC have high structural similarity. The intracellular domain of Trks possesses tyrosine kinase activity. TrkB and TrkC receptors have truncated forms which lack the tyrosine kinase domain. The low-affinity receptor, $p75^{NTR}$, has a short intracellular region containing the death domain, and belongs to the Fas/TNFR family of the receptors activation of PI3-kinase which in turn activates downstream molecules, e.g., Akt and Bad (Klesse and Parada 1999). On the other hand, in normal sympathetic neurons, the activation of PI3-kinase is mediated not by the tyrosine phosphorylation of the receptor but by the Ras activation which promotes neuronal survival, suggesting that the Trk intracellular signaling pathway might be deregulated in cancer cells. This is also the case in neuroblastoma. In the neuroblastoma cell lines with a single copy of *MYCN*, NGF can induce differentiation when exogenous TrkA is overexpressed (Eggert et al. 2000). In the cell lines with *MYCN* amplification, however, the NGF-stimulated TrkA receptors which were overexpressed cannot normally activate downstream signaling molecules, resulting in unresponsiveness to the ligand. Furthermore, it is surprising that BDNF/TrkB signaling appears to be functioning in the same cells by promoting survival (Nakagawara et al. 1994; Hishiki et al. 1998), although the signaling pathway might be different from that of sympathetic neurons (Klesse and Parada 1999).

5.2.2.3 GDNF Family Receptors

Neurotrophic factors of the glial cell line-derived neurotrophic factor (GDNF) family, which include GDNF, artemin and neurturin, are secreted by neuroblastoma cells as well as stromal cells and activate their receptor complex composed of Ret tyrosine kinase and the GFRα co-receptors expressed in neuroblastoma cells (Hishiki et al. 1998; Ichikawa et al. 2004). In contrast to NGF/TrkA and BDNF/TrkB, however, the GDNF/Ret/GFRα autocrine system is functioning in both favorable and unfavorable neuroblastomas to enhance the survival and differentiation of tumor cells (Hishiki et al. 1998).

5.2.2.4 Other Factors and Receptors

Neuroblastoma cells express other growth factors and receptors. Both pleiotrophin (PTN) and midkine (MK) are factors in the same family with neurotrophic function (Kadomatsu et al. 1990; Li et al. 1990; Kadomatsu and Muramatsu 2004). PTN is expressed significantly at high levels in favorable neuroblastomas, while MK is highly expressed in almost all neuroblastomas with a tendency to be expressed at high levels in tumors in advanced stages (Nakagawara et al. 1995). Neuroblastoma also expresses many other receptors, e.g., fibroblast growth factor receptor (FGFR; Schweigerer et al. 1991), insulin-like growth factor (IGFR; El-Badry et al. 1991), DCC (deleted in colon cancer) (Reale et al. 1996), and neuronal leucine-rich repeat receptors (NLRRs; Hamano et al. 2004), as well as a novel plasma membrane enzyme ECEL1, which is significantly highly expressed in favorable neuroblastomas (Kawamoto et al. 2003). The biological significance of these factors and receptors in neuroblastoma are not currently known.

5.2.3 Functional Role of p53 Family Genes

Recent lines of evidence suggest that both the p53 tumor suppressor protein and its related protein p73 are involved in the induction of programmed cell death and growth arrest in neuronal cells (Pozniak et al. 2000). p73 is a recently identified candidate tumor suppressor gene mapped to chromosome 1p36.2, a frequently deleted region in many human cancers including neuroblastoma and oligodendroglioma (Ichimiya et al. 1999; Billon et al. 2004). In cultured neonatal sympathetic neurons, p53 protein levels are increased in response to NGF withdrawal as well as $p75^{NTR}$ activation, and it functions downstream of c-Jun NH_2-terminal kinase (JNK) and upstream of Bax to induce apoptosis (Aloyz et al. 1998) (Fig. 5.6). Indeed, in $p53^{-/-}$ mice, naturally occurring sympathetic neuron death is inhibited. Pozniak et al. (2000) have also reported that p73 is primarily present in developing neurons as ΔNp73, an NH_2-terminally truncated isoform, whose level is decreased when sympathetic neurons undergo apoptosis after NGF withdrawal, and that p53 becomes activated to be pro-apoptotic. In contrast to the truncated form of p73, full-length p73 has induced neuronal differentiation in a mouse neuroblastoma cell line N1E115 (Laurenzi et al. 2000). These data suggest that the neuronal apoptosis induced by NGF withdrawal is at least partly regulated by a reciprocal balance between levels of pro-apoptotic p53 and anti-apoptotic ΔNp73.

Figure 5.6

A model of signaling pathway for survival and death in sympathetic neurons regulated by NGF. NGF depletion may induce activation of JNK/p53 pathway which could be modified by p73/ΔNp73 regulatory system. $p75^{NTR}$ activation, which sends signals of both survival and death, may also regulate downstream p53/p73/ΔNp73 pathway

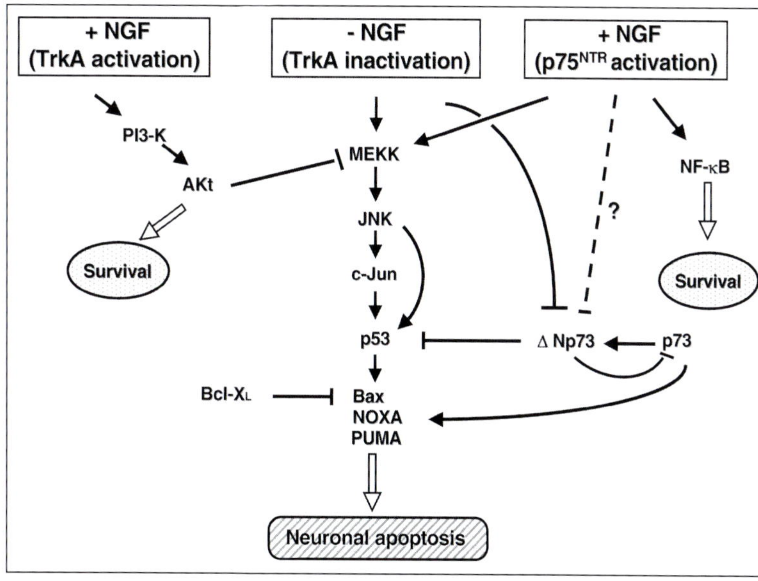

Figure 5.7

A possible signaling pathway regulating growth, differentiation and survival in neuroblastoma cells or sympathetic neurons. The NGF-triggered autophosphorylation of TrkA tyrosine kinase receptor induces activation of Ras/MAPK pathway, which in turn regulates nuclear pRB and Mdm2. In some poor-outcome neuroblastomas, p53, which is shuttling between cytosol and nucleus, is trapped in the cytosol by Parc, an anchoring protein of p53. *MYCN* induces expression of *Id-2* whose protein product in turn inhibits pRB. E2F1 negatively regulated by pRB directly induces expression of p73. p73 is regulated by ΔNp73 in a negative autoregulatory manner (Nakagawa et al. 2002), and ΔNp73 also inhibits p53

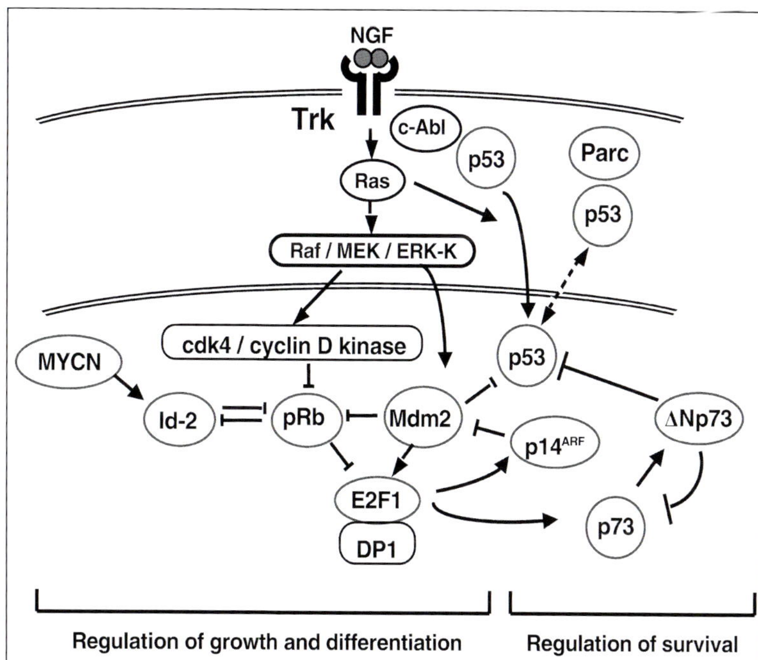

The importance of p53 and p73 has also been emphasized by the important observation that, in cultured neuroblastoma and other cancer cells, p73 directly transactivates the ΔNp73 gene by binding to its promoter after treating the cells with genotoxic reagents, e.g., cisplatin (Nakagawa et al. 2002). The induced ΔNp73 protein in turn interacts with either wild-type p53 or TAp73 and inhibits their proapoptotic function; thus, ΔNp73 can act as an oncogene and as an inhibitor of wild-type p53 and TAp73. The presence of this autoinhibitory feedback loop among p53, TAp73, and ΔNp73 may at least in part explain why there is no mutation of the p73 gene in cancers.

p53 is associated with TrkA via the proto-oncogene product c-Abl as an adaptor or bridging molecule, suggesting that it may also play a role in Trk signaling (Yano et al. 2000) (Fig. 5.7). The activation of Ras by NGF stimulation of the TrkA receptor induces p53 nuclear translocation and growth arrest in PC12 cells (Hughes et al. 2000). The c-Ha-Ras gene could be a target of p53, and protein products induce a positive feedback loop by activating $p14^{ARF}$ which counteracts the negative feedback loop mediated by mdm2 (Deguin-Chambon et al. 2000). These observations strongly suggest that p53 and p73 tumor suppressors function in neurotrophin signaling and modulate the growth, differentiation, and apoptosis of neurons.

In neuroblastoma and some other human cancers, wild type p53 is often localized in the cytoplasm (Moll et al. 1995). Although the regulatory mechanism of cellular localization of p53 and p73 is still unknown, activated Ras in NGF/TrkA signaling stimulates the nuclear translocation of p53 and leads to growth arrest by the induction of $p21^{WAF1}$ in PC12 cells (Hughes et al. 2000). Furthermore, some fractions of recurrent neuroblastomas and neuroblastoma cell lines acquire mutation of the p53 gene (Tweddle et al. 2001).

5.2.4 Apoptotic Signals in Neuroblastoma

To date, the spontaneous regression of neuroblastoma, has occurred only *in vivo*. Although this makes the analysis difficult, there are some important reports. An anti-apoptotic protein, Bcl-2, is expressed in primary neuroblastomas and neuroblastoma cell lines. The expression levels of Bcl-2 and Bcl-X_L are high in aggressive tumor cells but are low in regressing cells (Ikeda et al. 1995; Ikegaki et al. 1995). Caspase-1 and caspase-3 are expressed at significantly higher levels in favorable neuroblastomas (Nakagawara et al. 1997), and caspase-8 is silenced in aggressive neuroblastomas by the methylation of its promoter as one of mechanisms (Teitz et al. 2000). Silencing of caspase-8 is observed in 25–35% of primary neuroblastomas with a high frequency in more aggressive tumors (Teitz et al. 2000; Eggert et al. 2001; van Noesel et al. 2003). Survivin, a member of the inhibitors of apoptosis protein (IAP), is mapped to the long arm of chromosome 17. In neuroblastoma, survivin is highly expressed in high-risk tumors, and its overexpression inhibits cellular apoptosis (Islam et al. 2000). Kitanaka et al. (2002) have recently reported an interesting observation that "autophagy" may be involved in the regression of neuroblastoma cells.

5.3 Conclusions

Development of neuroblastoma may be triggered by a genetic event(s) that leads to chromosome and/or the genomic DNA abnormalities such as amplification of the *MYCN* gene and deletions or gains in chromosomal regions including 1p, 11q, and 17q. Together with other epigenetic mechanisms of gene activation or gene silencing, they affect gene and protein expression which in turn deregulate cellular signaling. In neuroblastoma the normal biology of developing neuronal cells and cancer biology appear to overlap. A further understanding of the mechanisms involved in the transformation of progenitors or the stem cells into neuroblastoma with significant cellular heterogeneity may provide clues for the development of novel therapeutic strategies for this often aggressive lethal disease.

Acknowledgements. I thank M. Ohira and T. Ozaki for reading the manuscript. I also thank K. Yagyu for preparing the figures.

References

Aloyz RS et al. (1998) p53 is essential for developmental neuron death as regulated by the TrkA and p75 neurotrophin receptors. J Cell Biol 143:1691–1703

Altaba ARi, Stecca B, Sanchez P (2004) Hedgehog-Gli signaling in brain tumors: stem cells and paradevelopmental programs in cancer. Cancer Lett 204:145–157

Axelson H (2004) The Notch signaling cascade in neuroblastoma: role of the basic helix-loop-helix proteins HASH-1 and HES-1. Cancer Lett 204:171–178

Azar CG, Scavarda NJ, Reynolds P, Brodeur GM (1990) Multiple defects of the nerve growth factor receptor in human neuroblastomas. Cell Growth Differ 1:421–428

Ball DW (2004) Achaete-scute homolog-1 and Notch in lung neuroendocrine development and cancer. Cancer Lett 159–169

Billon N et al. (2004) Roles for p53 and p73 during oligodendrocyte development. Development 131:1211–1220

Boon K et al. (2001) N-*MYC* enhances the expression of a large set of genes functioning in ribosome biogenesis and protein synthesis. EMBO J 20:1383–1393

Brodeur GM, Seeger RC, Schwab M, Varmus HE, Bishop JM (1984) Amplification of N-*MYC* in untreated human neuroblastomas correlates with advanced disease stage. Science 224:1121–1124

Canete A, Navarro S, Bermudez J, Pellin A, Castel V, Llombart-Bosch A (2000) Angiogenesis in neuroblastoma: relationship to survival and other prognostic factors in a cohort of neuroblastoma patients. J Clin Oncol 18:2789–2791

Deguin-Chambon V, Vacher M, Jullien M, May E, Bourdon JC (2000) Direct transactivation of c-Ha-Ras gene by p53: evidence for its involvement in p53 transactivation activity and p53-mediated apoptosis. Oncogene 19:5831–5841

Eggert A et al. (2000) Molecular dissection of TrkA signal transduction pathways mediating differentiation in human neuroblastoma cells. Oncogene 19:2043–2051

Eggert A et al. (2001) Resistance to tumor necrosis factor-related apoptosis-inducing ligand (TRAIL)-induced apoptosis in neuroblastoma cells correlates with a loss of caspase-8 expression. Cancer Res 61:1314–1319

El-Badry OM, Helman LJ, Chatten J, Steinberg SM, Evans AE, Israel MA (1991) Insulin-like growth factor II-mediated proliferation of human neuroblastoma. J Clin Invest 87: 648–657

Enomoto H et al. (1994) Identification of human DAN gene, mapping to the putative neuroblastoma tumor suppressor locus. Oncogene 9:2785–2791

Ernsberger U (2000) Evidence for an evolutionary conserved role of bone morphogenetic protein growth factors and phox2 transcription factors during noradrenergic differentiation of sympathetic neurons. Induction of a putative synexpression group of neurotransmitter-synthesizing enzymes. Eur J Biochem 267:6976–6981

Guillemot F, Lo LC, Johnson JE, Auerbach A, Anderson DJ, Joyner AL (1993) Mammalian achaete-scute homolog 1 is required for the early development of olfactory and autonomic neurons. Cell 75:463–476

Hamano S, Ohira M, Isogai E, Nakada K, Nakagawara A (2004) Identification of novel human neuronal leucine-rich repeat (hNLRR) family genes and inverse association of expression of Nbla10449/hNLRR-1 and Nbla10677/hNLRR-3 with the prognosis of primary neuroblastomas. Int J Oncol 24:1457–1466

Hishiki T et al. (1998) Glial cell line-derived neurotrophic factor/neurturin-induced differentiation and its enhancement by retinoic acid in primary human neuroblastomas expressing c-Ret, GFR-1 and GFR-2. Cancer Res 58:2158–2165

Huang EJ, Reichardt LF (2003) Trk receptors: roles in neuronal signal transduction. Annu Rev Biochem 72:609–642

Huber K, Combs S, Ernsberger U, Kalcheim C, Unsicker K (2002) Generation of neuroendocrine chromaffin cells from sympathoadrenal progenitors: beyond the glucocorticoid hypothesis. Ann NY Acad Sci 971:554–559

Hughes AL, Gollapudi L, Sladek TL, Neet KE (2000) Mediation of nerve growth factor-driven cell cycle arrest in PC12 cells by p53: simultaneous differentiation and proliferation subsequent to p53 functional inactivation. J Biol Chem 275: 37829–37837

Iavarone A, Lasorella A (2004) Id proteins in neural cancer. Cancer Lett 204:189–196

Ichikawa M, Murakumo Y, Takahashi M (2004) RET and neuroendocrine tumors. Cancer Lett 204:197–211

Ichimiya S et al (1999) p73 at chromosome 1p36.3 is lost in advanced stage neuroblastoma but its mutation is infrequent. Oncogene 18:1061–1066

Ichimiya S, Nimura Y, Seki N, Ozaki T, Nagase T, Nakagawara A (2001) Down-regulation of *hASH1* is associated with the retinoic acid-induced differentiation of human neuroblastoma cell lines. Med Pediatr Oncol 36:132–134

Ikeda H et al. (1995) Bcl-2 oncoprotein expression and apoptosis in neuroblastoma. J Pediatr Surg 30:805–808

Ikegaki N, Katsumata M, Tsujimoto Y, Nakagawara A, Brodeur GM (1995) Relationship between bcl-2 and *MYC* gene expression in human neuroblastoma. Cancer Lett 91:161–168

Islam A et al (2000) High expression of Survivin, mapped to 17q25, is significantly associated with poor prognostic factors and promotes cell survival in human neuroblastoma. Oncogene 19:617–623

Kadomatsu K, Muramatsu T (2004) Midkine and pleiotrophin in neural development and cancer. Cancer Lett 204:127–143

Kadomatsu K, Huang R-P, Suganuma T, Murata F, Muramatsu T (1990) A retinoic acid responsive gene MK found in the teratocarcinoma system is expressed in spatially and temporally controlled manner during mouse embryogenesis. J Cell Biol 110:607–616

Ziller 1993). More recently, restrictive signaling factors that promote commitment to particular cell fates in migratory and postmigratory neural crest precursor cells have been delineated (Lo et al. 2002; Hemmati et al. 2003; Luo et al 2003). For example, achaete–scute complex (e.g., HASH1) and atonal (ato) homologs (e.g., neurogenin) are required in vivo for development of autonomic and sensory neurons, respectively. By contrast, melanocytes are generated by Wnt signaling, while TGFβ promotes smooth muscle cell development. Finally, Notch and neuregulin promote satellite glial and Schwann cell differentiation.

6.3 Neuroblastoma Cellular Heterogeneity

Many of the cell phenotypes characteristic of the developing neural crest – neuroblasts, non-neuronal (Schwann, perineurial, or satellite) cells, and even melanocytes –are evident in the same NB (Shimada et al. 1999). Moreover, cellular heterogeneity and extent of maturation (e.g., stroma-rich and stroma-poor tumors or high- and low-risk tumors based on histological grade) correlate with clinical behavior and are useful for prognostication of the disease (see Chap. 7; Shimada et al. 1999).

This same cellular heterogeneity is seen in NB cell lines. Three distinct cellular phenotypic variants have been described (Rettig et al. 1987; Biedler et al. 1988, 1997): sympathoadrenal (N-type) neuroblasts; large flattened, substrate-adherent (S-type) cells; and morphologically intermediate (I-type) cells (Fig. 6.1). Studies over the past 25 years have shown that each phenotype represents a particular lineage within the neural crest. The availability of cell lines of the three cell types has led to an increased understanding of the differentiation and malignant potentials of each.

6.4 N-type Neuroblastic Cells

In vitro, the predominant neuroblastic (N) cells resemble sympathoadrenoblasts – immature neural/neuroendocrine precursors, with small rounded cell bodies and neuritic processes that vary widely in number and length. Cells adhere poorly to the underlying substrate but adhere well to each other to form cell clumps (pseudoganglia), achieving high saturation densities in culture (Rettig et al. 1987; Biedler et al. 1997; Spengler et al. 1997). Biochemically, they express proteins for synthesis, binding, and degradation of norepinephrine and acetylcholine (the two major neurotransmitters of the peripheral nervous system), as well as opioid and cholinergic receptors. They express the neuroectodermal stem cell intermediate filament nestin, as well as all three neurofilament proteins and chromogranin A (CgA) and secretogranin II (SgII), depending on their degree of differentiation (Biedler et al. 1997; Ross et al. 2002; Thomas 2003). In addition, they express dHAND and HASH-1, transcription factors that are markers of the early stages of neural crest development (Jögi et al. 2002).

Another transcription factor associated with NB and early neuronal development is *MYCN* (Chap. 4). Expression of the oncoprotein is associated with increased mitosis and a dedifferentiated state in neuroectodermal cells of the CNS. High-level expression requires a neuroblastic phenotype, as non-neuronal variants do not express the protein even in the cell lines with transcriptionally active, amplified *MYCN* genes (Spengler et al. 1997).

N-type cells are tumorigenic. They form colonies in soft agar and tumors in mice, with variable degrees of malignancy (Spengler et al. 1997); however, too few *MYCN*-nonamplified N-type cell lines have been tested to discern a relation between *MYCN* amplification status and malignant potential.

Experimental protocols can induce N-type cells to differentiate along either a neuronal or a neuroendocrine pathway or de-differentiate to an immature neural crest-like phenotype. Neuronal differentiation following addition of retinoids or cyclic AMP-elevating agents is characterized by decreases in cell division and amounts of CgA and *MYCN* protein and increases in SgII and neurofilament proteins and in the number and length of neurites (Ross et al. 2002). Neuroendocrine differentiation induced by synthetic glucocorticoids results in cell flattening, increases in CgA and *MYCN* levels, and decreases in neurite formation, SgII, and neurofilaments (Ross et al. 2002). Hypoxia has also been shown to affect neuroblastic

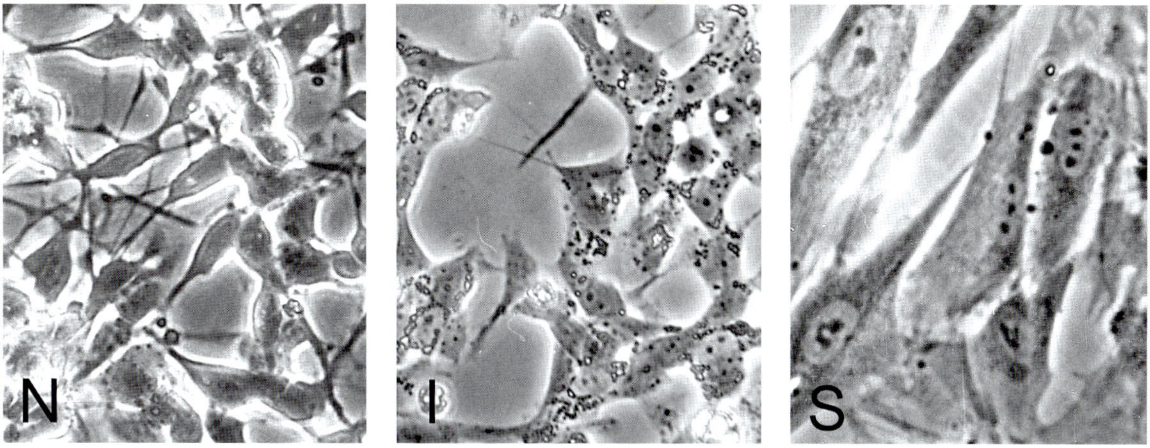

Figure 6.1

Phase-contrast photomicrographs of phenotypic cell variants derived from the LA-N-1 (*N*), SK-N-BE(2) (*I*), and SMS-KCN (*S*) neuroblastoma cell lines (magnification ×500)

differentiation. Growth of N-type cells under hypoxic conditions causes decreased expression of neuronal/ neuroendocrine-specific genes (e.g., CgA and neuropeptide Y) and increased expression of genes present in early neural crest development (c-kit, Notch-1, and HES-1) – indicators of de-differentiation (Jögi et al. 2002).

6.5 S-type Non-Neural Cells

In addition to neuroblasts, a second, clearly non-neuronal cell type is frequently observed in NB cell lines. Termed S, for "substrate adherent", it exhibits contact inhibition of growth, extensive migration on a substrate, and a limited lifespan in culture. Unlike the clearly defined neuronal lineage of N cells, the biochemical signature of S-type cells is more variable. Studies have identified melanocytic properties (tyrosinase, melanosomal glycoproteins, and melanosomes), Schwann or glial cell markers (chondroitin sulfate proteoglycans and large amounts of laminins and fibronectin), and/or smooth muscle cell features (alpha-smooth muscle actin and calponin) (Rettig et al. 1987; Tsokos et al. 1987; Jessen and Mirsky 1999; Sugimoto et al. 2000). All of these lineages are consistent with a neural crest origin for the S cell, as developing crest cells of the trunk give rise to non-neuronal Schwann, glial, melanocytic, and smooth muscle cell components in vivo. The presence of nestin in these cells is consistent with the S-cell phenotype as a neuroectodermal precursor of the non-neuronal lineages of the neural crest (Thomas 2003).

S cells differ from N cells in two other aspects. Firstly, S cells display markers for HLA class-I antigens and β2-microglobulin, which are absent on N-type cells (Rettig et al. 1987). Secondly, unlike N cells, S-type cells will not grow in soft agar or form tumors in nude mice (Biedler et al. 1988; Spengler et al. 1997).

The NB tumors with abundant stroma (stroma-rich) generally have a better prognosis than stroma-poor tumors (Ambros and Ambros 1995; Shimada et al. 1999; Brodeur 2003). The discovery that, in vitro, N and S cells arise from a common precursor suggested that, in vivo, stromal cells could be of tumor origin. One study, using paraffin nonisotopic in situ hybridization, concluded that stromal cells are of nontumor origin, presumably recruited by the neuroblasts in the tumor (Ambros and Ambros 1995). Subsequent studies, using short-term culture of bone marrow tumor cells or laser-capture microdissection with bicolor fluorescence in situ hybridization, showed that both neuroblasts and Schwann cells had identical genetic markers – strong evidence that they arise from a neoplastic precursor (Valent et al. 1999; Mora et al. 2001). This topic is still under debate.

Equally important is the extent of the interaction between Schwann (or S-type) cells and neuroblastic (or N-type) cells in the survival/proliferation/differentiation of each phenotype. In early experiments, N cells co-cultured with S cells were much more differentiated and grew more slowly (B.A. Spengler and J.L. Biedler, personal communication). Such results are consistent with studies of developing neurons and Schwann cells which show that reciprocal contact determines survival and differentiation (Jessen and Mirsky 1999). Also, conditioned medium from normal Schwann cells in culture increases NB cell survival and differentiation (Kwiatkowski et al. 1998) and contains a potent inhibitor of angiogenesis, thus providing a mechanistic basis for the benign behavior of stroma-rich tumors (Huang et al. 2000).

6.6 I-type Stem Cells

The I-type cell was initially identified in cultured cell lines because it appeared "intermediate" in morphology between N and S cells. It exhibits morphological features of both N-type cells (short neurite-like cell processes and growth to high saturation densities) and S-type cells (strong adhesion to and extensive migration over the substrate) (Biedler et al. 1997). These cells also express proteins of both differentiation pathways – noradrenergic biosynthetic enzymes, granins (CgA and SgII), and neurofilament proteins of neuroblasts as well as S cell proteins vimentin, EGF receptor, and CD44. Examples of I-type cells include the cell lines GOTO, NUB-7, BE(2)-C, SH-IN, and LA-N-2 (Biedler et al. 1988, 1997; Ross et al. 1995, 2002).

Continuing research indicates that this cell represents a unique cell type within the NB repertoire. Its ability to generate daughter cells with the same phenotype (self-renewal) and to differentiate bidirectionally along either neuroblastic or Schwann/glial pathways suggests that it is a neural crest cancer stem cell.

First demonstrated for BE(2)-C cell clones and subsequently for other I-type cell lines, I-type cells become neuroblastic when treated for 7–14 days with retinoic acid (RA), but differentiate into S-type cells following treatment with BUdR (Ross et al. 1995). Unlike N (or S) cells, I cells retain the ability to convert to two distinctly different cell lineages.

The most provocative finding regarding the NB I-type stem cell is its malignant potential. As a group, these stem cells are more malignant than neuroblastic variants; they have four- to fivefold higher colony-forming efficiencies in soft agar than N cells and have an over sixfold greater capacity to form tumors in nude mice (Ross et al. 2003; Spengler et al. 1986; Walton et al. 2004). Moreover, phenotype rather than *MYCN* amplification/overexpression determines malignancy; e.g., NB I-type stem cells lacking *MYCN* amplification are more tumorigenic than N-type cells which contain >150-fold amplified genes. Thus, research to date on cell lines suggests that the I-like stem cell could be the truly tumorigenic cell component of NB tumors.

Malignant stem cells in tumors could exert a significant negative effect on prognosis and long-term survival; however, distinguishing putative stem cells from those with a neuroblastic phenotype in tumor sections by routine hematoxylin–eosin analysis is difficult, if not impossible. To specifically search for I-like cells, tumor sections immunostained conjointly with antibodies specific for N or S cells were examined for the presence and frequency of double-labeled cells (Ross et al. 2003). In preliminary analyses, doubly labeled I-like cells were present in all tumors (Fig. 6.2). When the tumors were grouped as either good risk (typically local regional or stage 4s) or poor risk (stages 3 or 4), the frequency of I-like cells was significantly higher (~ fivefold) in the latter group (B.A. Spengler, personal communication). The characterization of this previously unnoticed NB cell type in cell lines and its potential role in refractory high-risk tumors may have identified an important new target for experimental therapeutics.

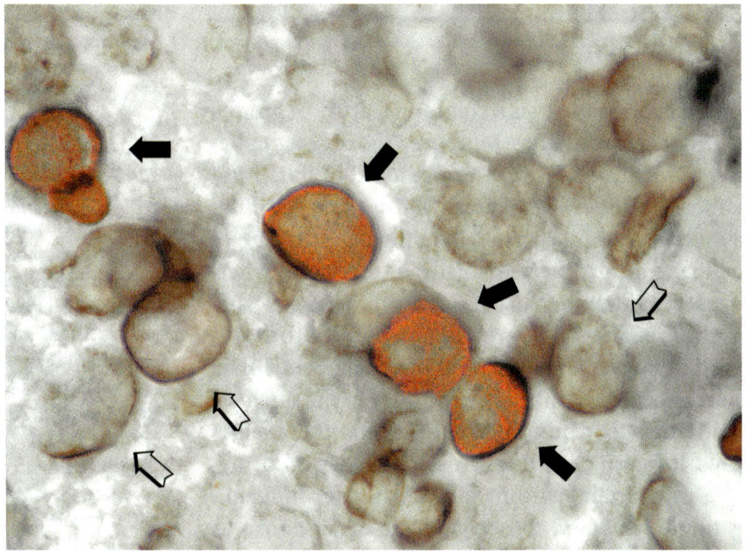

Figure 6.2

Neuroblastoma tumor section stained conjointly for expression of S100A6 (an S cell marker; *red*) and neurofilament 160 (an N-cell marker; *gray*). Examples of I-like cells expressing both proteins are indicated by *filled arrows*, whereas N cells expressing only neurofilament protein are denoted by *open arrows*

6.7 Transdifferentiation

Transdifferentiation is the process whereby cells change from one unique phenotype into another unique phenotype without going through a developmentally less mature stage (Liu and Rao 2003). This process has been reported for cells from all three germ layers and, in particular, for cells of the hematopoietic and neural systems. However, distinguishing de-differentiation/re-differentiation (a two-stage process involving reversion to a more immature stage before expression of the novel phenotype) from transdifferentiation is not easy, especially in heterogeneous populations of cells or those where the intermediate cell type is not readily identifiable (Liu and Rao 2003). In studies with SH-SY5Y (N-type) and SH-EP (S-type), clones of the SK-N-SH cell line, cells with morphological and biochemical features of the other phenotype arose spontaneously and were subcloned (Ross et al. 1995). Of importance, transdifferentiated subclones each have a marker chromosome unique to the clone of origin; therefore, these lines did not arise by clonal selection of pre-existing variants, as has been suggested (Cohen et al. 2003), but represent the conversion to a new cell phenotype. Similar phenotypic conversions have been seen for the LA-N-1 and SK-N-BE(2) cell lines: N-type LA1–55n arose spontaneously and was cloned from the S-type LA1–5s as were S-type LA1–19Bs cells from the N-type LA1–19n clonal cell line. Likewise, the twice-cloned BE(2)-M17 cell line gave rise to the BE(2)-M17F S-type clone. In all cases, the interconversion/transdifferentiation process occurred spontaneously and morphological, biochemical, and cytogenetic criteria were used to confirm the phenotype and cell of origin. Transdifferentiation is very rare and it is the ability to select for the different cell types in culture that has permitted its documentation. Whether the phenomenon observed in NB represents true transdifferentiation or a more complex process involving de-differentiation followed by differentiation along a second neural crest pathway has not been resolved. Nevertheless, the interconversion of N- and S-type cells in culture would suggest that it may occur in vivo. The evolution of quiescent S-type cells into highly proliferative N or I cells mimics the clinical picture of a rapidly recurrent neuroblastoma following a period of clinical remission.

later, vanillylmandelic acid (VMA) was identified as one of the main metabolites and tumor markers (Greenberg 1957; Stickler et al. 1959). In 1971 Evans et al. proposed the first internationally accepted staging system (Evans et al. 1971). Schwab and coworkers (1983) detected MYCN amplification as an important molecular feature of cell lines and primary tumors which proved to be a reliable marker for indicating rapid tumor progression (Seeger et al. 1985) and is now considered an essential parameter for risk estimation.

This chapter describes the clinical presentation of children with neuroblastoma and a comprehensive international perspective of the current criteria that are used for diagnosis, staging, and risk classification. The data regarding clinical presentation are derived from the German experience during the past 24 years. Greater than 95% of all German neuroblastoma patients known to the central children's tumor registry were enrolled in national trials during this time period, and only those with the wrong diagnosis were excluded from analysis; thus, these clinical data can be considered representative of neuroblastoma in a Western country.

7.2 Diagnosis

According to international agreement (Brodeur et al. 1993), the diagnosis of neuroblastoma is established if (a) unequivocal pathologic diagnosis is made from tumor tissue by light microscopy (with or without immunohistology, electron microscopy, increased urine, or serum catecholamine metabolites), or (b) bone marrow aspirate or trephine biopsy contain unequivocal tumor cells (e.g., syncytia or immunocytologically positive clumps of cells) *and* increased urine or serum catecholamine metabolites.

A "suspected clinical diagnosis" of neuroblastoma may be established in emergency situations based on its radiographic features together with distinctly elevated catecholamine metabolites and MIBG avidity. This diagnosis must be considered preliminary (because these tests do not rule out mature ganglioneuroma or pheochromocytoma) and incomplete; thus, tissue histology should always follow.

In addition to tumor histology and urinary catecholamines, the investigation of tumor tissue for genetic abnormalities can aid in the diagnosis of neuroblastoma and provide clinically relevant prognostic information. While certain genetic aberrations are characteristic of neuroblastoma (deletion of 1p36; *MYCN* amplification), specific tumor karyotypic abnormalities [e.g. (t11; 22) for Ewing's sarcoma, (t2;5), (t8;14) for non-Hodgkin's lymphoma, t(2;13) for rhabdomyosarcoma] exclude a diagnosis of neuroblastoma.

7.2.1 Diagnostic Tumor Tissue

Due to the considerable heterogeneity that can be present in neuroblastoma tumors, a single biopsy may not be representative of the tumor's histology or biology. Recently, specific guidelines for pathology and biology studies have been published (Ambros and Ambros 2001). It is recommended that at least two samples, each of 1×1×1 cm size from morphologically different appearing areas, be examined. For unresectable tumors, open biopsies are preferred and, if possible, two different areas should be biopsied by the surgeon. If only Tru-Cut biopsies are feasible, due to the poor general condition of the child, four samples from different areas are recommended (at least 1 cm long; 0.1 cm thick; needle size 18 G). Fine-needle aspiration cytology (22-G needle size; at least 10^5–10^6 cells) with or without ultrasound guidance do not provide an assessment of the tissue architecture and are not recommended but may be sufficient in some cases for cytological and molecular diagnosis.

To ensure the correct sampling and quick handling of the tumor tissue, the presence of an experienced pediatric oncologist in the operation room is highly recommended. Together with the pathologist, and optimally within 20 min from resection, touch preparations for cytology and fluorescence in situ hybridization (FISH) investigations are made before formalin fixation for the pathological examination. Pieces are snap frozen for molecular studies (e.g., Southern blot, PCR) and put in tissue culture medium for classic cytogenetic investigations and tissue culture studies. In the case of small specimens, histology with touch preparations and snap freezing should be priorities.

Figure 7.1 a,b

a A 6-week old girl with abdominal distension by massive liver enlargement (lower rim is marked) and bilateral adrenal primaries. Minimal bone marrow involvement (<1%), good general condition (stage 4S). **b** Blueberry appearance of subcutaneous metastases in a newborn with stage-4S disease

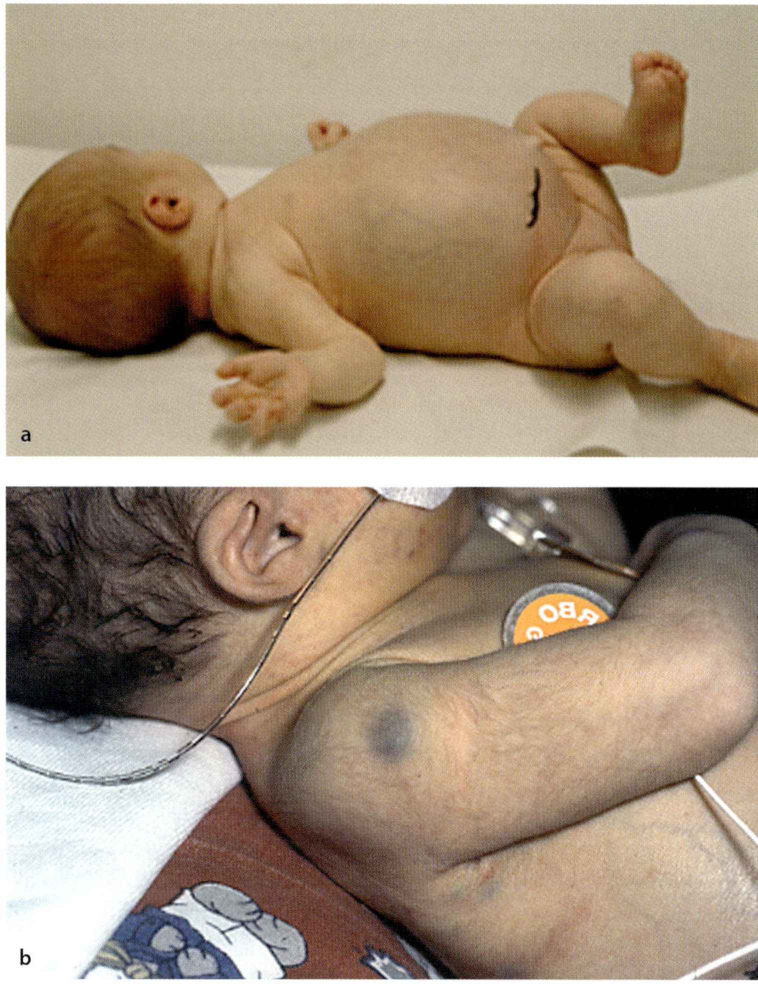

7.3 Clinical Presentation

7.3.1 Symptoms

7.3.1.1 Frequent Symptoms

Presenting signs and symptoms of children with neuroblastoma reflect both the location of the primary tumor and the extent of disease. The typical patient with neuroblastoma is an infant or a toddler. Pain from abdominal distension or metastases to bone is common (30%). Many patients fail to gain weight or have weight loss (11%). The characteristic bilateral periorbital ecchymosis, which is a sign of metastatic disease, is typically caused by intraorbital masses.

In contrast, infants with stage 4S commonly present with abdominal distension resulting from massive liver infiltration (Fig. 7.1a) and subcutaneous nodules (most of them better palpable than visible, sometimes blueberry appearance; Fig. 7.1b). The massive hepatomegaly can lead to respiratory distress, and kidney or bowel function can be impaired due to obstruction by the tumor. Their medical condition can rapidly deteriorate within hours or days (Berthold et al. 1990).

Table 7.1. Rare but characteristic symptoms of neuroblastoma (n=1878, trials NB90/97)

Symptom	Pathogenesis	Occurrence (%)	5-year survival (%)[a]
Transverse myelopathy	Dumbbell tumor with intraspinal, extradural extension	5.4	84±4
Treatment-resistant diarrhea	Vasointestinal peptide secretion by the tumor	3.9	55±7
Horner's syndrome	Cervical tumor with involvement of the cervical ganglion	2.4	79±7
Opsomyoclonus–ataxia syndrome	Unknown ("paraneoplastic")	1.3	87±8
Hypertension	Secretion of pressure active catecholamine metabolites by the tumor or compression of the renal artery	1.3	74±11

[a] The overall survival ratios reflect the data of the designated group. They have not been balanced according to risk factors such as age, stage, *MYCN* amplification, etc. The 5-year overall survival of the entire group was 71±1%

Patients with localized disease are often asymptomatic, and in many cases the diagnosis of neuroblastoma is made following a radiograph or ultrasound performed for unrelated reasons. The rate of incidental diagnosis has varied considerably between countries, even before screening programs were introduced. In Great Britain 7.7% of the neuroblastoma patients were diagnosed at visits for routine health examination or following an investigation of an unrelated condition, compared with 27.1% in Austria and 33.9% in Germany (Powell et al. 1998).

7.3.1.2 Rare but Characteristic Symptoms

Rare but characteristic symptoms of neuroblastoma are shown in Table 7.1.

Transverse Myelopathy

Transverse myelopathy can result from growth of a cervical, intrathoracic, or intraabdominal neuroblastoma through neural foramina into the spinal canal. Approximately half of the patients with dumbbell lesions initially present with neurological symptoms (Katzenstein et al. 2001), but myelopathy may develop soon afterwards, e.g., during surgery; thus, the degree of intraspinal tumor extension should be evaluated by MRI before surgery in order to avoid decompensation of a labile steady state. The neurological abnormalities associated with these tumors include motor deficit (>95%), radicular or back pain (54%), sphincter abnormalities, (34%), and sensory (12%) deficits (de Bernardi et al. 2001). The frequency of complete neurological recovery appears to be inversely correlated with the severity of the presenting neurological deficits (Katzenstein et al. 2001). Forty to 50% of the severely affected surviving children experience long-term neurological sequelae (Katzenstein et al. 2001; de Bernardi et al. 2001). There is a high likelihood of permanent neurological dysfunction in patients who experience neurological symptoms for more than 1 week prior to the initiation of treatment. Chemotherapy, radiotherapy, and surgical decompression with laminectomy have been shown to result in similar rates of neurological recovery, but chemotherapy may be associated with fewer long-term sequelae (Katzenstein et al. 2001; de Bernardi et al. 2001).

Opsomyoclonus–ataxia syndrome

The opsomyoclonus–ataxia syndrome (Kinsbourne syndrome) is characterized by rapid, irregular movements of the eyes ("dancing eyes"; may continue during sleep) and/or by myoclonus and ataxia of the limbs ("dancing feet"), the trunk, and the eyelids.

Many patients experience developmental delays including cognitive and motor delays, language deficits, and behavioral abnormalities (Russo et al. 1997; Rudnick et al. 2001). The pathogenesis is still unclear, although extensive lymphocytic infiltration of the tumor tissue (compared with neuroblastoma patients without opsomyoclonus) (Cooper et al. 2001) and the presence of anti-neuronal antibodies (Rudnick et al. 2001) suggest that the disorder is immunologically mediated. Removal of the primary tumor may not necessarily cure the neurological manifestation. The pharmacological treatment of the neurological symptoms includes glucocorticoids (prednisone or ACTH), high-dose immunoglobulins, and cytotoxic drugs. Anecdotal reports indicate that 60–80% of the patients respond to treatment, but long-term neurodevelopmental results are still poor (60–70% permanent handicaps). The survival rate of children with opsomyoclonus–ataxia syndrome is generally favorable, because the majority of them have localized tumors and present at a young age (Rudnick et al. 2001) (see Chaps. 11 and 13; Table 7.1).

Horner's Syndrome

Horner's syndrome (ptosis, miosis, enophthalmos) and heterochromia (difference in color between the two irises) is caused by disturbances of the cervical sympathetic ganglia which are responsible for normal eye color and development. An association has been found with neuroblastoma only and not with other tumors of the same area (Jaffe et al. 1984) indicating an intimate cooperation between the ganglia and the neuroblastoma development.

Treatment-Resistant Diarrhea

The association of treatment-resistant diarrhea, hypokalemia, and dehydration with neuroblastoma is observed in approximately 4% of patients and is thought to result from overproduction of the vasointestinal peptide (VIP) by maturing neuroblastomas (El Shafie et al. 1983) or ganglioneuromas. It usually resolves after surgical removal of the primary tumor. The use of chemically designed VIP antagonists is still in the preclinical phase (Lilling et al. 1994).

Hypertension

Hypertension is usually caused by tumor pressure on the renal artery with consequent stimulation of the renin–angiotensin system, rather than by tumor secretion of vasoactive catecholamine metabolites (dopamine, epinephrine, norepinephrine). With chemotherapy hypertension can worsen before it gets better. If α- and β-blockers or angiotensin-converting-enzyme inhibitors fail to control the blood pressure and the tumor remains unresectable, one may consider surgically freeing the renal artery without attempting tumor resection.

7.3.2 Tumor Markers

Neuroblastoma is one of the few pediatric tumors in which tumor markers have been shown to have a role in the diagnosis, prognosis, and disease monitoring. Generally, the frequency of abnormal levels increases with tumor burden (stage) and cell turnover (Table 7.2). The reference ranges are strongly age-dependent, with considerably higher values the newborn period and infancy.

Table 7.2. Stage dependence of abnormal tumor markers in neuroblastoma. *HVA* homovanillic acid, *VMA* vanillylmandelic acid, *INSS* International Neuroblastoma Staging System

Tumor marker	*N*	INSS stage			
		1–3 %	4 %	4S %	All %
HVA and/or VMA in urine and/or serum	1280	82	96	93	89
Neuron-specific enolase	1572	57	97	80	75
Lactate dehydrogenase	1809	38	88	45	58
Ferritin	1476	16	53	25	32

Table 7.4. Localization of metastases in patients with neuroblastoma stage 4 and stage 4S at diagnosis and at first recurrence

Disease localization	Stage 4 (%)		Stage 4S (%)	
	Initial[a]	First recurrence[b]	Initial[c]	First recurrence[d]
Bone marrow	87.3	35.2	61.5	19.2
Bone	66.1	46.6	0.0	15.1
Lymph nodes	18.6	8.9	0.0	7.7
Liver	17.4	7.5	76.0	38.5
Skin	2.8	0	12.5	7.7
Intracranial/cerebral	9.1	19.0	0.0	15.4
Lung/pleura	4.7	3.1	0.0	0
Paratesticular	1.0	0	2.6	11.5
Ovary	0.3	0	0.0	0
Isolated local recurrence		17.0		26.9
Isolated metastatic recurrence		58.1		30.7
Combined local and metastatic recurrence		24.9		42.4

[a] Evaluable patients: 725
[b] Evaluable patients: 358
[c] Evaluable patients: 192
[d] Evaluable patients: 26

sion of autologous stem cells, lung metastases are now observed. Moreover, with the use of more intensive induction chemotherapy and the monoclonal anti-GD2 antibody ch14.18 for consolidation, the number of patients with recurrences in the bone marrow has decreased (Simon et al. 2004). Thus, the distribution pattern of metastases after first-line therapy may vary depending on the therapeutic modalities used.

7.3.4.2 Bone Marrow Assessment

Because of the uneven distribution of metastases to the bone marrow, at least two marrow aspirates and two biopsies (trephines) from the iliac crests are recommended (Brodeur et al. 1993). Alternatively, four aspirates from four different sites of the iliac crest or in infants from the proximal tibial bone are sufficient to rule out gross marrow involvement. For an adequate biopsy at least 1 cm of marrow (not cartilage, not bone) is necessary (Brodeur et al. 1993) which may not be feasible in young infants. The bone marrow aspiration consists of three sampling steps per site:

- First aspiration (0.1–0.4 ml) for bone marrow smears
- Second aspiration (2–5 ml, anticoagulated with heparin) for immunocytology
- Third aspiration (2–3 ml, anticoagulated with EDTA or directly into extraction medium) for PCR investigations (Ambros and Ambros 2001).

Figure 7.2 demonstrates characteristic syncytia and immunocytologically positive clumps of cells as requested for the bone marrow diagnosis of neuroblastoma. Although consensus on the specific antibodies for marrow immunocytology has not yet been reached, commercially available anti-GD2 antibodies are widely accepted (Ambros and Ambros 2001) since very few neuroblastomas are GD2 negative. Complementary markers include the neural cell adhesion molecule (NCAM, CD56), NSE, chromogranin A, and

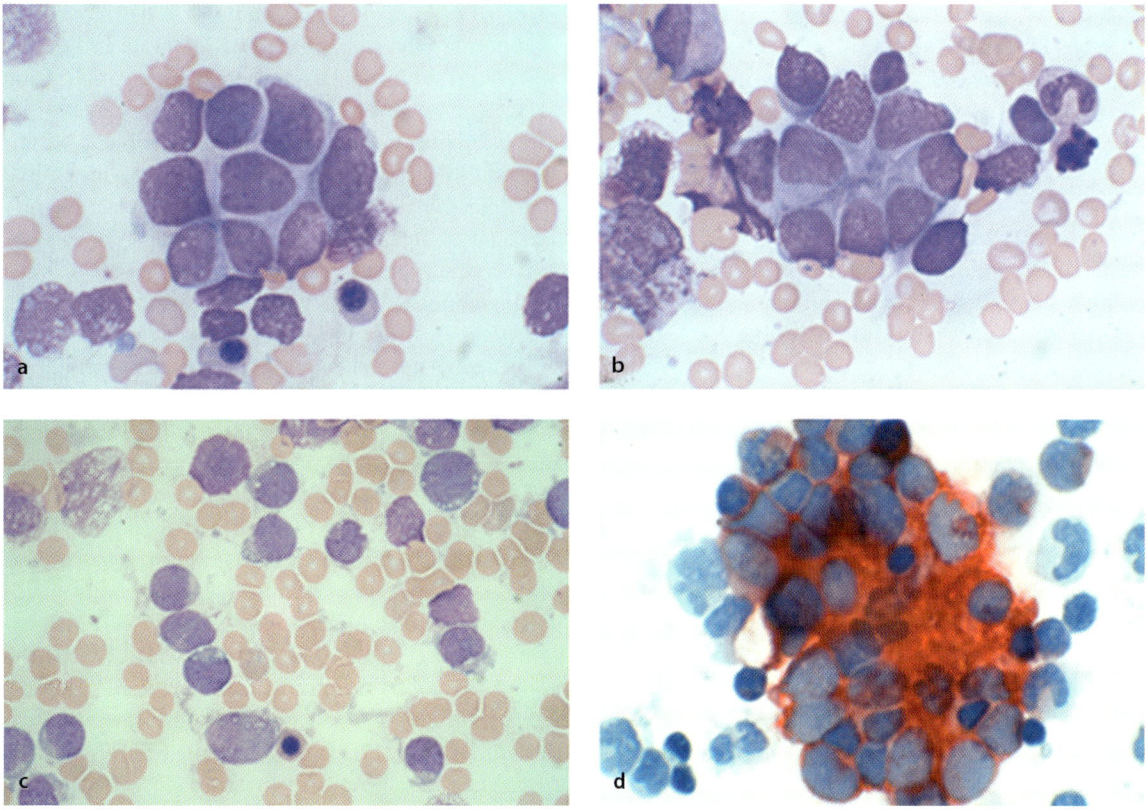

Figure 7.2 a–d

Neuroblastoma cells in bone marrow. **a** Characteristic clumps of cells (three to several hundred cells) closely adhering to each other. The cell size approximates two to three red blood cell diameters and appears a little bit larger and more polymorphic than hematopoietic blasts. High nucleus/cytoplasm ratio. The round-to-moderately oval nucleus contains fine grainy chromatin characteristically with small areas of higher density ("pepper-and-salt structure"). Nucleoli are not often visible. The basophilic cytoplasm is purely confined and the cell margins even invisible in cell clumps. Vacuoles are rarely seen, and granulation is never seen. Some neuroblastoma cells may demonstrate phagocytosis phenomena (not shown). **b** Homer-Wright rosette: typical neuroblastoma cells form a ring of cells around cytoplasmic material (neuropil) in the center. **c** Atypical "ALL like" neuroblastoma cells in bone marrow with many single cells of only one 1–2 red blood cell diameter size, but typical structure of the nucleus and ill-defined, fringed cytoplasm, no or only small clumps. **d** Small tumor clump consisting of cells with distinct membrane staining for GD2 (antibody 14G2a). Due to unspecific GD2 staining to other cell elements (e.g., some megakaryocytes, histocytes phagocytosing neuroblastoma cells), the morphology of the stained cell must be compatible with a neuroblastoma cell to be regarded as such. (Courtesy of R. Schumacher-Kuckelkorn, Cologne)

tyrosine hydroxylase. It is agreed that patients who meet the International Neuroblastoma Staging System (INSS) criteria for stages 1 – 3 should not be upstaged to stage 4 or stage 4S because of the detection of a few immunocytologically positive cells in the bone marrow in the absence of morphological evidence of disease by light microscopy (Brodeur et al. 1993).

The amount of marrow involvement in most infants with stage-4S disease is minimal (≤1% tumor cells per nucleated marrow cells). An upper limit of 10% has been defined. If this is exceeded, an upstaging from stage 4S to stage 4 is recommended (Brodeur et al. 1993).

7.3.4.3 Definition of Cortical Bone Metastases

Bone metastases discriminate between stage 4S and stage 4 and are considered more difficult to treat than other metastatic sites (Ladenstein et al. 1998); therefore, independent methods for defining cortical bone disease are desirable.

In the case of an MIBG-avid neuroblastoma without any focal distant lesion, no further investigation is generally necessary. If the primary tumor is MIBG negative, a technetium bone scan is recommended (in two-thirds of the cases the primary itself is taking up the technetium tracer) in order to detect MIBG negative distant bone metastases.

In lesions with focal MIBG uptake, controversy exists about the accuracy of MIBG in detecting cortical bone metastases (Suc et al. 1996). Some investigators have suggested evaluation of bone lesions by technetium bone scan (highly sensitive), while others rely on osteosclerotic or osteolytic changes in the plain X-ray radiographs (less sensitive).

7.4 Differential Diagnosis

7.4.1 Small Blue Round Cell Tumors

Neuronal differentiating features are present in most neuroblastomas; therefore, the histological diagnosis of neuroblastoma is unequivocal in the vast majority of the patients. In the case of a completely undifferentiated histological pattern, other small blue round cell tumors need to be ruled out; those include Ewing's sarcoma and other peripheral neuroectodermal tumors (PNET), rhabdomyosarcoma (RMS), desmoplastic small round cell tumor (DSRCT) and malignant non-Hodgkin's lymphoma (NHL). These tumors do not excrete elevated catecholamine metabolites and are not MIBG avid (Ewing's/ PNET tumors may demonstrate faint MIBG uptake). The locations of tumors may help to discriminate further [bone involvement in Ewing's sarcoma, ribs and thoracic wall in PNETs (Askin tumors), main soft tissue mass in rhabdomyosarcoma, peritoneal implants in DSRCT, and frequent lymphoblastic bone marrow infiltration in NHL]; however, one has to be reminded that dumbbell tumors with an intrathoracic/intraabdominal spindle mass extending into the intraspinal space has been described for (extraskeletal) Ewing's sarcoma as well as for NHL and for soft tissue sarcomas. Immunohistochemistry using a panel of antibodies is necessary to make the correct differential diagnosis in those cases. The histological diagnosis of neuroblastoma in an adult patient presenting with catecholamine-negative, MIBG-negative primary tumor and metastases only to the lung should raise suspicion. In the near future, the characteristic differences of gene expression between the small blue round cell tumors may help further distinguish these tumor types (Khan et al. 2001). Before small round blue cell tumor gene chips become readily available, already established tumor-specific translocations, such as *EWS-FLI1* (t11;22) (q24;q12) in the Ewing sarcoma family of tumors, *PAX3-FKHR* (t2;13) (q35;q14) in alveolar rhabdomyosarcoma, the *WT1-EWS* (t11;22) (p13;q12) in DSRCT, and the *cmyc* gene involving translocation (t8;14) (q24;q32) in Burkitt's lymphoma, may be helpful for differential diagnosis.

7.4.2 Adrenal Hemorrhage in the Newborn

The differentiation of necrotic/hemorrhagic neuroblastoma from bleeding residues of the adrenal during the newborn period may be difficult. The determination of urinary VMA/HVA levels rarely resolves the differential diagnosis because of the tumor is generally too small to produce abnormal marker levels. Since most patients are not in critical condition and the prognosis is favorable, histological investigation can be delayed for 1–3 months with close follow-up of tumor size and structure using ultrasonography. The majority of infants can be spared invasive diagnostic procedures using this wait-and-see approach. In a series of 53 infants with postnatal suprarenal masses, 58% were localized neuroblastomas with favorable outcome. All other cases showed spontaneous regression of the lesion (hemorrhage) or had a benign lesion (Sauvat et al. 2002).

7.4.3 Nephroblastoma

The European Wilms' tumor study has a long and successful tradition of preoperative chemotherapy where the initial diagnosis is based on radiological criteria only. Approximately 2% of 1603 histologically proven neuroblastomas have been pretreated wrongly according to the Wilms' tumor protocol (Hero et al. 2002). The poor outcome of these patients was related more to their unfavorable biological features than to the preoperative Wilms' chemotherapy. If the radiological criteria (Wilms' tumor: intrarenal, destruction of the renal pelvis; neuroblastoma: suprarenal, tumor calcifications) are unable to discriminate, careful observation of the tumor response to preoperative Wilms' tumor chemotherapy is important and, if inadequate, a strong indicator for misdiagnosis.

7.4.4 Esthesioneuroblastoma (Olfactory Neuroblastoma)

Esthesioneuroblastoma, a rare neoplasm of the superior nasal cavity, is believed to arise from basal progenitors of the olfactory epithelium. It is neither a neuroblastoma, as the name implies, nor a PNET, since in situ hybridization and PCR studies have not confirmed the 11;22 translocation for the majority of cases (Dulguerov et al. 2001); thus, esthesioneuroblastoma is considered a distinct clinical and molecular entity not to be confused with neuroblastoma.

7.4.5 Ganglioneuroma, Pheochromocytoma, Paraganglioma, Chemodectoma

These incomplete or complete ganglionic (ganglioneuroma) or chromaffin (adrenal pheochromocytoma, extraadrenal paraganglioma) differentiated tumors may secrete VMA and HVA or different vasoactive catecholamines [norepinephrine, dopamine by pheochromocytoma and paraganglioma, although most do not (ganglioneuroma) (Geoerger et al. 2001)]. The clinical presentation of the ganglioneuroma is similar to neuroblastoma, and many investigators believe that these tumors represent a mature variant of neuroblastoma. Pheochromocytoma and extraadrenal paraganglioma are very rare in childhood and present typically with the triad of episodic headache, sweating, and palpitation as a result of the release of stored catecholamines from the tumor. Non-chromaffin paragangliomas (e.g., paraganglioma carotis=chemodectoma) arise from parasympathetic ganglia, predominantly in the head and neck, and present with local mass effects such as cranial nerve palsies and tinnitus (Dluhy 2002). The potential differential diagnostic problem is usually solved by the equivocal histology.

7.5 Clinical and Laboratory Evaluation

7.5.1 Staging

Disease stage is a powerful prognostic factor in neuroblastoma (Table 7.5). In 1988 an international staging proposal was developed, which was further refined in 1993 (Brodeur et al. 1993). The INSS has been readily accepted worldwide; therefore, other staging systems that were used to determine extent of disease in the past, such as the Evans' staging system, the Pediatric Oncology Group staging system, and the TMN system, are not discussed in this chapter (Evans et al. 1971; Castleberry et al. 1994; Ng and Kingston 1993). The INSS is a surgical-based staging system (Table 7.6), although modern imaging tools together with the estimation of an experienced pediatric surgeon is likely to achieve the same stage category in almost all cases. The criterion "crossing the midline" for discriminating between stage 2 and stage 3 is described as the infiltrative contiguous extension beyond the opposite side of the vertebral bodies. Characteristically, these tumors encompass large vessels and other vital structures. A tumor just overhanging the midline (e.g., large adrenal tumors) would not be sufficient for stage-3 categorization.

Although it was anticipated that the introduction of new sensitive diagnostic techniques (e.g., of MIBG scintigraphy and immunocytology or PCR for

Table 7.5. International Neuroblastoma Staging System (INSS) (Brodeur et al. 1993)

Stage	Definition
Stage 1	Localized tumor confined to the area of origin. Complete gross resection with or without microscopic residual disease; identifiable ipsilateral and contralateral lymph node negative for tumor. Adherent lymph nodes in direct continuity with and removed with the tumor may be positive for the tumor. A *grossly resected* midline tumor without ipsilateral (with: stage 2A) or contralateral (with: stage 2B) lymph node involvement is considered stage 1
Stage 2A	Unilateral with incomplete gross resection; identifiable ipsilateral and contralateral lymph node negative for tumor
Stage 2B	Unilateral with complete or incomplete gross resection; with ipsilateral lymph node positive for tumor; identifiable contralateral lymph node negative for tumor
Stage 3	Tumor infiltrating across midline with or without regional lymph node involvement; or unilateral tumor with contralateral lymph node involvement or midline tumor with bilateral lymph node involvement
Stage 4	Dissemination of tumor to distant lymph nodes, bone marrow, liver, or other organs except as defined in stage 4S
Stage 4S	Localized primary tumor as defined for stage 1 or 2 with dissemination limited to liver, skin, and bone marrow (<10% of nucleated marrow cells are tumor cells)

Table 7.6. Variation of the relative stage incidence under and over 1 year of age in Japan (*J*; Ikeda et al. 2002), Germany (*G*) and United Kingdom (*UK*; Pearson and Philipp 2000), and North America (*NA*)

INSS stage	All ages				<1 year				≥1 year			
	J	G	UK	NA	J	G	UK	NA	J	G	UK	NA
No. of patients	644	670	1266	1253	485	271	332	450	159	399	934	803
	%	%	%	%	%	%	%	%	%	%	%	%
Stage 1	38	18	5	21	45	26	9	23	16	13	4	19
Stage 2	19	10	12	15	22	13	23	18	7	9	8	13
Stage 3	14	20	17	17	15	19	21	17	9	20	15	17
Stage 4S	6	11	6	6	8	27	22	18	–	–	–	–
Stage 4	23	41	60	41	9	15	25	24	67	58	73	51

Germany: 1 January 1990 to 31 March 1995; with INSS system and before the nationwide screening
UK is based on ENSG data
NA is based on COG data from study ANBL00B1, 1 April 2001 to 30 August 2003 (S.L. Cohn et al., unpublished results)

bone marrow evaluation) would enhance the ability to detect metastatic disease, the absolute number of stage-4 neuroblastoma per children <14 years of age in Germany has been remarkably constant over the past 15 years (Poisson regression for linear yearly trend of the stage-4 case incidence; per population, years 1988 – 2002; p=0.92; data courtesy of C. Spix, Mainz, Germany). Instead, an increase in the incidence of lower stages has been observed. One reason for this increase is the change of the staging system from Evans (more stage-3 patients) to INSS (more stage-1 patients). A second reason is the screening program that was introduced in Germany from 1995–2000.

Table 7.7. Biological types of neuroblastoma

Type	Presentation	Adverse molecular marker	Course of disease	Treatment approach	Current outcome
Regressive	Multilocular (stage 4S)	Absent	Progression(may be fast!) regression	Minimal therapy: inhibition of rapid tumor growth by "mild" chemotherapy; biopsy (resection)+observation only	80–85% survival
	Unilocular (stages 1–3)	Absent			
Progressive	Metastatic (stage 4)	Present or absent	Progression	Maximum therapy: polychemotherapy; megatherapy with stem cell support; surgery; radiotherapy; immunotherapy	20–30% survival
	Unilocular (stage 1–3)	Present			
Maturative	Unilocular (stage 1–3)	Absent	Maturation	No approach because this subtype can be identified only retrospectively	100% (?)

From Berthold F, Hero B (2000) Neuroblastoma: current drug therapy recommendations as part of the total treatment approach. Drugs 59:1261–1277

The INSS classification utilizes surgical resectability as one of the criteria for stage determination; thus, depending on the skills of an individual surgeon, the radiologically same midline neuroblastoma may be classified as stage 3 if incompletely resected or stage 1 if completely resected. Discussions of the participating institutions with the trial office in Germany demonstrated that the discrimination between stage 2 and stage 3 may also be difficult in selected cases. Another controversy relates to the stage-4S classification. While age over 1 year and the presence of bone metastasis is uniformly accepted to qualify for stage 4, the size of the primary tumor and the presence of metastases to sites other than bone marrow (<10%), liver, and skin are not. Some investigators believe that large stage-3 tumors and non-regional lymph node metastases may well be compatible with the biological characteristics of stage-4S neuroblastoma.

7.5.2 Biological Types of Neuroblastoma

The biological behavior of histologically identical neuroblastoma is extremely variable. At least three biological subtypes are known (Table 7.7).

7.5.2.1 Maturative Subtype

The maturative subtype can be identified only retrospectively after maturation to ganglioneuroma, and represents probably less than 5% of all peripheral neuroblastic tumors. A model of maturation suggests that neuroblastoma cells with spontaneous maturation capacity (not induced by cytotoxic agents) attract and recruit extratumoral Schwann cells that themselves inhibit neuroblastic proliferation and promote maturation (Ambros et al. 1996). So far, parameters that indicate an ongoing or future maturation process are lacking, and it is also unclear whether all gan-

of risk-based trials conducted in different regions of the world. While stage, age, and *MYCN* are generally accepted as key prognostic variables, a more refined system will have to wait for a better understanding of the biology underlying the diverse clinical types [regression/maturation/progression (fast/slowly)] underlying. It is also noted that risk factors are relevant only in the context of their respective treatments, since the latter can dramatically impact survival and may abolish even *MYCN* amplification as a risk factor (Kaneko et al. 2002).

In addition to stage and age, other clinical prognostic parameters include tumor markers (VMA/HVA; Laug et al. 1978; Berthold et al. 1992b), NSE (Zeltzer et al. 1983; Garaventa et al. 2002), Ferritin (Hann et al. 1981; Garaventa et al. 2002), LDH (Berthold et al. 1992a, 1994; Shuster et al. 1992; Lau 2002; Garaventa et al. 2002), chromogranin A (Hsiao et al. 1990), neuropeptide Y (Kogner et al. 1993), primary site and volume (Cotterill et al. 2000), and metastatic site (DuBois et al. 1999). An interdependence of the tumor markers has been demonstrated (Berthold et al. 1992a, 1994; Garaventa et al. 2002). A second set of clinical prognostic markers consists of response parameters like MIBG normalization as a consequence of chemotherapy (Hero et al. 2001; Ladenstein et al. 1998), clearing of tumor cell contaminated bone marrow (Chap. 11), response of tumor markers (Hero et al. 2001), and resectability of the primary tumor (Berthold et al. 1992a, 1994; Garaventa et al. 2002; von Schweinitz et al. 2002). Furthermore, the histological pattern of the tumor as defined by the mitosis-karyorrhexis index, the amount of Schwann cells, the neuroblastic differentiation and age has been used as prognostic parameter in particular in American trials (Shimada et al. 1984, 1999; Shimada and Roald 2000) (Table 7.8). In other series, the proliferation rate of neuroblastoma cells alone was of prognostic impact (Krams et al. 2002).

During the past 20 years a number of specific genetic changes have been found to be associated with biologic features, e.g., *MYCN* amplification and 1p36 deletion with the progressive type of neuroblastoma (Figure 7.5). Genetic investigation has become standard in most clinical trials, not for diagnostic purposes (Table 7.5) but rather for prognostic information (Brodeur et al. 1997; Mathew et al. 2001; Spitz et al. 2002, 2003a,b; Maris et al. 2001; White et al. 1995; Hallstensson et al. 1997; Vandesompele et al. 1998; Guo et al. 1999; Plantaz et al. 2001; Bown et al. 1999; Abel et al. 1999; Look et al. 1991; Ladenstein et al. 2001; Kramer et al. 1997; Combaret et al. 1996, 1997; Terpe et al. 1994; Norris et al. 1996) (Table 7.8). Genetic characteristics promise to reflect the natural course of the disease more directly than derived clinical parameters and present with a yes or no answer. Table 7.9 summarizes the factors that are believed to contribute to prognosis estimation. The incidence rates given for the unfavorable expression of the risk factors demonstrate that they describe only a fraction of the patients with unfavorable prognosis. Some factors are closely associated with each other, e.g., *MYCN* amplification and 1p36 alteration, deletion of 11q23 and 3p26, and loss of expression of trkA and CD44. Utilizing, for example, *MYCN*, del 1p, del 11q and del 3p together, 83 % of stage-4 and 30 % of stages 1 – 3 and stage-4S patients showed one or more of the chromosomal changes (Spitz et al. 2003a); however, the prediction of events of tumor progression in low-risk patients was possible roughly only in one-half using all the markers and their combinations listed in Table 7.9, while a substantial fraction of patients with chromosomal and/or immunohistological abnormalities in their tumors did not experience tumor progression (unpublished observation). Few of the listed molecular factors have been found unanimously to be of prognostic value. Contradictory results were obtained, for example, for *MYCN* amplification [lack of correlation with prognosis for localized (Cohn et al. 1995) and metastatic (Laug et al. 1978) neuroblastoma] and for 17q gain (Spitz et al. 2003b) which is likely to result from different treatment of the patients and different investigation methods in the lab. The suggested proposal for a standardized tumor tissue processing and analysis (Ambros and Ambros 2001) has been mentioned above. Apart from standardization issues, modern technologies that screen myriads of gene expression levels in small tumor biopsies are likely to define in the near future not only characteristic gene expression profiles (Sauvat et al. 2002), but also genetic key characteristics that allow the description of molecular risk categories. Using the Ewing's paradigm of seed growing in a soil,

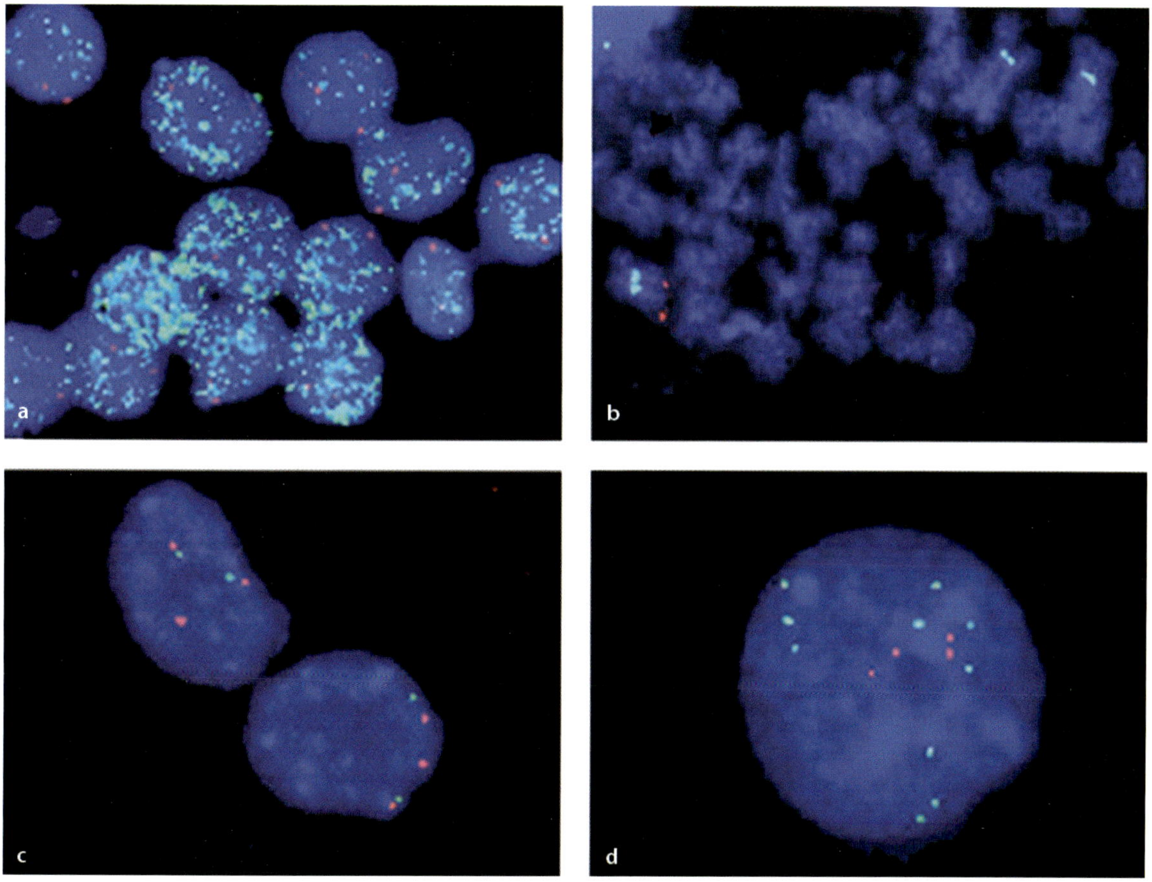

Figure 7.5 a–d

Interphase fluorescence in situ hybridization (FISH) studies of chromosomal loci frequently involved in neuroblastoma. **a** *MYCN* amplification (interphase FISH, tumor touch preparation): two red signals demonstrate centromeric regions of the two chromosome-2 copies. The dispersed green signals indicate multiple copies of the *MYCN* gene in 2p24. **b** Deletion in chromosome 1p (chromosomes of cell line IMR5): three chromosomes 1 demonstrate green centromeric signals (D1Z1), but only one derivative copy shows a red distal (1p36) signal. **c** Imbalance 11q: the nuclei show three red markings of chromosome 11 centromere, but only two green signals of the MLL-locus in 11q23. One of the three chromosome 11 alleles lost its distal long arm. **d** Gain 17q: the nucleus has four red dots of the chromosome 17, but ten green distal chromosome 17 signals (17q21). The distal part is overrepresented. (Courtesy of R. Spitz, Cologne)

understanding the genetic characteristics of the tumor (seed) in the context of the host (soil) should help define the natural history of neuroblastoma more directly than derived clinical parameters. Figure 7.4 shows an example of the relationship between clinical + molecular risk factors and survival. The observation group (surgery only) comprises 46% of all patients, the standard-risk group (four blocs of chemotherapy) 15%, and the high-risk group (all modalities) 40%.

Table 7.10. International neuroblastoma response criteria (INRG) (Brodeur et al. 1993)

Response	Primary tumor	Metastatic sites
CR	No tumor	No tumor; catecholamines normal
VGPR	Decreased by 90 – 99%	No tumor; catecholamines normal; residual ^{99}Tc bone changes allowed
PR	Decreased by >50%	All measurable sites decreased by >50%. Bones and bone marrow: no. of positive bone sites decreased by >50%, no more than one positive bone marrow site allowed
MR	No new lesions; >50% reduction of any measurable lesion (primary or metastases) with <50% reduction in any other; <25% increase in any existing lesion	
NR	No new lesions; <50% reduction, and <25% increase in any existing lesion	
PD	Any new lesion; increase of any measurable lesion by >25%; previous negative marrow positive for tumor	

7.5.4 Response Criteria

The evaluation of the tumor response to the treatment is mandatory; however, the correlation between initial response and long-term outcome is still weaker in neuroblastoma than prednisone response in acute lymphoblastic leukemia. The criteria for defining response (Brodeur et al. 1993) are shown in Table 7.10. All test results that were abnormal at diagnosis need to be reinvestigated after 3–4 months, after completion of each major therapeutic step (e.g., at the end of chemotherapy, after surgery). Most protocols require additional evaluations for disease response during the treatment period and following the completion of therapy (Therassa et al. 2000).

Currently, the response status is assessed using standard radiographic measurements to determine tumor size and evidence of metastases in addition to histological evaluation of the bone marrow. Many efforts of refinement are being undertaken such as PCR-based detection of minimal residual disease in the bone marrow (Chap. 11), *MYCN*-DNA levels in serum (Combaret et al. 2002), and antibody-based scintigraphy (Chap. 14). These studies need confirmation by other independent groups before they are adopted for standard response evaluation reporting.

7.6 Conclusions

Children with neuroblastoma have a wide range of presenting signs and symptoms. This cancer must be considered in every child with hepatomegaly, skin nodules, periorbital ecchymosis, bone pain, Horner's syndrome, opsoclonus–myoclonus, and/or transverse myelitis. Neuroblastoma is characterized by a diversity of clinical behavior, but to a large extent, outcome can be predicted by the stage of disease, the age at diagnosis, and the presence or absence of *MYCN* amplification. Additional factors, such as tumor pathology, DNA content, genetic abnormalities, and the presence of clinically threatening symptoms, have also been found to have prognostic value. Most countries have developed treatment strategies that are tailored according to patient risk; however, currently uniform criteria for risk-group stratification do not exist. An International Neuroblastoma Risk Classification System is needed so that treatment protocols performed in different regions of the world can be compared and optimal therapeutic strategies for patients with low-, intermediate-, and high-risk disease can be identified.

References

Abel F et al. (1999) Gain of chromosome arm 17q is associated with unfavourable prognosis in neuroblastoma, but does not involve mutations in the somatostatin receptor 2(SSTR2) gene at 17q24. Br J Cancer 81:1402–1409

Ambros I et al. (1996) Role of ploidy, chromosome 1p, and Schwann cells in the maturation of neuroblastoma. N Engl J Med 334:1505–1511

Ambros PF, Ambros IM (2001) Pathology and biology guidelines for resectable and unresectable neuroblastic tumors and bone marrow examination guidelines. Med Pediatr Oncol 37:492–504

Berthold F, Harms D, Lampert F, Niethammer D, Zieschang J (1990) Risk factors in neuroblastoma of infants. Contrib Oncol 41:101–117

Berthold F et al. (1992a) Prognostic factors in metastatic neuroblastoma. A multivariate analysis of 182 cases. Am J Pediatr Hematol Oncol 14:207–215

Berthold F et al. (1992b) Serum vanillylmandelic acid/homovanillic acid contributes to prognosis estimation in patients with localised but not with metastatic neuroblastoma. Eur J Cancer 28A:1950–1954

Berthold F et al. (1994) Multivariate evaluation of prognostic factors in localized neuroblastoma. Am J Pediatr Hematol Oncol 16:107–115

Berthold F et al. (1998) Are spontaenous regressions of neuroblastoma delayed embryofetal involutions? Sind Spontanregressionen beim Neuroblastom verspätete embryofetale Involutionen? In: Hein E, Schwarz, Stuttgard R (eds) Spontanremissionen in der Onkologie: theoretische Modelle und klinische Befunde. Schattauer, New York, pp 84–94

Bown N et al. (1999) Gain of chromosome arm 17q and adverse outcome in patients with neuroblastoma. N Engl J Med 340:1954–1961

Brodeur GM et al. (1993) Revisions of the international criteria for neuroblastoma diagnosis, staging, and response to treatment. J Clin Oncol 11:1466–1477

Brodeur GM et al. (1997) Biology and genetics of human neuroblastomas. J Pediatr Hematol Oncol 19:93–101

Castleberry RP et al. (1994) The Pediatric Oncology Group experience with the international staging system criteria for neuroblastoma. Member Institutions of the Pediatric Oncology Group. J Clin Oncol 12:2378–2381

Cohn SL et al. (1995) Lack of correlation of N-myc gene amplification with prognosis in localized neuroblastoma: a Pediatric Oncology Group study. Cancer Res 55:721–726

Combaret V et al. (1996) Clinical relevance of CD44 cell-surface expression and N-myc gene amplification in a multicentric analysis of 121 pediatric neuroblastomas. J Clin Oncol 14: 25–34

Combaret V et al. (1997) Clinical relevance of TRKA expression on neuroblastoma: comparison with N-MYC amplification and CD44 expression. Br J Cancer 75:1151–1155

Combaret V et al. (2002) Circulating MYCN DNA as a tumor-specific marker in neuroblastoma patients. Cancer Res 62:3646–3648

Cooper R et al. (2001) Opsoclonus-myoclonus-ataxia syndrome in neuroblastoma: histopathologic features – a report from the Children's Cancer Group. Med Pediatr Oncol 36:623–629

Cotterill SJ et al. (2000) Clinical prognostic factors in 1277 patients with neuroblastoma: results of The European Neuroblastoma Study Group "Survey" 1982–1992. Eur J Cancer 36:901–908

Cushing HSW (1927) The transformation of a malignant paravertebral sympathicoblastoma into a benign ganglioneuroma. Am J Pathol 3:203–216

De Bernardi B et al. (2001) Neuroblastoma with symptomatic spinal cord compression at diagnosis: treatment and results with 76 cases. J Clin Oncol 19:183–190

De la Monte SM et al. (1983) Nonrandom distribution of metastases in neuroblastic tumors. Cancer 52:915–925

Dluhy RG (2002) Pheochromocytoma: death of an axiom. N Engl J Med 346:1486–1488

DuBois SG et al. (1999) Metastatic sites in stage IV and IVS neuroblastoma correlate with age, tumor biology, and survival. J Pediatr Hematol Oncol 21:181–189

Dulguerov P et al. (2001) Esthesioneuroblastoma: a meta-analysis and review. Lancet Oncol 2:683–690

El Shafie M et al. (1983) Intractable diarrhea in children with VIP-secreting ganglioneuroblastomas. J Pediatr Surg 18:34–36

Evans AE et al. (1971) A proposed staging for children with neuroblastoma. Cancer 27:374–378

Evans AE et al. (1990) A comparison of four staging systems for localized and regional neuroblastoma: a report from the Childrens Cancer Study Group. J Clin Oncol 8:678–588

Garaventa A et al. (2002) Localized unresectable neuroblastoma: results of treatment based on clinical prognostic factors. Ann Oncol 13:956–964

Geoerger B et al. (2001) Metabolic activity and clinical features of primary ganglioneuromas. Cancer 91:1905–1913

Greenberg RE (1957) New diagnostic test for neural tumors in infancy: increased urinary excretion of 3-methoxy-4-hydroxymandelic acid and norepinephrin in a ganglioneuroma with chronic diarrhea. Pediatrics 24:683–684

Guo C et al. (1999) Allelic deletion at 11q23 is common in MYCN single copy neuroblastomas. Oncogene 18:4948–4957

Hallstensson K et al. (1997) Representational difference analysis and loss of heterozygosity studies detect 3p deletions in neuroblastoma. Eur J Cancer 33:1966–1970

Hann HW, Bombardieri E (2000) Serum markers and prognosis in neuroblastoma: Ferritin, LDH, NSE. In: Brodeur G, Sawada T, Tsuchida Y, Voute PA (eds) Neuroblastoma. Elsevier, Amsterdam, pp 371–381

Hann HW et al. (1981) Biologic differences between neuroblastoma stages IV-S and IV. Measurement of serum ferritin and E-rosette inhibition in 30 children. N Engl J Med 305:425–429

Hann HW et al. (1985) Prognostic importance of serum ferritin in patients with Stages III and IV neuroblastoma: the Childrens Cancer Study Group experience. Cancer Res 45: 2843–2848
Hero B et al. (2001) Evaluation of catecholamine metabolites, MIBG scan, and bone marrow cytology as response markers in stage 4 neuroblastoma. Med Pediatr Oncol 36:220–223
Hero B et al. (2002) Neuroblastoma preoperatively treated as nephroblastoma: Does inadequate therapy worsen the prognosis? Klin Padiatr 214:157–161
Hero B et al. (2000) Regression in stage 2 and 3 infant neuroblastoma: results of the prospective German neuroblastoma trial. Adv Neuroblastoma Res. Abstract, 15–18 May, Philadelphia, P20
Hsiao RJ et al. (1990) Chromogranin A in children with neuroblastoma. Serum concentration parallels disease stage and predicts survival. J Clin Invest 85:1555–1559
Hutchinson R (1907) On suprarenal sarcoma in children with metastases in the skull. Q J Med 1:33–38
Ikeda H et al. (2002) Experience with international neuroblastoma staging system and pathology classification. Br J Cancer 86:1110–1116
Jaffe R et al. (1984) The neuroectodermal tumor of bone. Am J Surg Pathol 8:885–898
Kaneko M et al. (2002) Intensified chemotherapy increases the survival rates in patients with stage 4 neuroblastoma with MYCN amplification. J Pediatr Hematol Oncol 24:613–621
Katzenstein HM et al. (2001) Treatment and outcome of 83 children with intraspinal neuroblastoma: the Pediatric Oncology Group experience. J Clin Oncol 19:1047–1055
Khan J et al. (2001) Classification and diagnostic prediction of cancers using gene expression profiling and artificial neural networks. Nat Med 7:673–679
Kogner et al. (1993) Neuropeptide Y in neuroblastoma: increased concentration in metastasis, release during surgery, and characterization of plasma and tumor extracts. Med Pediatr Oncol 21:317–322
Kramer K et al. (1997) Monoclonal antibody to human Trk-A: diagnostic and therapeutic potential in neuroblastoma. Eur J Cancer 33:2090–2091
Krams M et al. (2002) Proliferation marker KI-S5 discriminates between favorable and adverse prognosis in advanced stages of neuroblastoma with and without MYCN amplification. Cancer 94:854–861
Kushner BH et al. (1996) International neuroblastoma staging system stage 1 neuroblastoma: a prospective study and literature review. J Clin Oncol 14:2174–2180
Ladenstein R et al. (1998) Multivariate analysis of risk factors in stage 4 neuroblastoma patients over the age of one year treated with megatherapy and stem-cell transplantation: a report from the European Bone Marrow Transplantation Solid Tumor Registry. J Clin Oncol 16:953–965
Ladenstein R et al. (2001) Prognostic significance of DNA ditetraploidy in neuroblastoma. Med Pediatr Oncol 36:83–92
Lastowska M et al. (2001) Comprehensive genetic and histopathologic study reveals three types of neuroblastoma tumors. J Clin Oncol 19:3080–3090
Lau L (2002) Neuroblastoma: a single institution's experience with 128 children and an evaluation of clinical and biological prognostic factors. Pediatr Hematol Oncol 19:79–89
Laug WE et al. (1978) Initial urinary catecholamine metabolite concentrations and prognosis in neuroblastoma. Pediatrics 62:77–83
Lilling G et al. (1994) Inhibition of human neuroblastoma growth by a specific VIP antagonist. J Mol Neurosci 5:231–239
Look AT et al. (1991) Clinical relevance of tumor cell ploidy and N-myc gene amplification in childhood neuroblastoma: a Pediatric Oncology Group study. J Clin Oncol 9:581–591
Marchand F (1891) Beiträge zur Kenntnis der normalen und pathologischen Anatomie der Glandula carotica und der Nebennieren. Virchows Arch 5:578
Maris JM et al. (2001) Comprehensive analysis of chromosome 1p deletions in neuroblastoma. Med Pediatr Oncol 36:32–36
Mason GA, Hart-Mercer J, Miller E (1957) Adrenalin-secreting neuroblastoma in an infant. Lancet 273:322–325
Mathew P et al. (2001) Detection of MYCN gene amplification in neuroblastoma by fluorescence in situ hybridization: a pediatric oncology group study. Neoplasia 3:105–109
Mora J et al. (2001) Neuroblastic and schwannian stromal cells of neuroblastoma are derived from a tumoral progenitor cell. Cancer Res 61:6892–6898
Ng YY, Kingston JE (1993) The role of radiology in the staging of neuroblastoma. Clin Radiol 47:226–235
Nickerson HJ et al. (2000) Favorable biology and outcome of stage IV-S neuroblastoma with supportive care or minimal therapy: a Children's Cancer Group study. J Clin Oncol 18:477–486
Norris MD et al. (1996) Expression of the gene for multidrug-resistance-associated protein and outcome in patients with neuroblastoma. N Engl J Med 334:231–238
Pearson ADJ, Philipp T (2000) Prognosis of low-risk and high-risk neuroblastoma. In: Brodeur GM, Sawada T, Tsuchida Y, Voute PA (eds) Neuroblastoma. Elsevier, Amsterdam, pp 551–560
Pepper W (1901) A study of congenital sarcoma of the liver and suprarenal with the report of a case. Am J Med Sci 121: 287–299
Plantaz D et al. (2001) Comparative genomic hybridization (CGH) analysis of stage 4 neuroblastoma reveals high frequency of 11q deletion in tumors lacking MYCN amplification. Int J Cancer 91:680–686
Powell JE et al. (1998) Neuroblastoma in Europe: differences in the pattern of disease in the UK. SENSE. Study group for the Evaluation of Neuroblastoma Screening in Europe. Lancet 352:682–687

Rudnick E et al. (2001) Opsoclonus–myoclonus–ataxia syndrome in neuroblastoma: clinical outcome and antineuronal antibodies: a report from the Children's Cancer Group Study. Med Pediatr Oncol 36:612–622
Russo C et al. (1997) Long-term neurologic outcome in children with opsoclonus–myoclonus associated with neuroblastoma: a report from the Pediatric Oncology Group. Med Pediatr Oncol 28:284–288
Sauvat F et al. (2002) Outcome of suprarenal localized masses diagnosed during the perinatal period: a retrospective multicenter study. Cancer 94:2474–2480
Schilling FH et al. (2002) Neuroblastoma screening at one year of age. N Engl J Med 346:1047–1053
Schwab M et al. (1983) Amplified DNA with limited homology to MYCN cellular oncogene is shared by human neuroblastoma cell lines and neuroblastoma tumor. Nature 305: 245–248
Seeger RC, Brodeur GM, Sather H (1985) Association of multiple copies of N-myc oncogene with rapid progression in neuroblastoma. N Engl J Med 313:1111–1116
Shimada H, Roald B (2000) Histology: tumors of the neuroblastoma group. In: Brodeur GM, Sawada T, Tsuchida Y, Voute PA (eds) Neuroblastoma. Elsevier, Amsterdam, pp 341–354
Shimada H et al. (1984) Histopathologic prognostic factors in neuroblastic tumors: definition of subtypes of ganglioneuroblastoma and an age linked classification of neuroblastomas. J Natl Cancer Inst 73:405–416
Shimada H et al. (1999) The International Neuroblastoma Pathology Classification (the Shimada system). Cancer 86: 364–372
Shuster JJ et al. (1992) Serum lactate dehydrogenase in childhood neuroblastoma. A Pediatric Oncology Group recursive partitioning study. Am J Clin Oncol 15:295–303
Simon T et al. (2003) Tumour markers are poor predictors for relapse or progression in neuroblastoma. Eur J Cancer 39:1899–1903
Simon T et al. (2004) Consolidation treatment with chimeric anti-GD2-antibody ch14.18 in children older than 1 year with metastatic neuroblastoma. J Clin Oncol 22:3549–3557
Spitz R et al. (2002) Fluorescence in situ hybridization analyses of chromosome band 1p36 in neuroblastoma detect two classes of alterations. Genes Chromosomes Cancer 34:299–305
Spitz R et al. (2003a) FISH analyses for alterations in chromosomes 1, 2, 3, and 11 define high-risk groups in neuroblastoma. Med Pediatr Oncol 41:30–35
Spitz R et al. (2003b) Gain of distal chromosome arm 17q is not associated with poor prognosis in neuroblastoma. Clin Cancer Res 9:4835–4840
Stickler GB et al. (1959) Ganglioneuroma associated with chronic diarrhea and increased excretion of catecholamine. Proc Staff Meet Mayo Clin 34:548–549
Suc A et al. (1996) Metastatic neuroblastoma in children older than one year: prognostic significance of the initial metaiodobenzylguanidine scan and proposal for a scoring system. Cancer 77:805–811
Terpe HJ et al. (1994) Absence of CD44-standard in human neuroblastoma correlates with histological dedifferentiation, N-myc amplification and reduced survival probability. Death Differ 1:123–128
Therasse P et al. (2000) New guidelines to evaluate the response to treatment in solid tumors. European Organization for Research and Treatment of Cancer, National Cancer Institute of the United States, National Cancer Institute of Canada. J Natl Cancer Inst 92:205–216
Vandesompele J et al. (1998) Genetic heterogeneity of neuroblastoma studied by comparative genomic hybridization. Genes Chromosomes Cancer 23:141–152
Virchow R (1864) Hyperplasie der Zirbel und der Nebenniere. Die krankhaften Geschwulste, vols 11, 18. Vorlesung 7.2.1863. Hirschwald, Berlin, pp 148–150
Von Schweinitz D, Hero B, Berthold F (2002) The impact of surgical radicality on outcome in childhood neuroblastoma. Eur J Pediatr Surg 12:402–409
White PS et al. (1995) A region of consistent deletion in neuroblastoma maps within human chromosome 1p36.2–36.3. Proc Natl Acad Sci USA, 92:5520–5524
Woods WG et al. (2002) Screening of infants and mortality due to neuroblastoma. N Engl J Med 346:1041–1046
Wright J (1910) Neurocytoma or neuroblastoma, a kind of tumor not generally recognized. J Exp Med 12:556–561
Yamamoto K et al. (1998) Spontaneous regression of localized neuroblastoma detected by mass screening. J Clin Oncol 16:1265–1269
Zeltzer PM et al. (1983) Raised neuron-specific enolase in serum of children with metastatic neuroblastoma. A report from the Children's Cancer Study Group. Lancet 2:361–363

Pathology of Peripheral Neuroblastic Tumors

Hiroyuki Shimada, Inge M. Ambros

Contents

8.1 Introduction

Peripheral neuroblastic tumors (pNTs), which include neuroblastoma, ganglioneuroblastoma, and ganglioneuroma, are common pediatric tumors (Ross et al. 1996). These tumors are derived from immature sympathetic neuroblasts during embryonic, fetal, or early postnatal development, and their morphological features appear to recapitulate developmental stages of sympathetic ganglia. Their primary sites are anatomically related to the embryological distribution of neural crest cells, and include adrenal gland and structures of the sympathetic nervous system.

For many years pNTs were characterized as "enigmatic" because of their unexpected clinical behaviors, such as involution/spontaneous regression, maturation, or aggressive progression. Because of recent advances in clinical and basic research, pNTs now are considered to be biologically heterogeneous, and their individual molecular properties like account for their unique clinical behaviors (Brodeur and Maris 2002). Based primarily on their clinical biology, the International Neuroblastoma Pathology Classification (Shimada et al. 1999a,b) was established by adopting the concept of the original Shimada system (age-linked evaluation of the morphological features in this disease). In this chapter, histopathology of the pNTs is illustrated according to the Classification along with its biological relevance.

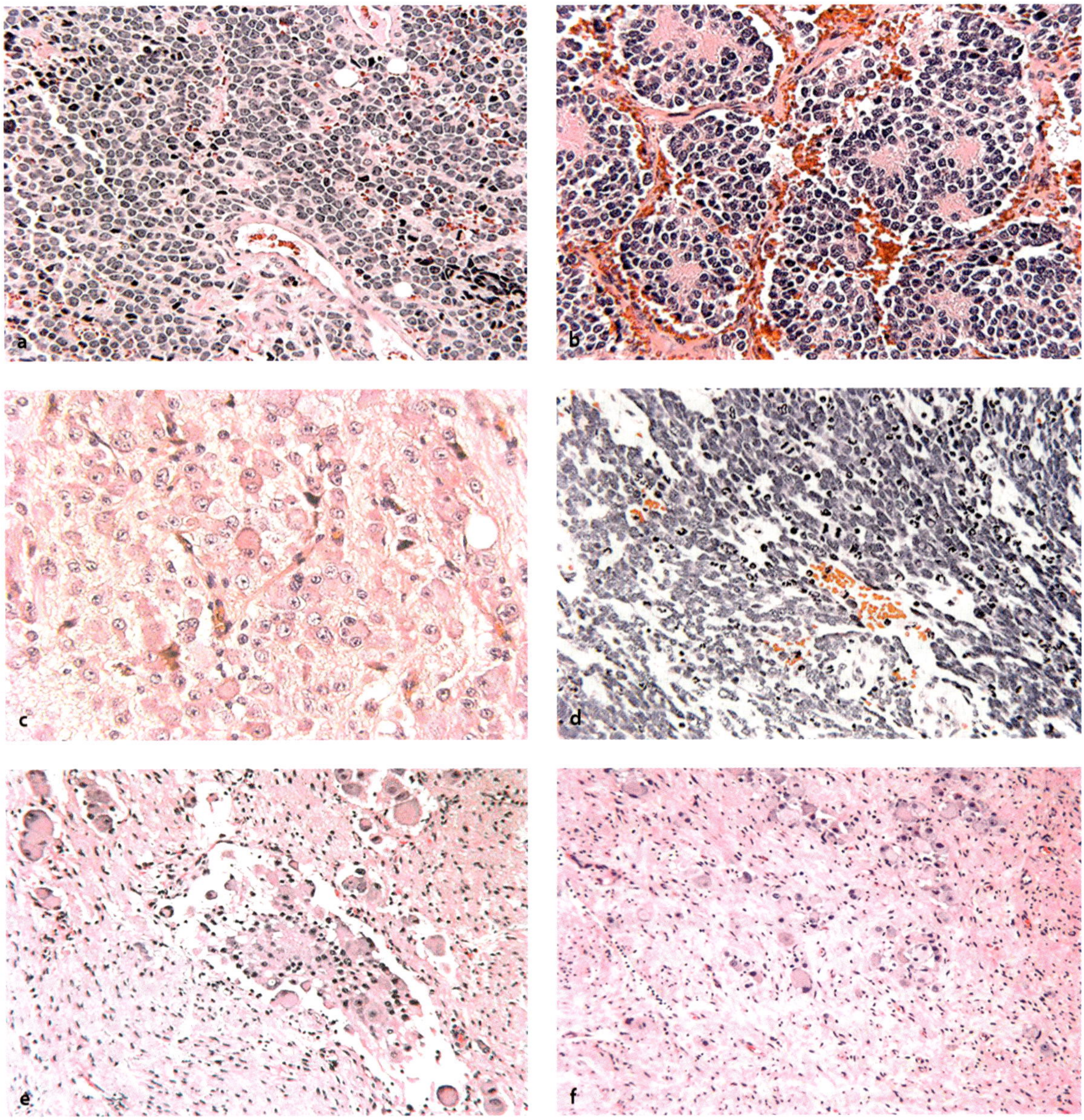

Figure 8.1 a–f

Histology of peripheral neuroblastic tumors. **a** Neuroblastoma (Schwannian stroma-poor), undifferentiated subtype. **b** Neuroblastoma (Schwannian stroma-poor), poorly differentiated subtype. **c** Neuroblastoma (Schwannian stroma-poor), differentiating subtype. **d** Neuroblastoma (Schwannian stroma-poor) with a high mitosis–karyorrhexis index. **e** Ganglioneuroblastoma, intermixed (Schwannian stroma-rich). **f** Ganglioneuroma (Schwannian stroma-dominant), maturing subtype.

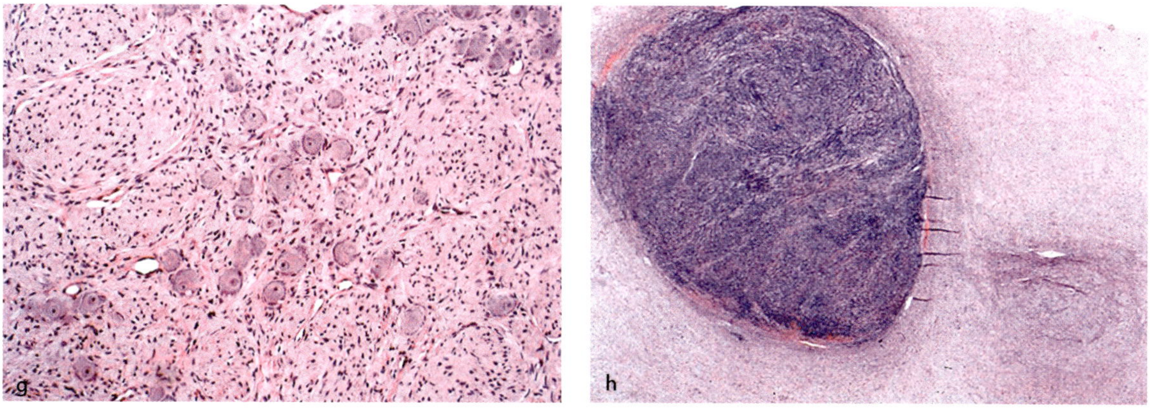

Figure 8.1 g–h

g Ganglioneuroma (Schwannian stroma-dominant), mature subtype. **h** Ganglioneuroblastoma, nodular (composite, Schwannian stroma-rich/stroma-dominant and stroma-poor)

nuclear material, usually accompanied by condensed eosinophilic cytoplasm. Simple hyperchromatic nuclei without chromatin fragmentation are not included in MKI counting.

8.3.2 Ganglioneuroblastoma, Intermixed (Schwannian Stroma-rich)

The international classification has stipulated that tumors having prominent Schwannian stromal development occupying more than 50% of the tumor tissue are upgraded to this category. Tumor histology is consistent with a transition to the full differentiation/maturation of ganglioneuroma (see below), but the process is not complete, as evidenced by scattered "residual" microscopic foci where neuroblastic cells in various stages of differentiation as well as varying numbers of maturing ganglion cells are found in the background of neuropil (Fig. 8.1 e).

8.3.3 Ganglioneuroma (Schwannian Stroma-dominant)

Tumors are predominantly composed of Schwannian stroma with individually distributed maturing/mature ganglion cells. Two subtypes, ganglioneuroma, maturing, and mature, are included in this category.

Ganglioneuroma, Maturing Subtype (Fig. 8.1 f): Tumor of this subtype was previously named "ganglioneuroblastoma, well differentiated" in the original Shimada classification. Some of the neuroblastic components appear to be on their way to fully mature ganglion cells and have appearances of differentiating neuroblasts and/or maturing ganglion cells.

Ganglioneuroma, Mature Subtype (Fig. 8.1 g): Tumor in this subtype is composed of fully developed Schwannian stroma and mature ganglion cells. Those mature ganglion cells are surrounded by satellite cells. Mature non-myelinating Schwann cells, the dominating component of tumor, characteristically form multiple fascicles covered with perineurial cells.

Tumors categorized as either ganglioneuroblastoma, intermixed, or ganglioneuroma have an elastic consistency, and their cut surfaces are always tan-yellow and homogenous with or without fibrous bands.

8.3.4 Ganglioneuroblastoma, Nodular (Composite, Schwannian Stroma-rich/ Stroma-dominant and Stroma-poor)

Tumor in this category is characterized by the presence of one or more macroscopic, usually hemorrhagic neuroblastomatous nodule(s) (stroma-poor component) coexisting with ganglioneuroblastoma, intermixed (stroma-rich component) or with gang-lioneuroma (stroma-dominant component; Fig. 8.1h). On microscopic examination, there is typically abrupt demarcation (pushing border or even fibrous pseudo-capsular formation) between the neuroblastomatous nodule(s) and the stroma-rich or stroma-dominant tumor tissue. Some nodules, however, are not clearly demarcated but rather have a zone of neuroblastic infiltration into the adjacent Schwannian stromal tissue. In rare cases the neuroblastomatous nodule becomes so large, dominating the tumor tissue, that one can recognize stroma-rich/stroma-dominant area only by light microscopic examination.

Nodular formation is usually considered to be a feature of the primary tumor, but it may be overlooked on gross examination; thus, those cases with ganglioneuroblastoma, intermixed or ganglioneuroma at the primary site and neuroblastoma at the metastatic site should be classified into this category.

8.4 Prognostic Classification

The International Neuroblastoma Pathology Classification (the Shimada system) distinguishes favorable and unfavorable histology groups (Shimada et al. 1999b). Tumors in the favorable histology group fall within a conceptual framework of age-linked maturational sequence from poorly differentiated subtype (<1.5 years of age at diagnosis) to differentiating subtype (<5 years of age) of neuroblastoma (Schwannian stroma-poor) to ganglioneuroblastoma, intermixed (Schwannian stroma-rich) to ganglioneuroma (Schwannian stroma-dominant). The neuroblastoma tumors in this group should have a low (for those patients <5 years of age) or an intermediate (for those <1.5 years of age) MKI. By contrast, tumors in the unfavorable histology group have immature histologies for patient's age and include undifferentiated subtype (at any age), poorly differentiated subtype (≥1.5 years of age), and all subtypes (≥5 years of age) of the neuroblastoma. Among the neuroblastoma tumors, those with a high MKI (at any age) or an intermediate MKI (≥1.5 years of age) also qualify as unfavorable histology. Ganglioneuroblastoma, intermixed and ganglioneuroma are classified into a favorable histology group regardless of the patients' age, although these tumors are usually diagnosed in older children. Ganglioneuroblastoma, nodular (composite, Schwannian stroma-rich/stroma-dominant and stroma-poor) can be divided into two subsets, favorable and unfavorable, by applying the same criteria of age-linked histopathological evaluation to the nodular (neuroblastomatous) component (Peuchmaur et al. 2003; Umehara et al. 2000).

While arriving at the proposed Classification, the International Neuroblastoma Pathology Committee tested other morphological indicators (calcification, mitotic rate) and classifications (original risk grouping by combination of mitotic rate, calcification, and age (Joshi et al. 1992); modified risk grouping by combination of MKI, calcification, and age (Joshi et al. 1996), and analyzed their prognostic effects (Shimada et al. 1999b). Although these indicators and classifications all had prognostic effects by univariate analysis, calcification and mitotic rate did not add any significant prognostic information to the International Neuroblastoma Pathology Classification in multivariate analysis. Furthermore, the Classification could provide significantly better prognostic information than those risk groupings. The Committee also examined the age factor of the Shimada system, and confirmed that the two cutoff points, i.e., 1.5 and 5 years of age at diagnosis, used in the Classification distinguished prognostic groups most significantly (Shimada et al. 1999b).

8.5 Biological Relevance

In this section, the biological relevance of International Neuroblastoma Pathology Classification (the Shimada system) is summarized.

8.5.1 Schwannian Development in Neuroblastic Tumors

Peripheral neuroblastic tumors consist of two main cell populations: neuroblastic/ganglionic cells and Schwann cells. As described above, the International Neuroblastoma Pathology Classification uses morphological features of both neuroblastic differentiation and Schwannian stromal development for defining maturational sequence of the pNTs. Based on embryological interactions between normal neuroblasts and Schwann cells (Reynolds and Woolf 1993), some postulate that neoplastic neuroblasts produce Schwann cell mitogens important for their proliferation and development (Ambros 2001). Schwann cells, in return, can secrete anti-proliferative and differentiation-inducing factors crucial to neuronal differentiation. This mutual interaction between neuroblastic cells and Schwannian stromal cells may explain the maturational processes of biologically favorable pNTs. In biologically unfavorable pNTs, there is generally less Schwannian component and limited tumor maturation. The origin of the tumor Schwann cells remains controversial. One study indicates that both cell types, i.e., neuroblastic/ganglionic cells and Schwann cells, arise from the same neoplastic neuroblastic clone or precursor cell (Mora et al. 2001); however, other studies present evidence to support that the Schwann cells in pNTs are reactive in nature and probably recruited from surrounding non-neoplastic tissue by tumor neuroblastic cells (Ambros et al. 1996).

8.5.2 Correlation of Histopathology with *MYCN* Amplification and trkA Expression

There is a reproducible correlation between the molecular event of *MYCN* amplification and the morphological manifestations in pNTs (Shimada et al. 1995; Goto et al. 2001). Those tumors with amplified *MYCN* typically are of the undifferentiated or poorly differentiated subtype of neuroblastoma (Schwannian stroma-poor) with markedly increased mitotic (proliferating) and karyorrhectic (apoptotic) activities (Shimada et al. 1995; Goto et al. 2001), an unfavorable histology group according to the International Neuroblastoma Pathology Classification. The presence of prominent nucleoli in neuroblastic cells of undifferentiated or poorly differentiated neuroblastoma, often associated with unfavorable prognosis (Ambros et al. 2002), can be an additional hallmark of *MYCN* amplification (own unpublished observations).

The balance appears to favor cellular proliferation (mitosis) more than cellular death (karyorrhexis) in a *MYCN* amplified tumor, which is well known to have a highly aggressive and rapidly progressive clinical behavior. In light microscopic sections from *MYCN* amplified tumors, however, the number of karyorrhectic cells always exceeds that of mitotic cells. This may be explained by the fact that the histologically visible stage of mitosis is much shorter than that of karyorrhexis (Bursch at al. 1991). Our preliminary data show that neuroblastoma tumors with favorable histology express significantly higher levels of trkA than those with unfavorable histology (Shimada et al. 2004). Favorable histology neuroblastoma tumors include both poorly differentiated and differentiating subtypes: although there is no difference in the level of trkA expression between these two histological subtypes, tumors of differentiating subtype are diagnosed in significantly older children (usually between 1 and 5 years of age) than those of poorly differentiated subtype (newborn to 1.5 years of age). This may suggest an in vivo latent period required for morphological evidence of neuroblastic differentiation among the neuroblastoma tumors in the favorable-histology group, and supports the concept of an age-linked Pathology Classification.

8.5.3 Composite Tumor

The term “composite” implies that the tumor is composed of histologically and, probably biologically, different clonal populations (Schmidt et al. 1993), a description possibly applicable to almost 10% of pNTs. In the International Neuroblastoma Pathology Classification, this composite form is designated as ganglioneuroblastoma, nodular (composite, Schwannian stroma-rich/stroma-dominant and stroma-poor). In this model the neuroblastic nodule(s) represents the evolution of one or multiple clones, either because of newly acquired genetic aberrations in late stage of tumor progression or the persistence of genetically and biologically distinct variants evolving early in tumor formation. Clinically, two-thirds of these composite tumors are aggressive (Peuchmaur et al. 2003; Umehara et al. 2000).

Table 10.3. Magnetic resonance imaging evaluation of patients with neuroblastoma. Suggested techniques, contrast, scan sequences, and anatomical sites

- Machine specifications
  - Magnet: 1.5-T unit
  - Coils: Body coils or phased-array coils are used for most pediatric patients. Head coils are used for neonates and infants
  - Slice thickness: ranges from 5-mm slice thickness with 0- to 1-mm intersection gaps to 8-mm slice thickness with 0- to 2-mm intersection gaps depending on the size of the patient
- Contrast
  - Gadolinium: 0.1 mm/kg
- Scan sequences
  - T1-weighted spin echo or T1-weighted gradient echo (in phase)
  - T2-weighted fat-suppressed fast spin echo
  - T1-weighted fat-suppressed spin echo or T1-weighted fat suppressed gradient echo (in phase) after IV injection of gadolinium
- Evaluation of anatomical sites
  - Pelvis and femurs to mid-femoral shafts for evaluation of marrow disease and pelvic involvement
    - Coronal T1-weighted spin-echo or gradient-echo (in phase) sequences
    - Transverse T2-weighted fat-suppressed fast spin-echo sequences
  - Chest and abdomen: to evaluate extent of disease
    - Coronal T1-weighted spin-echo or gradient-echo (in phase) sequence to include the neck for evaluation of possible neck nodes as a site for biopsy
    - Transverse T2-weighted fat-suppressed fast spin-echo sequence
    - Transverse T1-weighted fat-suppressed spin-echo or gradient-echo (in phase) sequence after injection of gadolinium
    - Coronal T1-weighted fat-suppressed spin-echo or gradient-echo (in phase) sequence after injection of gadolinium
  - Lumbar spine: to evaluate marrow disease
    - Sagittal T1-weighted spin-echo sequence
    - Sagittal T2-weighted fat-suppressed fast spin-echo sequence

10.2.3 Magnetic Resonance Imaging

Many investigators consider magnetic resonance imaging (MR; Table 10.3) the imaging modality of choice in the initial evaluation of NB (Siegel et al. 2002; Sofka et al. 1999). Magnetic resonance has distinct advantages over CT including (a) the absence of ionizing radiation, (b) the ability to evaluate neural foraminal and epidural involvement, and (c) the ability to detect bone marrow disease. In addition, MR is ideal for defining the precise extent of skeletal involvement, separating cortical bone from marrow involvement. Furthermore, invasion of the liver, kidney, and abdominal organs can readily be detected by MR imaging. This is particularly important in large, right-sided masses where separation of the mass from liver or kidney may be difficult by CT. By imaging in multiple planes, MR can usually demonstrate the relationship of the mass to adjacent organs. Gadolinium-enhanced scans can provide additional information in these cases (Kornreich et al. 1991). On MR neuroblastoma characteristically has prolonged

Table 10.4. Technetium-99m bone scintigraphy

Bone scanning principles	Scan technique
Image entire body with particular attention to patient position: knees and elbows should be as flat as obtainable to assess peri-articular uptake	Intravenous injection of 25 mCi Tc-99m-MDP/1.73 m^2, imaging begun 2–3 h after injection
Bladder should be empty for adequate visualization of the pelvis. In small children this may require bladder catheterization (if it can be safely done) or delayed images after voiding.	Multi-headed gamma camera with low-energy collimator preferred
	Computer acquisition
	Single photon emission CT as needed

T1 and T2 relaxation times, demonstrating heterogeneous low signal on T1 and high signal on T2. Bright signal in the mass on T1-weighted imaging sequences represents hemorrhage. Although calcifications are not as readily identified on MR as on CT, they are visualized as areas of signal void. Nevertheless, non-visualization of calcifications should not be a significant deterrent to using MR for the initial evaluation of NB.

10.2.4 Bone Scan

The bone scan (Table 10.4) has had a long-standing role for evaluating the entire skeleton for metastatic NB (Shulkin et al. 1992). In addition, many primary NBs also accumulate Tc-99m MDP because of their calcifications. The depiction of osseous lesions depends on the reaction of bone to the presence of tumor within bone. The bone scan provides a major diagnostic advantage over skeletal surveys in the assessment of bony NB lesions. Considerable attention to scan technique and positioning is critical to distinguish normal metaphyseal uptake from NB involvement, particularly when these lesions are symmetrical. Since NB frequently localizes in the metaphyseal region adjacent to the epiphyseal plates, sites of normally increased uptake of bone seeking tracers, metastatic involvement may be difficult to appreciate in these areas of normal high physiological accumulation.

10.2.5 MIBG Scintigraphy

Most NB tumors effectively concentrate tracers designed to image the sympathetic nervous system and other tracers with avidity for somatostatin receptors. Meta-iodobenzylguanidine (MIBG) scintigraphy was developed at University of Michigan in the late 1970s to image the adrenal medulla (Wieland et al. 1980), and was later successfully applied to functional imaging of pheochromocytoma (Sisson et al. 1981) and NB (Treuner et al. 1984; Geatti et al. 1985). MIBG is a tracer for the type-1 amine uptake and granular storage pathways (APUD: amine precursor uptake and decarboxylation). Once transported into the NB cell the majority of MIBG remains within the cytoplasm (Smets et al. 1989, 1990). In contrast to pheochromocytoma cells where MIBG is actively transported into catecholamine storage granules by a reserpine-sensitive pump, accumulation of MIBG in NBs depends on continued reuptake of the effluxed radiotracer. MIBG is not metabolized by the enzymes which metabolize catecholamines. Drugs that interfere with uptake of catecholamines and related compounds may impair visualization of NBs; these include over-the-counter non-prescription cough and cold preparations which contain pseudoephedrine or phenylpropanolamine, and labetolol, a beta-adrenergic antagonist. Before injection of the MIBG tracer, parents should be asked specifically about recent administration of all prescribed and over the counter drugs.

Table 10.5. MIBG imaging

Principles	Scan technique
Imaging of entire body	SSKI or other iodine solutions to block uptake of free radioiodine into the thyroid. Begin the day prior to injection and at minimum, 30 min prior to injection
I-123 MIBG produces images of much higher count density than I-131 MIBG. I-123 has less radiation hazard and requires less stringent thyroid protection	Intravenous injection of 10 mCi I-123-MIBG/1.73 m^2
Bladder should be empty for adequate visualization of the pelvis. In small children this may require bladder catheterization (if it can be safely done) or delayed images after voiding.	Whole-body imaging 18–24 h later, low-energy collimator
	Computer acquisition
	Single photon emission CT as needed

Review of 13 publications from eight countries on MIBG scintigraphy performed on 330 patients (Feine et al. 1987; Geatti et al. 1985; Heyman et al. 1988; Lumbroso et al. 1988; Schmiegelow et al. 1989; Shulkin and Shapiro 1990; Troncone et al. 1990) indicates that the sensitivity of disease detection is ~87% and the specificity is ~94%. The positive predictive value is ~98%, while the negative predictive value is ~70%. The majority of patients in the reported studies were evaluated with I-131 MIBG. Both I-131 and I-123 MIBG are excellent agents for imaging NB. In the United States both the I-131 and the I-123 labeled forms are commercially available, although I-123 MIBG has gained wider use in the past few years because of its superior scintigraphic properties and radiation safety considerations. The images obtained from I-123 MIBG studies have higher count densities and greater quality, and the sites of normal uptake are more readily recognized. In direct comparisons of the two compounds, one study showed that the same number of lesions were identified by both techniques, while another study suggested that more lesions were identified with I-123 MIBG scintigraphy (Gelfand 1996; Simon et al. 1992). High-quality single-photon-emission CT (SPECT) images can be obtained using I-123 MIBG. One study indicated that a greater number of abnormal sites of uptake can be detected by SPECT than by planar scintigraphy, with better anatomic localization of the lesions (Ruffini et al. 1996); however, other investigators did not find more lesions by SPECT, although an increase in the certainty that suspected abnormalities on planar imaging were indeed abnormal was reported (Gelfand et al. 1994).

MIBG is highly specific for NB in the usual pediatric context (Leung et al. 1997). The results of MIBG scintigraphy in 100 children with a variety of childhood tumors other than NB studied in five referral centers in three countries showed a specificity of >95%. In these studies, solid tumors of childhood, such as Wilms tumor and soft tissue sarcoma, failed to concentrate MIBG (0 of 14 and 0 of 15, respectively). The remainder of the patients also had negative scans except for 1 of 2 with infantile myofibromatosis, 1 of 2 with neuroendocrine carcinomas, 1 of 2 pancreatoblastomas, and 1 of 10 primitive neuroectodermal tumors; thus, MIBG is only rarely concentrated by non-neural crest tumors.

MIBG scans may also have prognostic value. A study by Suc and colleagues (1996) suggested that children older than 1 year with more than four deposits of MIBG avid NB at diagnosis were seven times less likely to achieve a complete remission after four courses of chemotherapy. Similar results have been reported by Perel and co-workers (1999). In addition, a recent study by Matthay et al. (2003) suggests that the number of MIBG-positive lesions identified after four cycles of induction therapy may be predictive of outcome.

10.2.6 Octreotide Scanning

Many neuroendocrine tumors express somatostatin receptors, and the currently available In-111DTPA-pentetreotide (Octreoscan) detects the majority of NBs and pheochromocytomas; however, this compound appears to be inferior to MIBG for imaging these tumor types (Lauriero et al. 1995; Manil et al. 1996; Sautter-Bihl et al. 1994). Visualization of NBs in the abdomen and pelvis can be impaired by the marked normal hepatic, splenic, renal, and bowel uptake of this agent. In contrast to specificity of MIBG, Octreoscan images many types of neuroendocrine tumors, including carcinoids, islet cell tumors, pituitary adenomas, and medullary carcinoma of the thyroid, and non-neuroendocrine tumors, such as lymphomas and small cell carcinoma of the lung. Inflammatory infiltrates may also show uptake.

10.2.7 Positron Emission Tomography Scanning

F-18 fluorodeoxyglucose (FDG) is concentrated by most NBs and pheochromocytomas (Fig. 10.2; Shulkin et al. 1996; Kushner et al. 2001). Unlike tracers specific for tissues of the adrenergic nervous system, FDG uptake does not depend on type-1 catecholamine uptake. Most NBs concentrate FDG and uptake prior to therapy is often intense, decreasing with treatment. FDG imaging in NBs is particularly valuable for monitoring those tumors which do not concentrate MIBG.

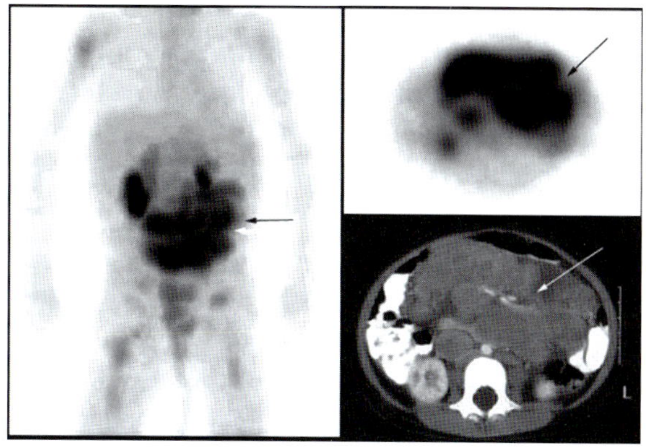

Figure 10.2

A 4-year-old with extensively treated neuroblastoma under consideration for bone marrow transplant. I-123 MIBG scan (not shown) showed no abnormal uptake. *Left panel:* Coronal image from PET-FDG scan shows large area of markedly increased uptake (*arrow*). Transverse image from PET-FDG scan (*right upper panel*) shows markedly increased uptake (*arrow*) occupying most of the abdomen. A CT scan of same area (*right lower panel*) shows the large abdominal mass (*arrow*) with mixed attenuation characteristics. The patient soon after died from progressive disease

10.2.8 Other Tracers

Gallium-67 is rarely used for imaging of NB. Although nearly 80% sensitivity for detection of the primary tumor has been reported, gallium imaging did not visualize skeletal involvement (Garty et al. 1989). Tl-201 has been useful for imaging a variety of soft tissue tumors, but this tracer localizes poorly in NB (Howman-Giles et al. 1995). A number of ligands similar to MIBG have also been used to study sympathetic innervation of the heart as well as to image neuroendocrine tumors. These include I-123 amino iodobenzylguanidine (AIBG), F-18 fluorodopamine, F-18 fluronorepinephrine, F-18 fluorometaraminol, C-11 hydroxyephedrine (HED), C-11 epinephrine (EPI), C-11 phenylephrine, and fluoro-metaiodobenzylguanidine (FIBG); only three have been investigated in patients with neuroendocrine tumors (Shulkin et al. 1986, 1996, 1999). FIBG has been shown to be concentrated by NB cells in culture (Vaidynathan et al. 1994b). Benzylguanidine labeled with the alpha particle emitter Astatine 211 has been proposed as a potential radiotherapeutic agent (Vaidyanathan et al. 1994a). These derivatives of MIBG rely on the type-1 uptake pathway for entry into the cell.

The I-131 labeled monoclonal antibody 3F8 specific for ganglioside GD2 has been used for radioimmunoscintigraphy and radioimmunotherapy of NB. Because of the abundance of this antigen on neuroblastoma ($5–10\times10^{-6}$ molecules per cell), high levels of radiolabel can be deposited selectively to tumor instead of normal tissues (Miraldi et al. 1986; Yeh et al. 1991). The I-124 labeled form has also been used to improve tumor dosimetry (Larson et al. 1992). Several other monoclonal antibodies that may prove to be useful in imaging NB are under investigation (see Chap. 14 for a detailed discussion of antibody-based radioimmunotherapy).

10.3 Disease Evaluation

10.3.1 Primary Site

Primary retroperitoneal NB tumors frequently infiltrate behind the aorta and IVC (inferior vena cava) displacing these vessels anteriorly. In addition, tumors commonly encase the aorta, IVC, renal arteries, renal veins, celiac axis, and superior mesenteric artery. When compared with CT, MR appears superior in evaluating vascular displacement and encasement (Tanabe et al. 1993a, b). Measurement of tumor volume as a quantitative response to therapy has become important study endpoints, for prognosis and follow-up. In some therapeutic protocols, the percentage of tumor shrinkage as determined by CT scan or MR imaging is critical to the continuation or abandonment of specific therapies (Wheatley et al. 1995).

10.3.2 Local Invasion

Extension of disease to lymph nodes adjacent to primary abdominal NB tumors in the renal hila, porta, and retroperitoneum is commonly seen. Separation of the primary tumor from the adjacent involved nodes is often not possible, regardless of the imaging modality utilized. Distant nodal disease, particularly in the neck where they are readily accessible to biopsy, should be identified on CT scans or on coronal MR scans in patients with large unresectable primary tumors, possibly sparing the patient an open biopsy (Abramson et al. 1996). Mediastinal, hilar, paratracheal, subcarinal, and azygoesophageal adenopathy can be due to direct extension of large thoracoabdominal primary tumors or may represent metastatic disease.

Direct invasion of abdominal organs, including liver and kidney, can occasionally be seen. Invasion of the psoas muscle is not uncommon. Pleural effusions are uncommon and are typically observed in the presence of tumor masses that are pleural based or rib lesions. Epidural involvement may be partially identified on CT. Magnetic resonance is necessary for full evaluation of foraminal and epidural tumor extension and possible cord compression (Sofka et al. 1999; Siegel et al. 1986) (Fig. 10.1).

10.3.3 Distant Metastases

10.3.3.1 Bone Metastases

Bone metastases may be detected by bone scintigraphy, MIBG scan, and PET scan. Symmetrical skeletal involvement is easier to interpret by MIBG than by bone scan. Furthermore, bone scan can remain abnormal for months even after the successful treatment of the tumor, whereas MIBG will not be taken up by healing bone; however, since bone and bone marrow are two distinct compartments with disparate prognostic importance (e.g., stage 4 vs stage 4S in infants), caution should be exercised in assigning bony involvement solely on MIBG. False-negative I-123 MIBG scans for skeletal involvement have been reported, prompting some investigators to recommend both I-123 MIBG plus bone scans for the evaluation of NB (Gordon et al. 1990). In stage-4 patients, where bony and bone marrow involvement usually go hand in hand, concordance between MIBG scanning and bone scanning is generally the rule (Shulkin et al. 1992); however, some studies have indicated that more skeletal lesions may be evident on MIBG scan compared with bone scan (Hadj-Djilani et al. 1995). Bone lesions may also be identified on CT; however, these lesions persist as abnormalities on CT for years, even in the face of bone and MIBG scans that have reverted to normal.

10.3.3.2 Bone-Based, Dural-Based, Leptomeningeal, and Brain Metastases

Computed tomography scan or MR imaging of skull metastases shows bony erosion or abnormal bone signal and soft tissue masses, which may extend into the soft tissues of the scalp or push through the inner table of the skull (Egelhoff and Zalles 1996). Dural

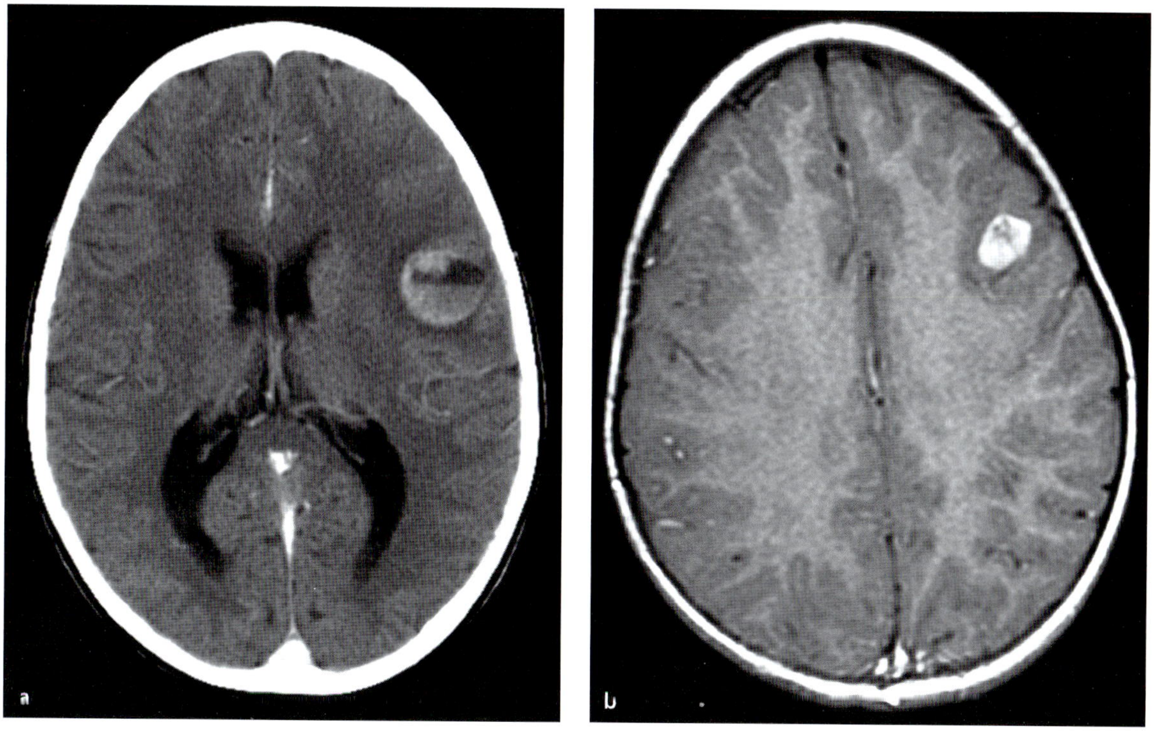

Figure 10.3 a,b

Intracerebral metastases. **a** Patient 1. Axial post-contrast CT of the brain reveals a hemorrhagic left posterior frontal brain metastasis. **b** Patient 2. Post-contrast axial T1-weighted image of the brain demonstrates a left frontal brain metastasis

disease, which is common, may be well demonstrated with either contrast-enhanced CT scan or MR imaging. Once through the dura, these tumors can impinge on the brain parenchyma. Sphenoid bone involvement may extend into the orbits as a soft tissue mass causing proptosis. Diffuse leptomeningeal disease may be visualized by CT (Sener 1993) or MRI. Although MR with gadolinium contrast has high sensitivity in detecting meningeal metastasis, occasionally false-positive results can be seen following general anesthesia and lumbar puncture. Intracerebral metastatic lesions are usually solid (Kramer et al. 2001) and occasionally hemorrhagic (Aronson et al. 1995) (Fig. 10.3) or cystic (Kenny et al. 1995). These cystic lesions may display contrast-enhancing rims and be confused with infection or inflammation.

10.3.3.3 Marrow Metastasis

Histological examination is the gold standard for the diagnosis of marrow metastasis. MIBG is the most efficient test to estimate the distribution and severity of bone marrow involvement (Fig. 10.4; Osmanagaoglu et al. 1993). Spotty marrow involvement can be missed by tissue biopsy. In addition, MIBG and MRI may show bone marrow involvement in areas not accessible to biopsy.

MRI may show more bone marrow lesions than MIBG (Corbett et al. 1991).

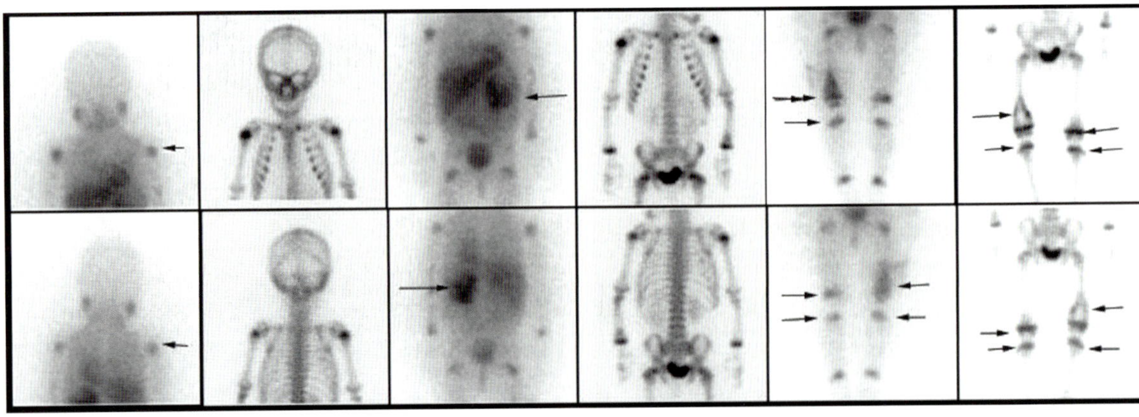

Figure 10.4

A 3-year-old with widespread neuroblastoma at presentation. Alternating panels of MIBG scan and bone scan. Foci of disease are much better delineated on the MIBG scan. *Top row* are anterior views, *bottom row* are posterior views. The MIBG scan shows extensive skeletal involvement: there is abnormal uptake in both shoulders (*arrows, panels 1 and 2*), both wrists (*panels 3 and 4*), the proximal femurs (*panels 3 and 4*), the distal right femurs (*panels 5 and 6*), both knees (*panels 5 and 6*), and ankles (*panel 5*). Ankles are seen on MIBG views only. A large left abdominal mass is seen on MIBG images (*panel 3*)

10.4 Prenatally Diagnosed Neuroblastoma

With the advent of routine prenatal ultrasonography, the diagnosis of fetal (Ho et al. 1993; Toma et al. 1994; Jennings et al. 1993) or congenital (Granata et al. 2000; Forman et al. 1990) neuroblastoma has become more common. The tumor may be solid or cystic (Atkinson et al. 1986; Hamada et al. 1999) and may be localized (stage 1) or associated with liver metastases (stage 4S; Toma et al. 1994). Subcutaneous nodules are frequently present. At birth, these findings can be confirmed by ultrasonography. In addition to NB, the differential diagnosis of an adrenal mass detected prenatally or at birth includes extralobar pulmonary sequestration (Curtis et al. 1997) and adrenal hemorrhage (Strouse et al. 1995; Burbige 1993). Many adrenal hemorrhages show shrinkage within 2 weeks after birth; however, shrinkage of an adrenal hemorrhage may sometimes take weeks to months. These masses therefore may be confused with tumor. On the other hand, regressing NB in a neonate can also mimic adrenal hemorrhage (Croitoru et al. 1992). In the absence of large tumor masses and organ compromise, observation rather than surgery is acceptable in an asymptomatic infant with a small adrenal mass (see Chap. 11). Follow-up ultrasonography is important, especially if there is liver involvement. If clinically indicated, the distinction between NB and adrenal hemorrhage can usually be made with MIBG scintigraphy.

10.5 Stage-4S Neuroblastoma

In the absence of adverse biological factors infants with stage-4S disease have a high incidence of spontaneous regression and an excellent prognosis (see Chaps. 7 and 10). In stage-4S disease the extent of disease is initially evaluated with CT or MR of the head, neck, chest, abdomen and pelvis, and MIBG scintigraphy; however, once the diagnosis is made and if good biology is confirmed, ultrasonography is a useful method of follow-up. The liver may show persistent heterogeneous echo texture, although focal nodules should eventually resolve (Fig. 10.5). If the mass

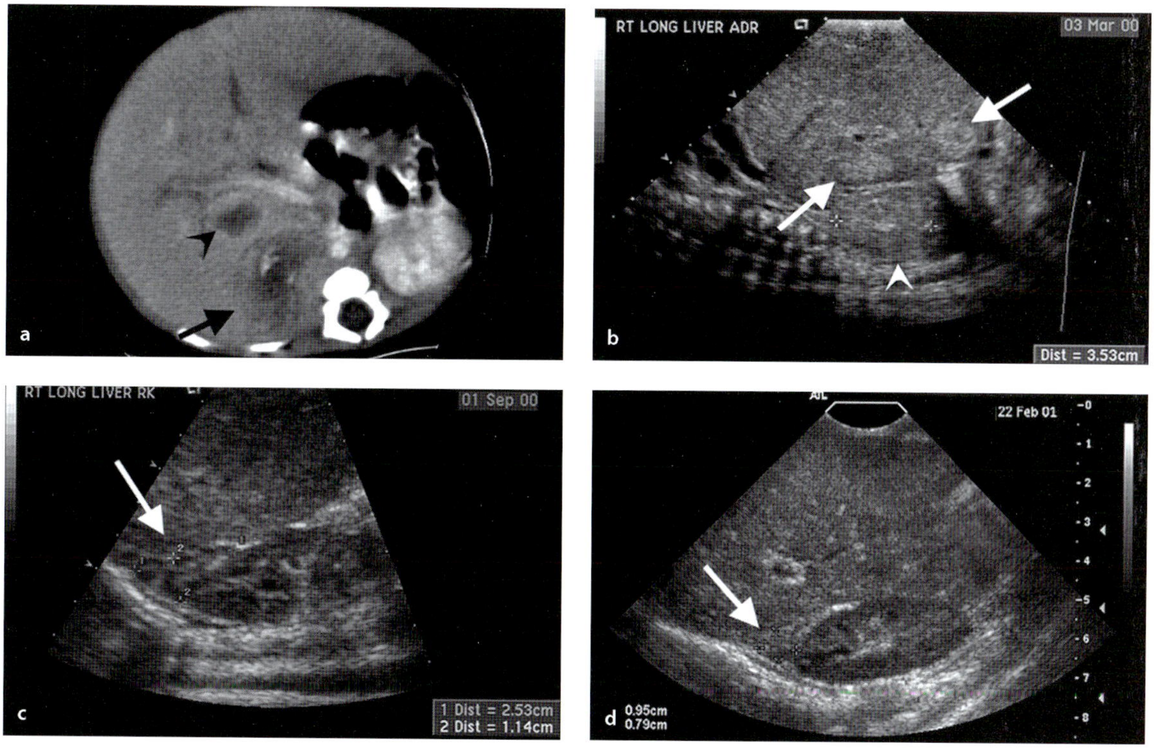

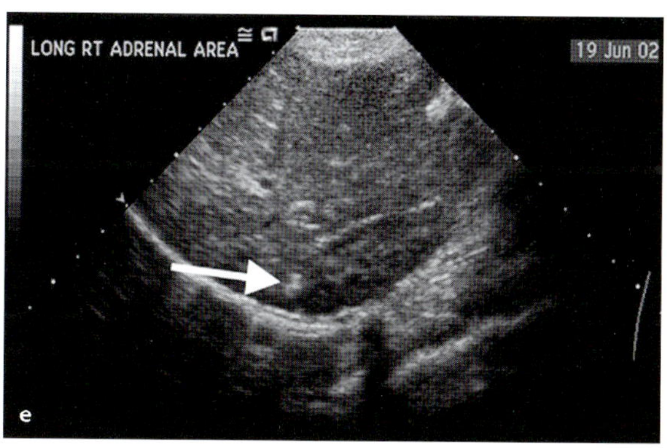

Figure 15.5 a–e

Stage-4S Neuroblastoma. Baby presented at 3 days of age. Bone and bone marrow were normal. The patient received no therapy. **a** Contrast-enhanced CT scan reveals a partially calcified right adrenal mass (*arrow*) and a low-attenuation liver metastasis (*arrowhead*). **b** Ultrasonography at diagnosis reveals a right adrenal mass (*arrowhead*) and several hepatic nodules (*arrows*). **c** Ultrasonography at 6 months of age demonstrates decrease in size of the right adrenal mass (*arrow*). **d** Ultrasonography at 11 months of age shows further decrease in size of the adrenal mass (*arrow*). The liver metastases have resolved. **e** Ultrasonography at 2 years 3 months shows only a residual hyperechoic area (calcification) in the region of the right adrenal gland (*arrow*)

increases in size or liver lesions progress, patients should be re-evaluated, and treatment may be indicated. Efforts to limit exposure to repeated ionizing radiation from follow-up CT examinations and routine MIBG studies in this group of young infants should be made.

10.6 Evaluation of Disease Response

According to the INSS, disease response should evaluated CT/MRI of the primary and metastatic sites, MR of epidural or CNS involvement, bone scan, and MIBG scan; however, it must be remembered that occasionally ganglioneuromas are detected by MIBG scintigraphy. Prior to second-look surgery, a repeat CT scan of the primary site is important for surgical planning. In addition to the primary tumor, adjacent lymph nodes in the thorax, retroperitoneum, and pelvis should be evaluated. Small lymph nodes are better identified on CT than MR, and may be too small to characterize on MIBG scanning.

For patients with intermediate- and high-risk disease, CT/MRI examinations are typically performed in conjunction with MIBG scans at 3- to 6-month intervals during treatment and for 1–2 years following the completion of therapy. Routine scanning after this time should be continued only for those patients with persistent abnormalities. Routine follow-up bone scans do not yield much extra information, unless progression is suspected and or local radiation is planned. Equivocal findings can be further evaluated with FDG-PET scans (Fig. 10.2).

10.7 Conclusion

Imaging plays a critical role in evaluating the extent of disease at diagnosis and in assessing response to therapy. A variety of imaging modalities are available, and each can provide unique information. Radiation exposure, scanning protocols, and sedation times are significant factors that should be taken into account in determining which studies should be used. Minimizing radiation exposure is of paramount importance in the follow-up of neonates and young infants with favorable biology NB. At the present time, several different imaging studies are needed to optimally evaluate the primary tumor, and the presence and location of metastatic disease. New imaging modalities may improve our ability to evaluate NB with less risk of radiation exposure.

References

Abramson SJ (1997) Adrenal neoplasms in children. Radiol Clin North Am 35:1415–1453

Abramson SJ, Berdon W, Stolar C et al (1996) Stage IV N neuroblastoma: MRI diagnosis of left supraclavicular "Virchow's" nodal spread. Pediatr Radiol 26:717–719

Aronson MR, Smoker WR, Oetting GM (1995) Hemorrhagic intracranial parenchymal metastases from primary retroperitoneal neuroblastoma. Pediatr Radiol 25:284–285

Atkinson GS, Zaatari GTS, Lorenzo RI (1986) Cystic neuroblastoma in infants: radiographic and pathologic features. AJR 146:113–117

Burbige K (1993) Prenatal adrenal hemorrhage confirmed by postnatal surgery. J Urol 150:1866–1869

Cohen M (1992) Endocrine tumors. In: Cohen M (ed) Imaging of children with cancer. Mosby Yearbook, St. Louis

Corbett R, Olliff J, Fairley N, Moyes J, Husband J, Pinkerton R, Carter R, Treleaven J, McElwain T, Meller S (1991) A prospective comparison between magnetic resonance imaging, meta-iodobenzylguanidine scintigraphy and marrow histology/cytology in neuroblastoma. Eur J Cancer 27: 1560–1564

Croitoru D, Sinksy A, Laberge J (1992) Cystic neuroblastoma. J Pediatr Surg 27:1320–1321

Curtis MR, Mooney DP, Vaccaro TJ et al. (1997) Prenatal ultrasound characterization of the suprarenal mass: distinction between neuroblastoma and subdiaphragmatic extralobar pulmonary sequestration. J Ultrasound Med 16: 75–83

Egelhoff JC, Zalles C (1996) Unusual CNS presentation of neuroblastoma. Pediatr Radiol 26:51–54

Feine U, Muller-Schauenburg W, Treuner J, Klingebiel T (1987) Metaiodobenzylguanidine (MIBG) labeled with 123I/131I in neuroblastoma diagnosis and follow-up treatment with a review of the diagnostic results of the International Workshop of Pediatric Oncology held in Rome, September 1986. Med Pediatr Oncol 15:181–187

Forman HP, Leonidas JC, Berdon WE et al. (1990) Congenital neuroblastoma. Evaluation with multimodality imaging. Radiology 175:365–369

Garty I, Friedman A, Sandler MP, Kedar A (1989) Neuroblastoma: imaging evaluation by sequential Tc-99m MDP, I-131MIBG, and Ga-67 citrate studies. Clin Nucl Med 14: 515–522

Geatti O, Shapiro B, Sisson JC, Hutchinson RJ, Mallette S, Eyre P, Beierwaltes WH (1985) Iodine-131 metaiodobenzylguanidine scintigraphy for the location of neuroblastoma: preliminary experience in ten cases. J Nucl Med 26:736–742

Gelfand MJ (1996) I-123-MIBG and I-131-MIBG imaging in children with neuroblastoma. J Nucl Med 37:35P

Gelfand MJ, Elgazzar AH, Kriss VM, Masters P, Golsch GJ (1994) Iodine-123-MIBG SPECT versus planar imaging in children with neural crest tumors. J Nucl Med 35:1753–1757

Gordon I, Peters AM, Gutman A, Morony S, Dicks-Mireaux C, Pritchard J (1990) Skeletal assessment in neuroblastoma: the pitfalls of iodine-123-MIBG scans. J Nucl Med 31:129–134
Granata C, Fagnani AM, Gambini C et al. (2000) Features and outcome of neuroblastoma detected before birth. J Pediatr Surg 35:88–91
Hadj-Djilani NL, Lebtahi NE, Delaloye AB, Laurini R, Beck D (1995) Diagnosis and follow-up of neuroblastoma by means of iodine-123 metaiodobenzylguanidine scintigraphy and bone scan, and the influence of histology. Eur J Nucl Med 22:322–329
Hamada Y, Ikebururo K, Sato M et al. (1999) Prenatally diagnosed cystic neuroblastoma. Pediatr Surg Int 15:71–74
Heyman S, Evans AE, D'Angio GJ (1988) I-131 metaiodobenzylguanidine: diagnostic use in neuroblastoma patients in relapse. Med Pediatr Oncol 16:337–340
Ho PTC, Estroff JA, Kozakewich H et al. (1993) Prenatal detection of neuroblastoma: a ten-year experience from the Dana-Farber Cancer Institute and Children's Hospital. Pediatrics 92:358
Howman-Giles R, Uren RF, Shaw PJ (1995) Thallium-201 scintigraphy in pediatric soft-tissue tumors. J Nucl Med 36:1372–1376
Jennings RW, LaQuaglia MP, Leong K et al. (1993) Fetal neuroblastoma: prenatal diagnosis and natural history. J Pediatr Surg 28:1168–1174
Kenny B, Pizer B, Duncan A et al. (1995) Cystic metastatic cerebral neuroblastoma. Pediatr Radiol 25:97–98
Kornreich G, Horev C, Kaplinsky N et al. (1991) Neuroblastoma: evaluation with contrast enhanced MR imaging. Pediatr Radiol 21:566–569
Kramer K, Kushner B, Heller G, Cheung NK (2001) Neuroblastoma metastatic to the central nervous system: the Memorial Sloan-Kettering Cancer Center experience and a literature review. Cancer 91:1510–1519
Kushner BH, Yeung HW, Larson SM, Kramer K, Cheung NK (2001) Extending positron emission tomography scan utility to high-risk neuroblastoma: Fluorine-18 fluorodeoxyglucose positron emission tomography as sole imaging modality in follow-up of patients. J Clin Oncol 19:3397–3405
Larson SM, Pentlow KS, Volkow ND, Wolf AP, Finn RD, Lambrecht RM, Graham MC, Resta G di, Bendriem B, Daghighian F, Yeh SDJ, Wang GJ, Cheung NKV (1992) PET scanning of iodine-124-3F8 as an approach to tumor dosimetry during treatment planning for radioimmunotherapy in a child with neuroblastoma. J Nucl Med 33:2020–2023
Lauriero F, Rubini G, D'Addabbo F, Rubini D, Schettini F, D'Addabbo A (1995) I-131 MIBG scintigraphy of neuroectodermal tumors. Comparison between I-131 MIBG and In-111 DTPA-octreotide. Clin Nucl Med 20:243–249
Leung A, Shapiro B, Hattner R et al. (1997) The specificity of radioiodinated MIBG for neural crest tumors in childhood. J Nucl Med 38:1352–1357
Lumbroso JD, Guermazi F, Hartmann O, Coornaert S, Rabarison Y, Leclere JG, Couanet D, Bayle C, Caillaud JM, Lemerle J et al. (1988) Meta-iodobenzylguanidine (mIBG) scans in neuroblastoma: sensitivity and specificity, a review of 115 scans. Prog Clin Biol Res 271:689–705
Manil L, Edeline V, Lumbroso J, Lequen H, Zucker JM (1996) Indium-111-pentetreotide scintigraphy in children with neuroblast-derived tumors. J Nucl Med 37:893–896
Matthay KK, Edeline V, Lumbroso J, Tanguy ML, Asselain B, Zucker JM, Valteau-Couanet D, Hartmann O, Michon J (2003) Correlation of early metastatic response by 123I-metaiodobenzylguanidine scintigraphy with overall response and event-free survival in stage IV neuroblastoma. J Clin Oncol 21:2486–2491
Miraldi FD, Nelson AD, Kraly C, Ellery S, Landmeier B, Coccia PF, Strandjord SE, Cheung NK (1986) Diagnostic imaging of human neuroblastoma with radiolabeled antibody. Radiology 161:413–418
Osmanagaoglu K, Lippens M, Benoit Y, Obrie E, Schelstraete K, Simons M (1993) A comparison of iodine-123 metaiodobenzylguanidine scintigraphy and single bone marrow aspiration biopsy in the diagnosis and follow-up of 26 children with neuroblastoma. Eur J Nucl Med 20:1154–1160
PerelY, Conway J, Kletzel M, Goldman J, Weiss S, Feyler A, Cohn SL (1999) Clinical impact and prognostic value of metaiodobenzylguanidine imaging in children with metastatic neuroblastoma. J Pediatr Hematol Oncol 21:13–18
Ruffini V, Fisher GA, Shulkin BL, Sisson JC, Shapiro B (1996) 123I-MIBG imaging of neuroblastoma; utility of SPECT and delayed imaging. J Nucl Med 37:1464–1468
Ruzal-Shapiro C, Berdon W, Cohen M et al. (1991) MR imaging of diffuse bone marrow replacement in pediatric patients with cancer. Radiology 181:587–589
Sautter-Bihl ML, Dorr U, Schilling F, Treuner J, Bihl H (1994) Somatostatin receptor imaging: a new horizon in the diagnostic management of neuroblastoma. Semin Oncol 21 (Suppl 13):38–41
Schmiegelow K, Simes MA, Agertoft L, Berglund G, Storm-Mathisen I, Andreassen M, Salmi TT, Nygard R, Wiebe T, Kreuger A et al. (1989) Radio-iodobenzylguanidine scintigraphy of neuroblastoma: conflicting results, when compared with standard investigations. Med Pediatr Oncol 17: 127–130
Sener RN (1993) CT of diffuse leptomeningeal metastasis from primary extracerebral neuroblastoma. Pediatr Radiol 23: 402–403
Shulkin B, Shapiro B, Tobes M, Shen S-W, Wieland D, Meyers L, Lee H, Petry N, Sisson J, Beierwaltes W (1986) ^{123}I-4-Amino-3-iodobenzylguanidine (^{123}I-AIBG), a new sympatho-adrenal imaging agent: Comparison with ^{123}I-meta-iodobenzylguanidine (^{123}I-MIBG). J Nucl Med 27:1138–1142
Shulkin BL, Shapiro B, Hutchinson RJ (1992) Iodine-131-metaiodobenzylguanidine and bone scintigraphy for the detection of neuroblastoma. J Nucl Med 33:1735–1740

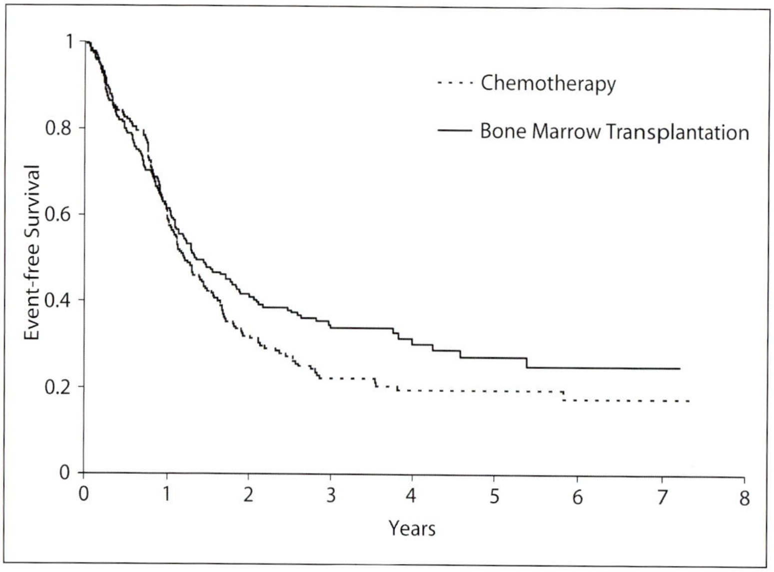

Figure 11.3.1

Results of CCG-3891, a randomized study of myeloablative chemoradiotherapy with purged autologous bone marrow transplantation vs intensive non-myeloablative therapy. A second randomization was performed on all consenting patients completing the consolidation therapy without progression to test the efficacy of 13-*cis*-retinoic acid for minimal residual disease. (From Matthay et al. 1999). **a** Improved EFS with myeloablative therapy compared with standard dose chemotherapy. The difference in EFS for the 379 randomized patients was 34 vs 22% at 3 years (*P*=0.034).

later continues to show a significant difference in EFS (Reynolds et al. 2002). Further follow-up will be required to see if high-dose therapy with hematopoietic support has truly made an impact on long-term cure rate in this disease (Matthay et al. 1999).

At present, pilot studies have led to the approach currently used in ongoing studies both in Europe and the U.S. of further increase in chemotherapy dose intensity by eliminating total body irradiation, and instead using higher doses of chemotherapy and local irradiation, with an EFS of 62% at 3 years (Villablanca et al. 1999). Intensification may also be achieved using a tandem transplant approach, with two or three consecutive myeloablative courses (Grupp et al. 2000; Philip et al. 1993; Frappaz et al. 2000; Kletzel et al. 2002). These studies have demonstrated feasibility with good engraftment, although toxicity prevented proceeding to the subsequent myeloablative course in some cases. Further cooperative randomized studies are necessary to determine the relative risks and benefits of the tandem approach.

Allogeneic hematopoietic cell transplant may obviate the possible risk from tumor cell contamination of autologous peripheral blood stem cells or bone marrow, but presents other problems, including graft-vs-host disease, difficulty finding an HLA match, and much higher toxic death rates in the previously reported studies.

11.3.5 Therapy of Minimal Residual Disease

Early and late relapse continue to occur at a high rate, although the newer, dose-intensive induction and myeloablative therapies have considerably prolonged survival and improved EFS (Matthay et al. 1999). Relapse is most common in bone and bone marrow, and sites of hypoxic and microscopic residual disease (DuBois et al. 1999). For this reason it has become increasingly important to find new approaches to eliminate minimal residual disease with agents that will be tolerable following myeloablative therapy, when disease is likely to be minimal. This provides the ideal window of time to eradicate resistant clones that are still present using novel therapies not dependent upon standard cytotoxic mechanisms (see Chaps. 14–16); these include differentiating agents such as 13-*cis*-retinoic acid (Matthay et al. 1999), fenretinide (Delia et al. 1993; Maurer et al. 1999; Garaventa et al. 2003; Basniewski et al. 1999), anti-GD_2 monoclonal antibodies (Ozkaynac et al. 2000), immunocytokines (Lode et al. 1997), genetically engineered vaccines (Bowman et al. 1998; Davidoff et al. 1999), anti-angiogenic therapy (Stern et al. 2001), small molecule inhibitors of tyrosine kinase genes (Evans et al. 1999; Smith et al. 2004), or histone deacetylase inhibitors (Huang et al. 2002).

11.3.6 Conclusion

High-risk neuroblastoma presents a continuing therapeutic challenge. Progress thus far in combination chemotherapy, local control, myeloablative consolidation therapy, and treatment with differentiating agents for microscopic residual disease has improved the overall prognosis. Although the 3-year event-free survival for children with stage-4 disease has improved from <10 to >40% in the past two decades, late relapses continue to be a challenge such that the overall cure rate for stage-4 patients diagnosed at age greater than 18 months with neuroblastoma remained less than 25%.

Dose-intensive induction protocols coupled with gross total resection are expected to achieve near complete remission (CR or VGPR) rates in excess of 70% of patients. In addition, primary site recurrence can now be effectively reduced with surgery combined with ~20 Gy hyperfractionated radiation. Although tumors cannot be detected by histologic examinations or functional nuclear imaging, MRD remains the final hurdle. Myeloablative therapy while prolonging progression-free survival may only have a small effect on the long-term cure rate. Relapses in the CNS plus secondary leukemia can be other serious adverse events. Although their prevalence is <10% among survivors, these late effects of intensive chemotherapy and radiation therapy are expected to surface as patients live longer.

The challenges therefore are multiple. Since treatment induced cancer (e.g., leukemia) is a function of dose (Le Deley et al. 2003), can CR/VGPR rates be maintained by reducing dose without sacrificing dose intensity for subsets of patients? Can new cytotoxic drugs be incorporated into induction therapy for the subset of patients whose tumors are resistant to standard agents? Should myeloablative therapy be applied to only those at higher risk for relapse? New methods to detect MRD suggest that this often persists even when patients are in clinical complete remission, and may predict relapse. Can MRD measurement provide surrogate markers of disease such that different consolidation strategies can be objectively compared, and earlier treatment intervention be initiated? Finally, other approaches to eliminate MRD need to be explored urgently. Novel strategies to overcome drug resistance and to attack sanctuary sites of disease are necessary. Such approaches may include targeted radiotherapy, differentiating agents, immunologic therapies, agents to inhibit important transduction pathways, or drugs to inhibit tumor angiogenesis and invasion.

References

Abemayor E (1992) The effects of retinoic acid on the in vitro and in vivo growth of neuroblastoma cells. Laryngoscope 102:1133–1149

Adkins ES, Sawin R, Gerbing RB, London WB, Matthay KK, Haase GM (2004) Efficacy of complete resection for high-risk neuroblastoma: a Children's Cancer Group study. J Pediatr Surg 39:931–936

August CS, Serota FT, Koch PA et al. (1984) Treatment of advanced neuroblastoma with supralethal chemotherapy, radiation, and allogeneic or autologous marrow reconstitution. J Clin Oncol 2:609–616

Basniewski PG, Reid JM, Villablanca JG, Reynolds CP, Ames MM (1999) A phase I pharmacokinetic study of fenretinide (HPR) in chldren with high-risk solid tumors. A Children's Cancer Group (CCG) study. Proc Am Assoc Cancer Res 40:92

Bowman L, Grossmann M, Rill D et al. (1998) IL-2 adenovector-transduced autologous tumor cells induce antitumor immune responses in patients with neuroblastoma. Blood 92:1941–1949

Burchill SA, Lewis IJ, Abrams KR et al. (2001) Circulating neuroblastoma cells detected by reverse transcriptase polymerase chain reaction for tyrosine hydroxylase mRNA are an independent poor prognostic indicator in stage 4 neuroblastoma in children over 1 year. J Clin Oncol 19:1795–1801

Castel V, Canete A, Navarro S et al. (2001) Outcome of high-risk neuroblastoma using a dose intensity approach: improvement in initial but not in long-term results. Med Pediatr Oncol 37:537–542

Castleberry RP, Cantor AB, Green AA et al. (1994) Phase II investigational window using carboplatin, iproplatin, ifosfamide, and epirubicin in children with untreated disseminated neuroblastoma: a Pediatric Oncology Group study (see comments). J Clin Oncol 12:1616–1620

Cheung IY, Lo Piccolo MS, Kushner BH, Kramer K, Cheung NK (2003) Quantitation of GD2 synthase mRNA by real-time reverse transcriptase polymerase chain reaction: clinical utility in evaluating adjuvant therapy in neuroblastoma. J Clin Oncol 21:1087–1093

Cheung NV, Heller G (1991) Chemotherapy dose intensity correlates strongly with response, median survival, and median progression-free survival in metastatic neuroblastoma (see comments). J Clin Oncol 9:1050–1058

Cheung NK, Miraldi FD (1988) Iodine 131 labeled GD2 monoclonal antibody in the diagnosis and therapy of human neuroblastoma. Prog Clin Biol Res 271:595–604

Cheung NK, Burch L, Kushner BH, Munn DH (1991) Monoclonal antibody 3F8 can effect durable remissions in neuroblastoma patients refractory to chemotherapy: a phase II trial. Prog Clin Biol Res 366:395–400

Cheung NK, Kushner BH, Yeh SJ, Larson SM (1994) 3F8 monoclonal antibody treatment of patients with stage IV neuroblastoma: a phase II study. Prog Clin Biol Res 385:319–328

Cheung NK, Kushner BH, Cheung IY et al. (1998a) Anti-G(D2) antibody treatment of minimal residual stage 4 neuroblastoma diagnosed at more than 1 year of age. J Clin Oncol 16: 3053–3060

Cheung NK, Kushner BH, Yeh SDJ, Larson SM (1998b) 3F8 monoclonal antibody treatment of patients with stage 4 neuroblastoma: a phase II study. Int J Oncol 12:1299–1306

Cheung NK, Kushner BH, La Quaglia MP et al. (2001a) N7: a novel multi-modality therapy of high risk neuroblastoma (NB) in children diagnosed over 1 year of age. Med Pediatr Oncol 36:227–230

Cheung NK, Kushner BH, Kramer K (2001b) Monoclonal antibody-based therapy of neuroblastoma. Hematol Oncol Clin North Am 15:853–866

Coze C, Hartmann O, Michon J et al. (1997) NB87 induction protocol for stage 4 neuroblastoma in children over 1 year of age: a report from the French Society of Pediatric Oncology. J Clin Oncol 15:3433–3440

Davidoff AM, Kimbrough SA, Ng CY, Shochat SJ, Vanin EF (1999) Neuroblastoma regression and immunity induced by transgenic expression of interleukin-12. J Pediatr Surg 34:902–907

Delia D, Aiello A, Lombardi L et al. (1993) N-(4-hydroxyphenyl)retinamide induces apoptosis of malignant hemopoietic cell lines including those unresponsive to retinoic acid. Cancer Res 53:6036–6041

Dini G, Philip T, Hartmann O et al. (1989) Bone marrow transplantation for neuroblastoma: a review of 509 cases. EBMT Group. Bone Marrow Transplant 4 (Suppl 4):42–46

Dini G, Lanino E, Garaventa A et al. (1991) Myeloablative therapy and unpurged autologous bone marrow transplantation for poor-prognosis neuroblastoma: report of 34 cases. J Clin Oncol 9:962–969

Dopfer R, Berthold F, Einsele H et al. (1989) Bone marrow transplantation in children with neuroblastoma. Folia Haematol Int Mag Klin Morphol Blutforsch 116:427–436

DuBois SG, Kalika Y, Lukens JN et al. (1999) Metastatic sites in stage IV and IVS neuroblastoma correlate with age, tumor biology, and survival (see comments). J Pediatr Hematol Oncol 21:181–189

Evans AE, August CS, Kamani N et al. (1994) Bone marrow transplantation for high risk neuroblastoma at the Children's Hospital of Philadelphia: an update. Med Pediatr Oncol 23:323–327

Evans AE, Kisselbach KD, Yamashiro DJ et al. (1999) Antitumor activity of CEP-751 (KT-6587) on human neuroblastoma and medulloblastoma xenografts. Clin Cancer Res 5:3594–3602

Faulkner LB, Garaventa A, Paoli A et al. (2000) In vivo cytoreduction studies and cell sorting – enhanced tumor-cell detection in high-risk neuroblastoma patients: implications for leukapheresis strategies. J Clin Oncol 18:3829–3836

Finklestein JZ, Krailo MD, Lenarsky C et al. (1992) 13-cis-retinoic acid (NSC 122758) in the treatment of children with metastatic neuroblastoma unresponsive to conventional chemotherapy: report from the Childrens Cancer Study Group. Med Pediatr Oncol 20:307–311

Frappaz D, Michon J, Coze C et al. (2000) LMCE3 treatment strategy: results in 99 consecutively diagnosed stage 4 neuroblastomas in children older than 1 year at diagnosis. J Clin Oncol 18:468–476

Frei E III, Teicher BA, Holden SA, Cathcart KN, Wang YY (1988) Preclinical studies and clinical correlation of the effect of alkylating dose. Cancer Res 48:6417–6423

Frost JD, Hank JA, Reaman GH et al. (1997) A phase I/IB trial of murine monoclonal anti-GD2 antibody 14.G2a plus interleukin-2 in children with refractory neuroblastoma: a report of the Children's Cancer Group. Cancer 80:317–333

Garaventa A, Rondelli R, Lanino E et al. (1996) Myeloablative therapy and bone marrow rescue in advanced neuroblastoma. Report from the Italian Bone Marrow Transplant Registry. Italian Association of Pediatric Hematology-Oncology, BMT Group. Bone Marrow Transplant 18:125–130

Garaventa A, Luksch R, Piccolo MS et al. (2003) Phase I trial and pharmacokinetics of fenretinide in children with neuroblastoma. Clin Cancer Res 9:2032–2039

George R, London WB, Maris JM, Cohn SL, Diller L, Look AT (2003) Age as a continuous variable in predicting outcome for neuroblastoma patients with metastatic disease: impact of tumor biological features. Proc Am Soc Clin Oncol 22:799

Graham-Pole J, Casper J, Elfenbein G et al. (1991) High-dose chemoradiotherapy supported by marrow infusions for advanced neuroblastoma: A Pediatric Oncology Group study. J Clin Oncol 9:152–158

Grupp SA, Stern JW, Bunin N et al. (2000) Tandem high-dose therapy in rapid sequence for children with high-risk neuroblastoma. J Clin Oncol 18:2567–2575

Haase GM, Meagher DP Jr, McNeely LK et al. (1994) Electron beam intraoperative radiation therapy for pediatric neoplasms. Cancer 74:740–747

Haas-Kogan DA, Fisch BM, Wara WM et al. (2000) Intraoperative radiation therapy for high-risk pediatric neuroblastoma. Int J Radiat Oncol Biol Phys 47:985–992
Haas-Kogan DA, Swift PS, Selch M et al. (2003) Impact of radiotherapy for high-risk neuroblastoma: a Children's Cancer Group study. Int J Radiat Oncol Biol Phys 56:28–39
Handgretinger R, Baader P, Dopfer R et al. (1992) A phase I study of neuroblastoma with the anti-ganglioside GD2 antibody 14.G2a. Cancer Immunol Immunother 35:199–204
Hartmann O, Benhamou E, Beaujean F et al. (1987) Repeated high-dose chemotherapy followed by purged autologous bone marrow transplantation as consolidation therapy in metastatic neuroblastoma. J Clin Oncol 5:1205–1211
Hartmann O, Valteau-Couanet D, Vassal G et al. (1999) Prognostic factors in metastatic neuroblastoma in patients over 1 year of age treated with high-dose chemotherapy and stem cell transplantation: a multivariate analysis in 218 patients treated in a single institution. Bone Marrow Transplant 23:789–795
Hero B, Kremens B, Klingebiel T et al. (1997) Does megatherapy contribute to survival in metastatic neuroblastoma? A retrospective analysis. German Cooperative Neuroblastoma Study Group. Klin Padiatr 209:196–200
Huang Y, Tan M, Gosink M, Wang KK, Sun Y (2002) Histone deacetylase 5 is not a p53 target gene, but its overexpression inhibits tumor cell growth and induces apoptosis. Cancer Res 62:2913–2922
Ikeda H, August CS, Goldwein JW, Ross AJ, D'Angio GJ, Evans AE (1992) Sites of relapse in patients with neuroblastoma following bone marrow transplantation in relation to preparatory "debulking" treatments. J Pediatr Surg 27:1438–1441
Kamani N, August CS, Bunin N et al. (1996) A study of thiotepa, etoposide and fractionated total body irradiation as a preparative regimen prior to bone marrow transplantation for poor prognosis patients with neuroblastoma. Bone Marrow Transplant 17:911–916
Kaneko M, Tsuchida Y, Uchino J et al. (1999) Treatment results of advanced neuroblastoma with the first Japanese study group protocol. Study Group of Japan for Treatment of Advanced Neuroblastoma (see comments). J Pediatr Hematol Oncol 21:190–197
Kemshead JT, Heath L, Gibson FM et al. (1986) Magnetic microspheres and monoclonal antibodies for the depletion of neuroblastoma cells from bone marrow: experiences, improvements and observations. Br J Cancer 54:771–778
Keshelava N, Seeger RC, Groshen S, Reynolds CP (1998) Drug resistance patterns in human neuroblastoma cell lines derived from patients at different phases of therapy. Cancer Res 58:5396–5405
Kletzel M, Abella EM, Sandler ES et al. (1998) Thiotepa and cyclophosphamide with stem cell rescue for consolidation therapy for children with high-risk neuroblastoma: a phase I/II study of the Pediatric Blood and Marrow Transplant Consortium. J Pediatr Hematol Oncol 20:49–54
Kletzel M, Katzenstein HM, Haut PR et al. (2002) Treatment of high-risk neuroblastoma with triple-tandem high-dose therapy and stem cell rescue: results of the Chicago Pilot II Study. J Clin Oncol 20:2284–2292
Kohler JA, Imeson J, Ellershaw C, Lie SO (2000) A randomized trial of 13-Cis retinoic acid in children with advanced neuroblastoma after high-dose therapy. Br J Cancer 83:1124–1127
Kreissman S, Seeger R, Sender L et al. (2000) Peripheral blood stem cell (PBSC) support for multiple cycles of dose intensive chemotherapy for stage IV neuroblastoma (NB) is feasible with little risk of tumor contamination: a Children's Cancer Group report. Proc Am Soc Clin Oncol
Kremens B, Klingebiel T, Herrmann F et al. (1994) High-dose consolidation with local radiation and bone marrow rescue in patients with advanced neuroblastoma. Med Pediatr Oncol 23:470–475
Kretschmar CS, Kletzel K, Murray K, Smith EI, Marcus R, Castleberry R (1995) Phase II therapy with taxol and topotecan in untreated children (>365 days) with disseminated (INSS stage 4) neuroblastoma (NB). A POG study. Med Pediatr Oncol 24:243
Kushner BH, O'Reilly RJ, Mandell LR, Gulati SC, La Quaglia MP, Cheung NK (1991) Myeloablative combination chemotherapy without total body irradiation for neuroblastoma. J Clin Oncol 9:274–279
Kushner BH, Yeh SD, Kramer K, Larson SM, Cheung NK (2003) Impact of metaiodobenzylguanidine scintigraphy on assessing response of high-risk neuroblastoma to dose-intensive induction chemotherapy. J Clin Oncol 21:1082–1086
La Quaglia MP, Kushner BH, Heller G, Bonilla MA, Lindsley KL, Cheung NK (1994) Stage 4 neuroblastoma diagnosed at more than 1 year of age: gross total resection and clinical outcome. J Pediatr Surg 29:1162–1166
Ladenstein R, Lasset C, Hartmann O et al. (1994) Comparison of auto versus allografting as consolidation of primary treatments in advanced neuroblastoma over one year of age at diagnosis: report from the European Group for Bone Marrow Transplantation. Bone Marrow Transplant 14:37–46
Ladenstein R, Philip T, Lasset C et al. (1998) Multivariate analysis of risk factors in stage 4 neuroblastoma patients over the age of one year treated with megatherapy and stem cell transplantation: a report from the European Bone Marrow Transplantation Solid Tumor Registry. J Clin Oncol 16:953–965
Le Deley MC, Leblanc T, Shamsaldin A et al. (2003) Risk of secondary leukemia after a solid tumor in childhood according to the dose of epipodophyllotoxins and anthracyclines: a case-control study by the Societe Francaise d'Oncologie Pediatrique. J Clin Oncol 21:1074–1081
Lode HN, Xiang R, Varki NM, Dolman CS, Gillies SD, Reisfeld RA (1997) Targeted interleukin-2 therapy for spontaneous neuroblastoma metastases to bone marrow. J Natl Cancer Inst 89:1586–1594

Mastrangelo S, Tornesello A, Diociaiuti L et al. (2001) Treatment of advanced neuroblastoma: feasibility and therapeutic potential of a novel approach combining 131-I-MIBG and multiple drug chemotherapy. Br J Cancer 84:460–464
Matsumura M, Atkinson JB, Hays DM et al. (1988) An evaluation of the role of surgery in metastatic neuroblastoma. J Pediatr Surg 23:448–453
Matthay KK (1997) Neuroblastoma: biology and therapy. Oncology 11:1857–1866; discussion 1869–1872, 1875
Matthay KK, Yamashiro D (2000) Neuroblastoma. In: Bast RC, Kufe DW, Pollock RE, Weichselbaum RR, Holland JF, Frei E (eds) Cancer medicine. Decker, London, pp 2185–2197
Matthay KK, Atkinson JB, Stram DO, Selch M, Reynolds CP, Seeger RC (1993) Patterns of relapse after autologous purged bone marrow transplantation for neuroblastoma: a Childrens Cancer Group pilot study. J Clin Oncol 11:2226–2233
Matthay KK, Seeger RC, Reynolds CP et al. (1994) Allogeneic versus autologous purged bone marrow transplantation for neuroblastoma: a report from the Childrens Cancer Group. J Clin Oncol 12:2382–2389
Matthay KK, Villablanca JG, Seeger RC et al. (1999) Treatment of high-risk neuroblastoma with intensive chemotherapy, radiotherapy, autologous bone marrow transplantation, and 13-cis-retinoic acid. Children's Cancer Group. N Engl J Med 341:1165–1173
Matthay KK, Edeline V, Lumbroso J et al. (2003) Correlation of early metastatic response by 123I-metaiodobenzylguanidine scintigraphy with overall response and event-free survival in stage IV neuroblastoma. J Clin Oncol 21:2486–2491
Maurer BJ, Metelitsa LS, Seeger RC, Cabot MC, Reynolds CP (1999) Fenretinide (4-HPR) induces ceramide in neuroblastoma and 4-HPR cytotoxicity is increased by modulators of ceramide metabolism. Med Pediatr Oncol 33:227
Melino G, Thiele CJ, Knight RA, Piacentini M (1997) Retinoids and the control of growth/death decisions in human neuroblastoma cell lines. J Neurooncol 31:65–83
Ohnuma N, Takahashi H, Kaneko M et al. (1995) Treatment combined with bone marrow transplantation for advanced neuroblastoma: an analysis of patients who were pretreated intensively with the protocol of the Study Group of Japan. Med Pediatr Oncol 24:181–187
Ozkaynak MF, Sondel PM, Krailo MD et al. (2000) Phase I study of chimeric human/murine anti-ganglioside G(D2) monoclonal antibody (ch14.18) with granulocyte-macrophage colony-stimulating factor in children with neuroblastoma immediately after hematopoietic stem cell transplantation: a Children's Cancer Group Study. J Clin Oncol 18:4077–4085
Philip T, Bernard JL, Zucker JM et al. (1987) High-dose chemoradiotherapy with bone marrow transplantation as consolidation treatment in neuroblastoma: an unselected group of stage IV patients over 1 year of age. J Clin Oncol 5:266–271
Philip T, Zucker JM, Bernard JL et al. (1991) Improved survival at 2 and 5 years in the LMCE1 unselected group of 72 children with stage IV neuroblastoma older than 1 year of age at diagnosis: is cure possible in a small subgroup? J Clin Oncol 9:1037–1044
Philip T, Ladenstein R, Zucker JM et al. (1993) Double megatherapy and autologous bone marrow transplantation for advanced neuroblastoma: the LMCE2 study. Br J Cancer 67:119–127
Pinkerton CR (1991) ENSG 1-randomised study of high-dose melphalan in neuroblastoma. Bone Marrow Transplant 7 (Suppl 3):112–113
Pinkerton CR, Blanc Vincent MP, Bergeron C, Fervers B, Philip T (2000) Induction chemotherapy in metastatic neuroblastoma: Does dose influence response? A critical review of published data standards, options and recommendations (SOR) project of the National Federation of French Cancer Centres (FNCLCC). Eur J Cancer 36:1808–1815
Pole JG, Casper J, Elfenbein G et al. (1991) High-dose chemoradiotherapy supported by marrow infusions for advanced neuroblastoma: a Pediatric Oncology Group study (published erratum appears in J Clin Oncol 1991, 9:1094). J Clin Oncol 9:152–158
Reynolds CP, Seeger RC, Vo DD, Black AT, Wells J, Ugelstad J (1986) Model system for removing neuroblastoma cells from bone marrow using monoclonal antibodies and magnetic immunobeads. Cancer Res 46:5882–5886
Reynolds CP, Kane DJ, Einhorn PA et al. (1991) Response of neuroblastoma to retinoic acid in vitro and in vivo. Prog Clin Biol Res 366:203–211
Reynolds CP, Villablanca JG, Gerbing RB, Stram DO, Seeger RC, Matthay KK (2002) 13-cis-retinoic acid improves overall survival following myeloablative therapy for high-risk neuroblastoma: a randomized Children's Cancer Group (CCG) study. ASCO Annual Meeting, abstract #1564
Schmidt ML, Lal A, Seeger RC et al. (2003) Favorable prognosis for patients ages 12–18 months with stage 4 MYCN-non-amplified neuroblastoma: a Children's Cancer Group Study. Proc Am Soc Clin Oncol 22:800
Seeger RC, Reynolds CP, Gallego R, Stram DO, Gerbing RB, Matthay KK (2000) Quantitative tumor cell content of bone marrow and blood as a predictor of outcome in stage IV neuroblastoma: a Children's Cancer Group Study. J Clin Oncol 18:4067–4076
Seeger RC, Villablanca JG, Matthay KK et al. (1991) Intensive chemoradiotherapy and autologous bone marrow transplantation for poor prognosis neuroblastoma. Prog Clin Biol Res 366:527–533
Seeger RC, Reynolds CP (1991) Treatment of high-risk solid tumors of childhood with intensive therapy and autologous bone marrow transplantation. Pediatr Clin North Am 38:393–424
Shorter NA, Davidoff AM, Evans AE, Ross A Jr, Zeigler MM, O'Neill JA Jr (1995) The role of surgery in the management of stage IV neuroblastoma: a single institution study. Med Pediatr Oncol 24:287–291

Shuster JJ, Cantor AB, McWilliams N et al. (1991) The prognostic significance of autologous bone marrow transplant in advanced neuroblastoma (see comments). J Clin Oncol 9:1045–1049
Smith BD, Levis M, Beran M et al. (2004) Single agent CEP-701, a novel FLT3 inhibitor, shows biologic and clinical activity in patients with relapsed or refractory acute myeloid leukemia. Blood 63:5559–5563
Stern JW, Fang J, Shusterman S et al. (2001) Angiogenesis inhibitor TNP-470 during bone marrow transplant: safety in a preclinical model. Clin Cancer Res 7:1026–1032
Stram DO, Matthay KK, O'Leary M et al. (1996) Consolidation chemoradiotherapy and autologous bone marrow transplantation versus continued chemotherapy for metastatic neuroblastoma: a report of two concurrent Children's Cancer Group studies (see comments). J Clin Oncol 14:2417–2426
Tweddle DA, Pinkerton CR, Lewis IJ, Ellershaw C, Cole M, Pearson AD (2001) OPEC/OJEC for stage 4 neuroblastoma in children over 1 year of age. Med Pediatr Oncol 36:239–242
Villablanca JG, Khan AA, Avramis VI et al. (1995) Phase I trial of 13-cis-retinoic acid in children with neuroblastoma following bone marrow transplantation. J Clin Oncol 13:894–901
Villablanca JG, Reynolds CP, Swift PS et al. (1998) Phase I trial of carboplatin, etoposide, melphalan and local irradiation (CEM-LI) with purged autologous marrow transplantation for children with high risk neuroblastoma. Proc Am Soc Clin Oncol 17:533a
Villablanca JG, Matthay KK, Swift PS et al. (1999) Phase I trial of carboplatin, etoposide, melphalan and local irradiation (CEM-LI) with purged autologous bone marrow transplantation for children with high risk neuroblastoma. Med Pediatr Oncol 33:170
Wheatley JM, Rosenfield NS, Heller G, Feldstein D, La Quaglia MP (1995) Validation of a technique of computer-aided tumor volume determination. J Surg Res 59:621–626
Wolden SL, Gollamudi SV, Kushner BH et al. (2000) Local control with multimodality therapy for stage 4 neuroblastoma. Int J Radiat Oncol Biol Phys 46:969–974
Yu AL, Uttenreuther-Fischer MM, Huang CS et al. (1998) Phase I trial of a human-mouse chimeric anti-disialoganglioside monoclonal antibody ch14.18 in patients with refractory neuroblastoma and osteosarcoma. J Clin Oncol 16:2169–2180

11.4 The Role of Surgery in the Treatment of Neuroblastoma

Michael P. La Quaglia

11.4.1 Introduction

The surgeon has a crucial role in the management of neuroblastoma. Initial diagnosis and assessment of *MYCN* amplification, histopathology, DNA index (ploidy), and other parameters are dependent on close collaboration between the surgical oncologist, pediatric oncologist, and pathologist. In particular, the surgeon must obtain an adequate tumor sample for both histopathology and molecular studies. During surgical resection of the primary tumor, efforts should be made to preserve normal organs, such as the kidney. Furthermore, the surgeon must evaluate the status of both ipsilateral and contralateral lymph nodes and accurately describe the extent of primary tumor resection to ensure accurate assignment of stage and risk status. Finally, supportive procedures, including institution of reliable vascular access and management of treatment-related complications like typhlitis, bowel obstructions, and others are important in the surgical management of neuroblastoma patients. This chapter describes the role of surgical intervention in the management of this heterogeneous and challenging tumor.

11.4.2 History

In 1953 Robert E. Gross noted for neuroblastoma in infancy and childhood that "extensive and radical surgery has a definite place under certain circumstances and can lead to permanent cure" (Gross 1953). In 1955 C. Everett Koop described the positive effect of tumor de-bulking on outcome in a book he authored entitled, "Neuroblastoma in Childhood. Survival after Major Surgical Insult to the Tumor" (Koop et al. 1955). These were among the first publications in which a role for surgical resection in neuroblastoma was reported. In 1968 Koop analyzed the impact of surgical interventions depending on whether the tumor was resectable, non-resectable, or

Table 11.4.1 High-risk neuroblastoma: review of the surgical literature

Positive effect of primary site resection Reference	 Number/stages	Little or no effect of surgical resection Reference	 Number/stages
Koop and Schnaufer (1975)	X/1–4	Kiely (1993)	80/3,4
Rosen et al. (1984)	136/1–4	Losty et al. (1993)	57/1–4
Le Tourneau et al. (1985)	130/1–4	Shorter et al. (1995)	79/1–4
Carlsen et al. (1986)	253/1–4	Kaneko et al. (1997)	14/4
Moss et al. (1987)	21/4	Kaneko et al. (1998)	36/1–4, 4s
Matsumara et al. (1988)	320/4	Castel et al. (2002)	98/4
Haase et al. (1989)	58/3	Von Schweinitz et al. (2002) (surgery effective only in MYCN amplified disease)	878/4
Hata et al. (1990)	76/1–4	Olgun et al. (2003)	1–4, 4 s
Nakadate et al. (1990)	25/4		
Haase et al. (1991)	118/2–4		
Shamberger et al. (1991)	60/3, 4		
Philip et al. (1991)	62/4		
Tsuchida et al. (1992)	121/3, 4		
Berthold et al. (1992)	308/4		
La Quaglia et al. (1992)	70; 4		
Chamberlain et al. (1995)	24/4		
De Cou et al. (1995)	99/4		
Strother et al. (1995)	88/4		
Yokoyama et al. (1995)	8/4		
Mugishima et al. (1995)	36/4		
Powis et al. (1996)	202/3		
Matthay et al. (1998)			
Kaneko et al. (1999)	157/3, 4		
Kawa et al. (1999)	66/3, 4, 4s (all *MYCN* amplified		
Wolden et al. (2000)	47/4		
Castel et al. (2002)	72/3, 4		
Tsuchida et al. (2002)	66/3, 4, 4s		
Kuroda et al. (2003)	33/3, 4		
La Quaglia et al. (2004)			
Adkins et al. (2004)			

metastatic (Koop 1968a), essentially an early attempt to define risk status. During the 1960s workers in both Japan and Europe also described their experience with neuroblastoma resection (Kasai and Watanabe 1968; Menjyo 1968; Schenga 1969; Zittel and Wuttke 1969). With the introduction of adjuvant chemotherapy in 1965 (James et al. 1965), plus major advances in pediatric imaging, surgery, anesthesia, blood banking, and critical care (Harrison et al. 1974; Hollmann and Lampert 1975; Stephen 1977; Tsunooka 1972), and the establishment of the pediatric oncology cooperative groups in the 1970s, multi-institution data became available and the number of surgical reports on neuroblastoma has steadily increased. Retrospective studies from the Children's Cancer Study Group (CCSG) on the role of surgery in disseminated neuroblastoma and localized neuroblastomas were published in 1983 and 1985, respectively (O'Neill et al. 1985; Sitarz et al. 1983). In 1988 investigators from the Pediatric Oncology Group (POG) published a prospective study (Nitschke et al. 1988) showing that certain localized neuroblastomas could be effectively treated with surgery alone despite regional nodal involvement. Furthermore, the authors noted that overall survival was excellent, even in patients who developed relapses; however, comparisons between cooperative group experiences were hampered by lack of a uniform staging system. This was remedied by the establishment of the International Neuroblastoma Staging System (INSS) in 1988 and its revision in 1993 (Brodeur et al. 1988, 1993).

During the 1980s and early 1990s controversy arose as to the efficacy of primary tumor resection in patients with advanced-stage disease. Table 11.4.1 compares surgical reports supporting surgical resection of the primary tumor in high-risk neuroblastoma with those that do not. Despite doubts as to the feasibility, safety, and efficacy of surgical resection in high-risk neuroblastoma, the present consensus in the Children's Oncology Group (COG), and European and Japanese cooperative groups is that an aggressive resection of loco-regional disease should be attempted. Surgery has an even more important role in low- and intermediate-risk disease.

11.4.3 Staging

Staging systems for pediatric solid tumors have traditionally placed great weight on surgical removal of the primary tumor and regional nodal involvement (Evans et al. 1976a) The present INSS was devised as a synthesis of the previous systems (Kiely 1993; Evans et al. 1990). This staging system has been adopted by the Children's Oncology Group USA (COG), as well as cooperative groups in Europe and Japan. It is worthwhile to review each staging system to illustrate the impact of surgery on stage and consequently risk status and treatment.

11.4.3.1 Stage 1

The classification of a stage-1 tumor is dependent not only on primary tumor resection, but also on microscopic evaluation of regional nodes. It is imperative that the surgeon seek and biopsy lymph nodes in the main draining lymphatic echelons at the time of primary tumor removal. For adrenal primaries the ipsilateral peri-caval nodes on the right, or peri-aortic nodes on the left, should be sampled. The surgeon should also evaluate interaortocaval lymph nodes located in the space between the abdominal aorta and inferior vena cava, as well as those located either supra-renally or infra-renally, or both. In assessing these nodes, the surgeon should separate the aorta and vena cava and visualize the spine posteriorly. Finally, an assessment of contralateral lymph nodes and those at the base of the mesentery should be performed. For a right-sided adrenal primary, examination and biopsy of the contralateral peri-aortic nodes should be done. Conversely, contralateral peri-caval lymph nodes should be sampled for left-sided primaries. If these nodes cannot be identified, the surgeon must comment on this in the operative note documenting that they were actively sought.

For thoracic primaries, peri-aortic nodes on the left and peri-azygous nodes on the right should be assessed, and any abnormal nodes running along the intercostals vessels should be excised. It is helpful to biopsy normal-appearing nodes in these regions when feasible. In the case of pelvic primaries the lymph nodes running along the iliac vessels should

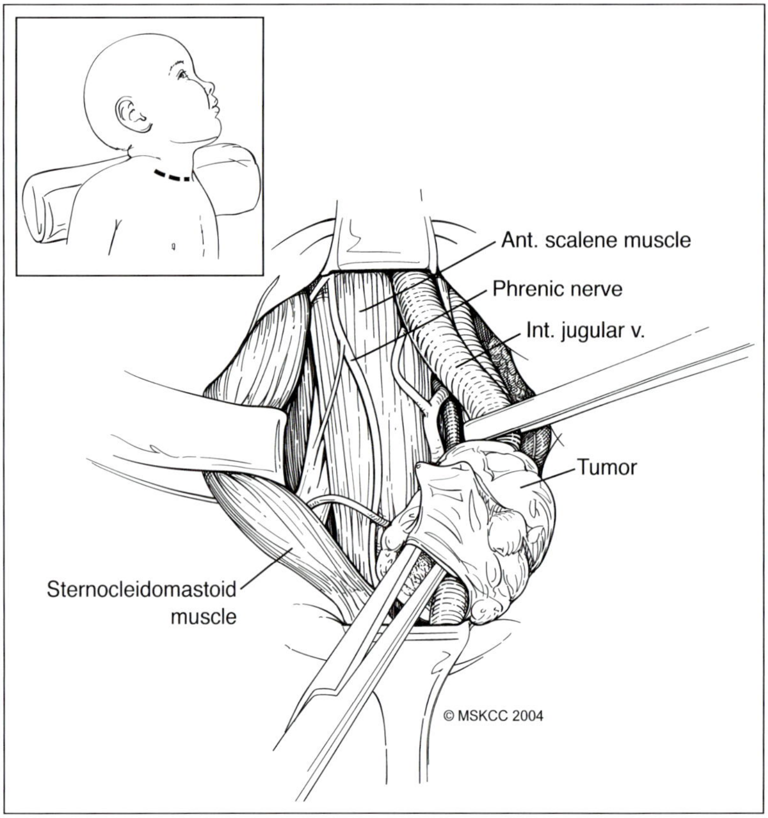

Figure 11.4.1

Resection of a cervical neuroblastoma. A transverse neck incision followed by dissection of the carotid sheath contents was done. Division of the tumor over blood vessels is a characteristic of neuroblastoma surgery

be sampled as well as those in the lower peri-aortic and peri-caval regions. The level II–IV jugulo-digastric lymph nodes are sampled with cervical primaries(Figs. 11.4.1–11.4.3).

11.4.3.2 Stage 2

The criteria for stage 2 focus on the extent of primary tumor resection and on the microscopic assessment of ipsilateral lymph nodes. The contralateral region is explored and identifiable lymph nodes are sampled. If thorough review of pre-operative imaging and intraoperative exploration fails to identify contralateral lymph nodes, then this should be documented in the operative note.

11.4.3.3 Stage 3

Stage-3 disease crosses the midline and is usually associated with encasement of the great vessels. In the abdomen, the aorta and/or vena cava, as well as the celiac axis, superior mesenteric artery, and renal arteries, may be involved. In the mediastinum encasement of the thoracic aorta or azygous vein can occur. Vascular encasement prevents or complicates gross total resection; however, on occasion, tumors that appear to be stage 3 by imaging studies obtained pre-operatively can at times be completely resected (gross total resection), thus down-staging the patient to stage 1, thereby improving prognosis and eliminating the need for further therapy. The ability for tumor surgery to change risk classification, should not be underestimated. Haase et al. (1989) reported an improved survival in Evans stage-III

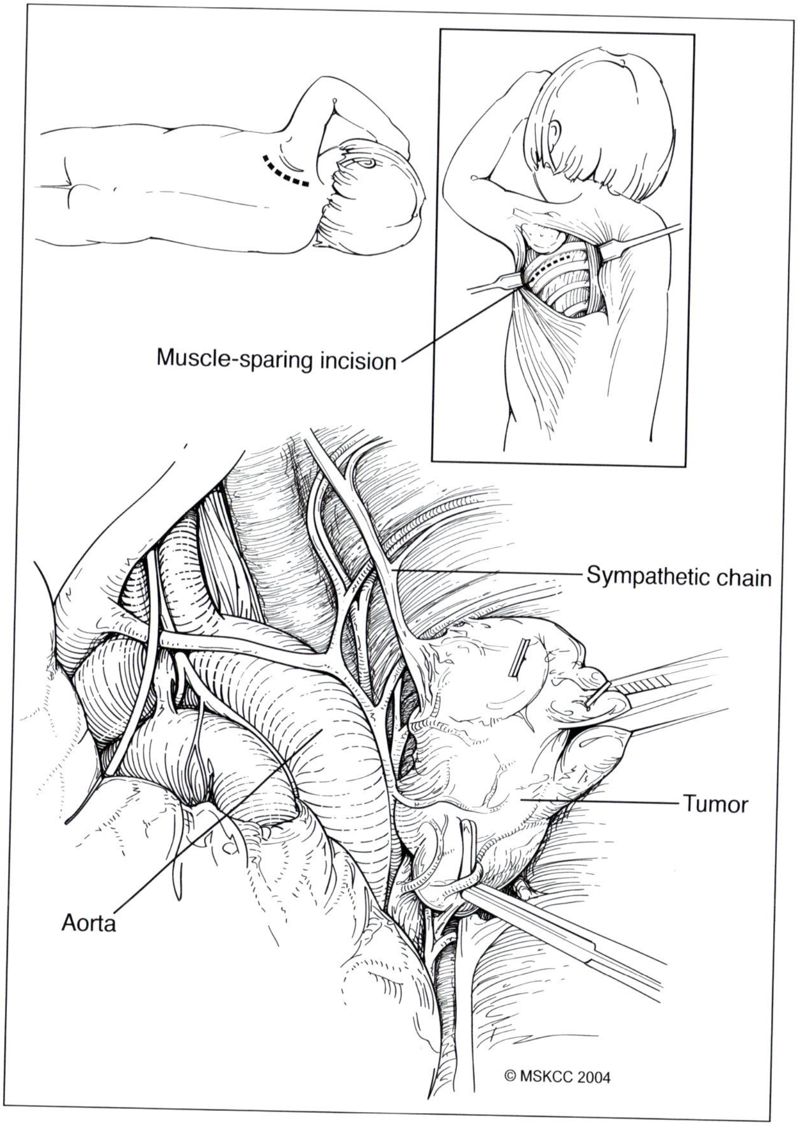

Figure 11.4.2

The approach for posterior mediastinal tumors. A muscle-sparing technique can be used for small lesions. Infiltration through spinal foramina may require foraminotomy.

patients who underwent gross total resection. A similar finding was noted by Matthay et al. (1998).

11.4.3.4 Stage 4

In the past, the role of surgery in stage-4 disease was limited. Presently, besides playing a key role in establishing the diagnosis, the surgical oncologist can ensure the procurement of adequate tissue for assessing relevant biologic parameters, even in cases where the diagnosis can be made solely based on urinary catecholamines plus bone marrow studies. It is recommended that at least 1 cm^3 of viable tumor tissue be obtained at initial biopsy, although this volume requirement is likely to be substantially reduced with future refinements in various molecular techniques. Foremost among biological parameters is determination of the *MYCN* proto-oncogene copy number. Tu-

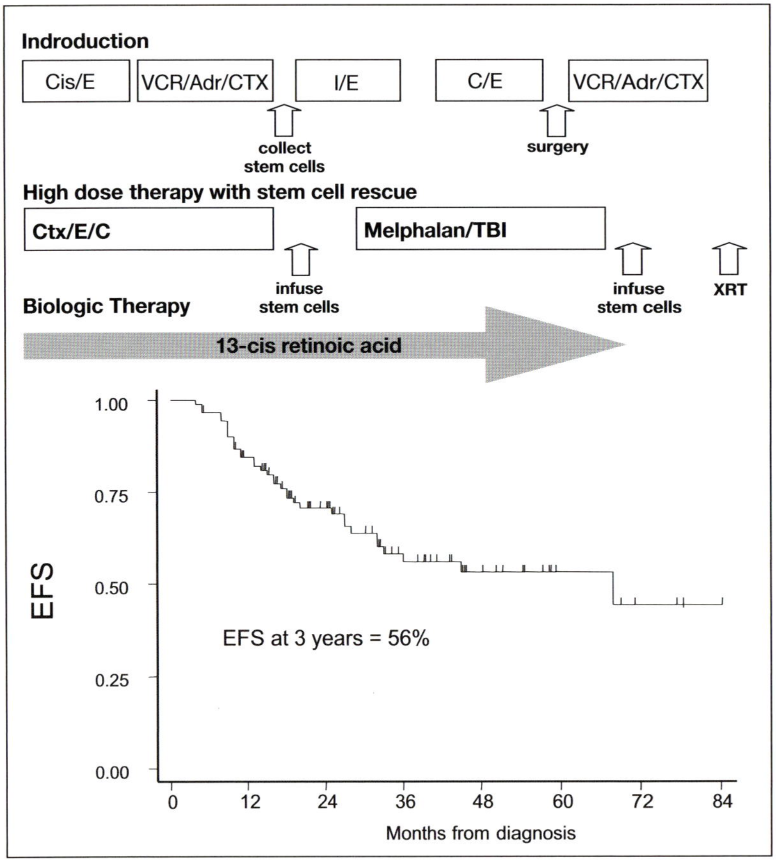

Figure 11.6.1

Top panel. Schema of the CHOP/DFCI tandem transplant study. Bottom panel. Event-free survival (*EFS*) from diagnosis. *C* carboplatin, *E* etoposide, *Cis* cisplatin, *I* ifosfamide, *VCR* vincristine, *Adr* adriamycin, *CTX* cyclophosphamide, *TBI* total body irradiation

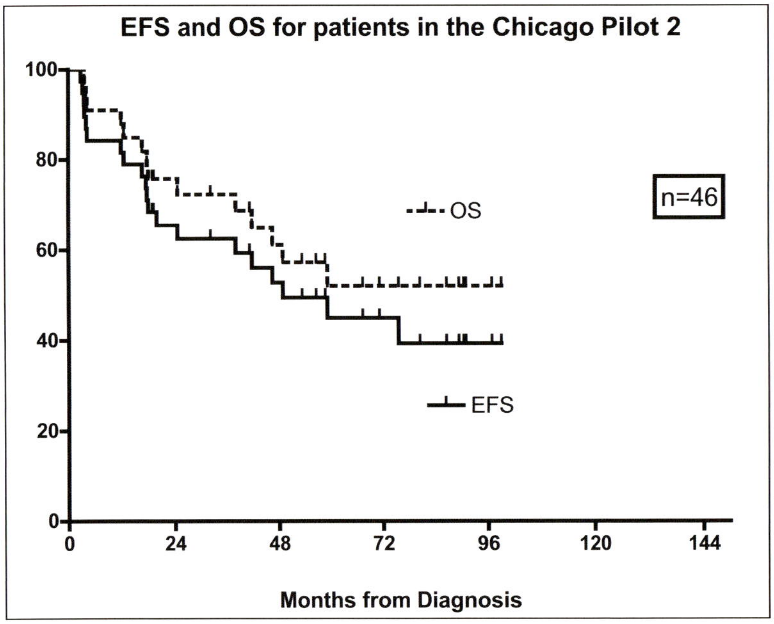

Figure 11.6.2

Event-free survival (*EFS*) from diagnosis on the Chicago "triple tandem" transplant study. *OS* overall survival

Two other experimental approaches to transplantation are worthy of mention. Combining therapeutic doses of [^{131}I-m]IBG with high-dose chemotherapy showed preliminary evidence of efficacy in high-risk patients (Klingebiel et al. 1998; Yanik et al. 2002). Another experimental approach to NB transplant is the use of allogeneic transplant. A graft-vs-tumor effect, thought to accompany the graft-vs-host response, has been demonstrated in leukemias, especially chronic myelogenous leukemia. This effect has not convincingly been demonstrated in the setting of solid tumors (Srinivasan et al. 2004). Retrospective analyses of conventional allogeneic BMT for NB have failed to show any benefit over standard therapy (Matthay et al. 1994; Philip et al. 1997). With the advent of nonmyeloablative transplant regimens, the interest in allogeneic transplant in NB has been revived, with the hope that reduced intensity will reduce TRM in order to detect a therapeutic benefit. At this point, there are no data to justify this approach in children undergoing their primary treatment for high-risk NB.

11.6.3 PBSC Collection

There are a variety of techniques to mobilize more stem and progenitor cells circulating in the peripheral blood. Apheresis separates specific blood components from a patient continuously by centrifugation. Any component can be targeted for relatively specific removal – plasma, red cells, platelets, or white cells. After venous blood is collected and processed through the apheresis device, the nontargeted components are returned to the patient.

11.6.3.1 Vascular Access

To allow continuous blood processing for PBSC collection two ports of vascular access are necessary. In adults this requires two antecubital lines. In 5–10% of adults and most children, percutaneous antecubital large-bore access is not possible and a pheresis catheter is used instead. A veno-arterial approach, utilizing an arterial line to draw blood and a conventional venous catheter to return it to the patient, has also been described (Takaue et al. 1995). Although there are many configurations, a pheresis catheter is generally a two-lumen catheter with offset proximal and distal ports and side holes along the tip of the catheter. This offset configuration minimizes mixing of processed and unprocessed blood and maximizes the efficiency of the collection. Since apheresis machines can draw 70 cc per min, conventional Broviac-type catheters can be difficult for patients <35 kg, because the lumen collapses under the negative pressure used to draw blood at 2 ml/kg min^{-1}. A pheresis catheter is designed to allow faster draw rates using a combination of larger lumen size, shorter catheter length, and stiffer walls.

Pheresis catheters are available both for temporary and tunneled insertion. Small patients (approx. 10–30 kg) may require an 8 F cuffed tunneled pheresis catheter (MedComp). Smaller patients may require femoral line placement. The concern in smaller patients is threefold: (a) the risk of partial or complete vessel occlusion with the catheter; (b) the risk of vessel erosion and perforation, which may be greater with stiffer catheters in small vessels (Welch et al. 1997); and (c) the difficulty in placing an offset catheter in a short vessel where, if the proximal port is in adequate position, the distal port may be too far advanced. Femoral catheters are short, allowing faster collect rates for a given diameter; however, a patient with a percutaneous nontunneled femoral catheter cannot walk, necessitating admission to the hospital for what is otherwise an outpatient procedure. Also, the perceived risk of complication (especially infection) with a femoral catheter is higher (Merrer et al. 2001). For both of these reasons, femoral catheters are generally only placed temporarily, except in unusual circumstances (Chow et al. 2001). Another approach used at some institutions is to place a single lumen 7F Broviac-type central venous catheter on the opposite side of the patient's existing double lumen catheter. The single lumen line is then used as the draw line and the smaller double lumen catheter is used as the return line.

11.6.3.2 Collection

Even in a mobilized patient, the number of stem cells circulating in the entire blood volume may be inadequate to provide engraftment; thus, processing of multiple blood volumes, often over more than 1 day, is required for some patients (Rowley et al. 2001). This is typical for patients who have been extensively pre-treated with chemotherapy. The minimum required for most patients is one large-volume leukapheresis (LVL), which represents approximately 20 l in an adult or three to four blood volumes in a child. This volume is a typical goal for a single apheresis session, although some physicians will pherese for a total of six or more blood volumes.

There are two issues in PBSC collection that require special consideration in children. First is the issue of priming. Even using devices that minimize extracorporeal volume, smaller children require priming of the apheresis machine with red cells. This prevents unacceptable dilutional anemia. Second is the issue of anticoagulation. In older patients, anticoagulation required for the apheresis procedure is accomplished using ACD. Although rapidly reversible, ACD creates a higher risk of symptomatic hypocalcemia in young patients. These patients are managed with a combination of ACD and heparin to achieve anticoagulation, or receive a calcium infusion in the apheresis return line.

11.6.3.3 Techniques for Stem Cell Mobilization

Large increases in the number of circulating stem and progenitor cells occur during recovery from myelosuppressive chemotherapy, typically when the absolute neutrophil count (ANC) has reached 1000/µl and rapidly rising. The exact point of maximal stem cell mobilization is difficult to predict and highly patient dependent (see 11.6.3.4). Commonly, cyclophosphamide (a total dose of 4 g/m^2 over 2 days) has been used. Multiple-drug regimens as part of the primary treatment can also be used to induce a nadir after which PBSC collection is possible. Because of the concern that the DNA damage may occur in hematopoietic stem cells, and hence increased risk of secondary (treatment-related) leukemia, topoisomerase inhibitors (e.g., etoposide) are often not used to induce the nadir. In one study, use of PBSC collected after etoposide resulted in a 7- to 12-fold relative risk of secondary leukemia (Krishnan et al. 2000), with other studies also demonstrating an increased risk attributable more to the prior chemotherapy than to the preparative regimen used for the stem cell transplant (Kollmannsberger et al. 1998). This effect, together with the observation that multiple cycles of chemotherapy reduce yields of PBSC collection (Jerjis et al. 2000), argue that PBSC should be collected as early in treatment as possible, but after sufficient therapy (usually two to three cycles of chemotherapy) to clear circulating tumor (Faulkner et al. 2000; Moss et al. 1990).

The use of chemotherapy to mobilize PBSC may not be possible or desirable in every patient, has a risk of toxicity during the nadir, and is clearly not appropriate for normal allogeneic donors in whom the chemotherapy has no potential benefit. An alternative approach of using hematopoietic growth factors (HGF) is in widespread use. Donors are placed on a daily regimen of HGF injections, followed by initiation of PBSC collection on day 4–5 of treatment. The HGF treatment continues until the apheresis is complete. There are several choices of HGF doses and regimens (Table 11.6.3). Filgrastim (rhuG-CSF) is the most common HGF used for this purpose. Doses given vary widely. There is a modest dose-response effect between 2 and 16 µg/kg of G-CSF. Although doses as high as 24 µg/kg day^{-1} have been used for mobilization, there is little evidence that these very high doses are more efficacious and they have the disadvantage of greater cost and higher incidence of side effects, especially bone pain.

Sargramostim (rhuGM-CSF) is an alternative. Comparisons of G-CSF and GM-CSF as single agents reveal either no significant advantage of one HGF over the other in terms of PBSC collection efficiency or extent of progenitor cell mobilization (Gazitt 2002), or a modest advantage for G-CSF (Weaver et al. 2001). Laboratory studies have suggested that PBSC collected after G-CSF mobilization may have a polarization in T-cell response toward the more suppressive T-helper lymphocyte type 2 (Th2) response (Sloand et al. 2000). This may have a theoretical

Table 11.6.3 Regimens for PBSC mobilization

Cyclophosphamide 2000 mg/m^2 day^{-1} over 2 days, followed by G-CSF 5 µg/kg day^{-1} SQ from day 3 to the end of pheresis
G-CSF 5 µg/kg day^{-1} SQ for 3–4 days, followed by pheresis on days 4–5 and subsequently
GM-CSF 250 µg/m^2 day^{-1} SQ for 3–4 days, followed by pheresis on days 4–5 and subsequently
Combination of G-CSF 5–10 µg/kg day^{-1} (SQ in AM) and GM-CSF 250 µg/m^2 day^{-1} (SQ in PM) for 4 days, pheresis starting on day 5
Other chemotherapy/HGF combinations

advantage for (a) recovery of cellular immunity after SCT, and (b) the risk of graft-vs-host disease after allogeneic SCT. The combination of G-CSF and GM-CSF may be superior to either alone, although one pediatric study failed to show an advantage for the combination.

The one setting in which the combination of G-CSF plus GM-CSF may be superior is when a patient has had inadequate numbers of stem cells collected over several aphereses. In these so-called poor mobilizers, combination HGF regimens may improve the likelihood that adequate PBSC can be collected (Stiff 1999). Other HGF have been tested as PBSC mobilizers, including stem cell factor and thrombopoietin, but there is no evidence to suggest superiority in terms of clinical outcome during transplant over the standard use of G-CSF, even when higher numbers of CD34+ cells are collected. On the other hand, collection of higher numbers of CD34+ cells has the potential to reduce the number of LVL a donor must undergo, which is a benefit in terms of cost, convenience, and potential donor exposure, especially in children. Balanced against this is the high cost of HGF, and the fact that adding a second HGF doubles this cost. In patients who are receiving myelosuppressive chemotherapy, HGF such as filgrastim are often used to improve recovery. The concurrent use of chemotherapy and an HGF improve PBSC mobilization as well (Knudsen et al. 1996; Levine and Boxer 2002), although a randomized trial did not show this improved mobilization to have an impact on survival or engraftment (Narayanasami et al. 2001). Thus, any patient receiving chemotherapy after which PBSC collection is planned should be placed on an HGF, even if similar courses during the treatment are not supported by an HGF.

11.6.3.4 Target Dose for PBSC Infusion

When bone marrow is collected, most operators target a final volume, or more commonly, a volume and a nucleated cell dose. Because of the high variability in stem and progenitor cell content in PBSC, a more direct assay is needed to assure that adequate numbers for reliable engraftment have been collected. There is no well-established assay for human stem cells, although stem cell activity is likely to be found in a portion of cells that are detected by the long-term culture initiating cell assay or the SCID mouse repopulating cell assay. Progenitor cell content can be assessed by the colony-forming unit granulocyte/monocyte (CFU-GM) assay. The presence of $2–10\times10^4$ CFU-GM/kg of recipient weight is predictive of engraftment, but the assay is laborious, expensive, and difficult to standardize. It also takes 14 days to complete, making it useless to assess PBSC collections in real time. For all these reasons, most centers have moved away from CFU-GM assays.

A major advance in the use of PBSC was the recognition that most (although not all) (Goodell et al. 1997) of the cells in the hematopoietic stem- and progenitor cell compartment bear the antigen CD34, regardless of lineage. Enumeration of CD34+ cells allows for more accurate assessment of engraftment potential provided by a given number of mononuclear cells. There is a threshold for reliable engraftment and a rough correlation between number of CD34+ cells above this threshold and engraftment (Table 11.6.4). The threshold for reliable engraftment is generally thought to be 1×10^6 CD34+ cells/kg (Shpall et al. 1998). Below this threshold, the likelihood of delayed engraftment of neutrophils and especially platelets increases (Weaver et al. 1997). Increasing the minimum acceptable number to $2–2.5\times10^6$ CD34+ cells/kg decreases this likelihood somewhat further, and this is the threshold that most transplant centers attempt to achieve. Some authors

Table 11.6.4 Choosing doses of PBSC for stem-cell transplantation

Dose level	CD34+ cells/kg of recipient weight	Notes
Minimum	1×10^6	At this dose, there is a risk of prolonged neutropenia and extended platelet transfusion requirements
Optimum	$2–2.5 \times 10^6$	Threshold dose for many centers
Ideal	5×10^6	There is a limited dose-response effect at doses $>2.5 \times 10^6$ cells, and this target may increase number of phereses needed and cost

have advocated a goal (rather than a minimum) of 5 to up to 15×10^6 CD34+ cells/kg (Stiff 1999). This higher goal is unrealistic in a number of patients, especially patients who have been treated with multiple cycles of chemotherapy prior to collection, and has the potential to significantly increase the cost and length of apheresis.

CD34+ cells in the bone marrow can range from 1 to 4%, while CD34+ cells in mobilized pheresis products can range from 0.1% (in a poor mobilizer) to >1%. The assay for CD34+ cells is a flow cytometric assay (Sutherland et al. 1996; Trischmann et al. 1993), and this technique is inherently inaccurate at low percentages. This means that the number of CD34+ cells based on a measured frequency of 0.1% could easily be off by twofold in either the direction of more or fewer cells, and this must be borne in mind when assessing when to stop apheresis in patients with poor collections. In collections that have undergone CD34 selection (see 11.6.3.5), the CD34 purity is generally >60% and these determinations are extremely accurate. Another consideration is that low CD34 PBSC collections often may have a higher granulocyte content, which can complicate freezing/thawing and therefore have an impact on yield of cells actually infused after storage.

There are many different approaches to determining when a donor will be most successfully pheresed for the highest number of PBSC. The goals are to get adequate numbers of PSBC as defined above, preferably in a single collection procedure. When HGF regimens alone are used, timing is simple: the donor is pheresed on either the fourth or fifth day of HGF administration. After chemotherapy, the point at which the best collection can be obtained in more difficult to predict. Peripheral WBC count is a poor predictor of stem cell mobilization (Yu et al. 1999). There is some theoretical concern for donor safety and possible hyperleukocytosis at WBC counts of more than 70×10^9/l, and some advocate G-CSF dose reductions for donors whose WBC reaches this level. Many centers use some variation on the following algorithm: 1–3 days after the rising ANC reaches 1000, at a point where there is some evidence of platelet recovery, stem cell collection begins. Rather than using a rising neutrophil count to trigger apheresis, some centers with access to rapid-turnaround, quantitative (or "absolute") CD34+ cell counts use the rise in peripheral CD34+ cells to time initiation of collection. Detection of <5 CD34+ cells/µl of blood is highly predictive of poor PBSC collection, whereas >10–20 CD34+ cells/µl correlates well with the likelihood of collecting $>2.5\times10^6$ CD34 cell/kg in a single LVL procedure (Yu et al. 1999).

11.6.3.5 Processing and Storage of PBSC

Most PBSC products collected to support transplant procedures are autologous and must be cryopreserved for later use. In the allogeneic setting, products can be collected prior to starting pretransplant conditioning in the recipient or they can be collected on the day of intended infusion. In addition to cryopreservation, other processing options exist, depending on the purpose for which the PBSC will be used. Specific engineering of the graft is possible to remove or expand desired cell populations

After collection, the PBSC product is taken to the stem cell processing lab. This is where procedures to ensure quality of the product take place, including determination of CD34+ cell content (see 11.6.3.4), viability determinations, mononuclear cell counts, and confirmation of sterility. Stem cell practice has attracted more regulatory attention recently. The Foundation for the Accreditation of Cell Therapy has been established to provide uniform standards for collection and processing of stem cell products, as well as the clinical care of both donors and recipients (Rowley 2002). The various procedures involved in stem cell processing have also attracted more scrutiny from the Food and Drug Administration. Options for stem cell processing include (a) depletion of granulocytes by density gradient centrifugation (Rowley et al. 1990), (b) depletion of potential tumor cells by a direct purging technique or CD34 selection (Civin et al. 1990), and (c) depletion of T cells in an allogeneic product to decrease the risk of graft-vs-host disease. Many of the stem cell processing steps described here and below, with the notable exception of CD34 selection, were developed using marrow products and all are made somewhat more complicated by the considerably higher number of cells found in PBSC compared with bone marrow.

11.6.3.6 Tumor Cell Purging

All of these processing procedures either depend on negative selection (removal of the cell type that is unwanted) or positive selection (selection of stem/progenitor cells, leaving all other cells behind). CD34 selection is the primary positive selection technique available to stem cell labs. CD34 is a cellular antigen that is expressed on stem cells, as well as progenitor cells of all hematopoietic lineages. Automated processes that select the CD34+ cell population (Strauss et al. 1991) away from the 99% of PBSC that are irrelevant for engraftment are available, and one of these technologies, the Isolex 300i device, is FDA approved. An alternative device, the Miltenyi CliniMACS device (Schumm et al. 1999), is approved in Europe and may soon become available in the United States. In general, CD34 selection will result in a product that is 60–95% CD34+, removing more than 99% of T cells (Beelen et al. 2000) and tumor cells (Donovan et al. 2000; Klein et al. 2001; Mohr et al. 2001), providing that the tumor cells do not express the CD34 antigen. Hematopoietic tumors, such as acute leukemias, often express CD34 and are therefore not depleted by CD34 selection. CD34 selection has been used to purge stem cell products in patients with NB, but concerns have been raised that some NB cells or cell lines may express CD34 or express surface epitopes that cross-react with monoclonal antibodies (MoAbs) that recognize CD34 (Hafer et al. 1999; Voigt et al. 1997). Our data have not confirmed expression of CD34 on NB (Donovan et al. 2000), and we and others have shown purging of NB cells from PBSC products in the clinical setting (Kanold et al. 2000). These data suggest that CD34 selection may be a purging alternative for PBSC products obtained from NB patients.

Negative selection procedures, by contrast, are tumor- or cell-type specific. For example, many techniques have been developed to negatively select T cells or T-cell subsets away from stem and progenitor cells in bone marrow and PBSC (see Ho and Soiffer 2002 for a recent review). These include: (a) a variety of monoclonal antibodies directed against T cells; (b) counterflow centrifugal elutriation (Wagner et al. 1990), which separates out lymphocytes based on physical characteristics; (c) sheep red blood cell rosetting (Reisner et al. 1981); and (d) immunomagnetic removal of T cells. Some of these procedures allow for more specific graft engineering by removing specific T-cell subsets such as CD8+ T cells or T cells expressing activation markers such as CD25 or CD69 (Fehse et al. 2000).

It is also possible to deplete tumor cells using specific anti-tumor monoclonal antibodies, relying on complement (Stein et al. 1988) plus cell-mediated cytotoxicity (Cheung et al. 2002), or more often an immunomagnetic depletion method (Reynolds et al. 1986). This approach has been proven to purge tumor cells from stem cell products collected from patients with B-cell lymphomas (Freedman et al. 1999). That tumor-contaminating stem cell products may contribute to relapse was shown in gene-marking studies in NB patients undergoing autologous bone marrow transplant. In these studies, a bone marrow aliquot was transfected with a marker gene and infused after transplant. Tumor cells at sites of relapse were found to con-

Matthay KK, Seeger RC, Reynolds CP, Stram DO, O'Leary MC, Harris RE, Selch M, Atkinson JB, Haase GM, Ramsay NK (1994) Allogeneic versus autologous purged bone marrow transplantation for neuroblastoma: a report from the Childrens Cancer Group. J Clin Oncol 12:2382–2389

Matthay KK, Harris R, Reynolds CP, Shimada H, Black T, Stram DO, Seeger RC (1998) Improved event-free survival for autologous bone marrow transplantation vs chemotherapy in neuroblastoma: a Childrens Cancer Group study. Med Pediatr Oncol 31:191–207

Matthay KK, Villablanca JG, Seeger RC, Stram DO, Harris RE, Ramsay NK, Swift P, Shimada H, Black CT, Brodeur GM et al. (1999) Treatment of high-risk neuroblastoma with intensive chemotherapy, radiotherapy, autologous bone marrow transplantation, and 13-cis-retinoic acid. N Engl J Med 341:1165–1173

Merrer J, De Jonghe B, Golliot F, Lefrant JY, Raffy B, Barre E, Rigaud JP, Casciani D, Misset B, Bosquet C et al. (2001) Complications of femoral and subclavian venous catheterization in critically ill patients: a randomized controlled trial. J Am Med Assoc 286:700–707

Mohr M, Dalmis F, Hilgenfeld E, Oelmann E, Zuhlsdorf M, Kratz-Albers K, Nolte A, Schmitmann C, Onaldi-Mohr D, Cassens U et al. (2001) Simultaneous immunomagnetic CD34+ cell selection and B-cell depletion in peripheral blood progenitor cell samples of patients suffering from B-cell non-Hodgkin's lymphoma. Clin Cancer Res 7:51–57

Moss TJ, Sanders DG, Lasky LC, Bostrom B (1990) Contamination of peripheral blood stem cell harvests by circulating neuroblastoma cells. Blood 76:1879–1883

Narayanasami U, Kanteti R, Morelli J, Klekar A, Al-Olama A, Keating C, O'Connor C, Berkman E, Erban JK, Sprague KA et al. (2001) Randomized trial of filgrastim versus chemotherapy and filgrastim mobilization of hematopoietic progenitor cells for rescue in autologous transplantation. Blood 98:2059–2064

Philip T, Ladenstein R, Zucker JM, Pinkerton R, Bouffet E, Louis D, Siegert W, Bernard JL, Frappaz D, Coze C (1993) Double megatherapy and autologous bone marrow transplantation for advanced neuroblastoma: the LMCE2 Study. Br J Cancer 67:119–127

Philip T, Ladenstein R, Lasset C, Hartmann O, Zucker JM, Pinkerton R, Pearson AD, Klingebiel T, Garaventa A, Kremens B et al. (1997) 1070 myeloablative megatherapy procedures followed by stem cell rescue for neuroblastoma: 17 years of European experience and conclusions. European Group for Blood and Marrow Transplant Registry Solid Tumour Working Party. Eur J Cancer 33:2130–2135

Powell JL, Bunin NJ, Callahan C, Aplenc R, Griffin G, Grupp SA (2004) An unexpectedly high incidence of Epstein-Barr virus lymphoproliferative disease after CD34+ selected autologous peripheral blood stem cell transplant in neuroblastoma. Bone Marrow Transplant 33:651–657

Reisner Y, Kapoor N, Kirkpatrick D, Pollack MS, Dupont B, Good RA, O'Reilly RJ (1981) Transplantation for acute leukaemia with HLA-A and B nonidentical parental marrow cells fractionated with soybean agglutinin and sheep red blood cells. Lancet 2:327–331

Reynolds CP, Seeger RC, Vo DD, Black AT, Wells J, Ugelstad J (1986) Model system for removing neuroblastoma cells from bone marrow using monoclonal antibodies and magnetic immunobeads. Cancer Res 46:5882–5886

Rill DR, Santana VM, Roberts WM, Nilson T, Bowman LC, Krance RA, Heslop HE, Moen RC, Ihle JN, Brenner MK (1994) Direct demonstration that autologous bone marrow transplantation for solid tumors can return a multiplicity of tumorigenic cells. Blood 84:380–383

Rowley SD (2002) Regulation of hematopoietic stem cell processing and transplantation. Int J Hematol 75:237–245

Rowley SD, Anderson GL (1993) Effect of DMSO exposure without cryopreservation on hematopoietic progenitor cells. Bone Marrow Transplant 11:389–393

Rowley SD, Davis JM, Piantadosi S, Jones RJ, Yeager AM, Santos GW (1990) Density-gradient separation of autologous bone marrow grafts before ex vivo purging with 4-hydroperoxycyclophosphamide. Bone Marrow Transplant 6:321–327

Rowley SD, Donaldson G, Lilleby K, Bensinger WI, Appelbaum FR (2001) Experiences of donors enrolled in a randomized study of allogeneic bone marrow or peripheral blood stem cell transplantation. Blood 97:2541–2548

Schumm M, Lang P, Taylor G, Kuci S, Klingebiel T, Buhring HJ, Geiselhart A, Niethammer D, Handgretinger R (1999) Isolation of highly purified autologous and allogeneic peripheral CD34+ cells using the CliniMACS device. J Hematother 8:209–218

Shpall EJ, Champlin R, Glaspy JA (1998) Effect of CD34+ peripheral blood progenitor cell dose on hematopoietic recovery. Biol Blood Marrow Transplant 4:84–92

Sloand EM, Kim S, Maciejewski JP, van Rhee F, Chaudhuri A, Barrett J, Young NS (2000) Pharmacologic doses of granulocyte colony-stimulating factor affect cytokine production by lymphocytes in vitro and in vivo. Blood 95:2269–2274

Somlo G, Sniecinski I, ter Veer A, Longmate J, Knutson G, Vuk-Pavlovic S, Bhatia R, Chow W, Leong L, Morgan R et al. (1999) Recombinant human thrombopoietin in combination with granulocyte colony-stimulating factor enhances mobilization of peripheral blood progenitor cells, increases peripheral blood platelet concentration, and accelerates hematopoietic recovery following high-dose chemotherapy. Blood 93:2798–2806

Srinivasan R, Barrett J, Childs R (2004) Allogeneic stem cell transplantation as immunotherapy for nonhematological cancers. Semin Oncol 31:47–55

Stein J, Strandjord S, Saarinen U, Warkentin P, Gerson S, Lazarus H, von Hoff D, Coccia P, Cheung NK (1988) In vitro treatment of autologous bone marrow for neuroblastoma patients with anti GD2 monoclonal antibody and human complement: a pilot study. Prog Clin Biol Res 271:237–248

Stiff PJ (1999) Management strategies for the hard-to-mobilize patient. Bone Marrow Transplant 23 (Suppl 2):S29–S33
Strauss LC, Trischmann TM, Rowley SD, Wiley JM, Civin CI (1991) Selection of normal human hematopoietic stem cells for bone marrow transplantation using immunomagnetic microspheres and CD34 antibody. Am J Pediatr Hematol Oncol 13:217–221
Sutherland DR, Anderson L, Keeney M, Nayar R, Chin-Yee I (1996) The ISHAGE guidelines for CD34+ cell determination by flow cytometry. International Society of Hematotherapy and Graft Engineering. J Hematother 5:213–226
Takaue Y, Kawano Y, Abe T, Okamoto Y, Suzue T, Shimuzu T, Saito S, Sato J, Makimoto A, Nakagawa R et al. (1995) Collection and transplant of peripheral blood stem cells in very small children weighing 20 kg or less. Blood 85:372–380
Trischmann TM, Schepers KG, Civin CI (1993) Measurement of CD34+ cells in bone marrow by flow cytometry. J Hematother 2:305–313
Voigt A, Hafer R, Gruhn B, Zintl F (1997) Expression of CD34 and other haematopoietic antigens on neuroblastoma cells: consequences for autologous bone marrow and peripheral blood stem cell transplantation. J Neuroimmunol 78:117–126
Wagner JE, Santos GW, Noga SJ, Rowley SD, Davis J, Vogelsang GB, Farmer ER, Zehnbauer BA, Saral R, Donnenberg AD (1990) Bone marrow graft engineering by counterflow centrifugal elutriation: results of a phase I–II clinical trial. Blood 75:1370–1377
Weaver CH, Potz J, Redmond J, Tauer K, Schwartzberg LS, Kaywin P, Drapkin R, Grant B, Unger P, Allen C et al. (1997) Engraftment and outcomes of patients receiving myeloablative therapy followed by autologous peripheral blood stem cells with a low CD34+ cell content. Bone Marrow Transplant 19:1103–1110
Weaver CH, Schulman KA, Buckner CD (2001) Mobilization of peripheral blood stem cells following myelosuppressive chemotherapy: a randomized comparison of filgrastim, sargramostim, or sequential sargramostim and filgrastim. Bone Marrow Transplant 27 (Suppl 2):S23–S29
Welch RH, Gravenstein N, Blackshear RH (1997) Multilumen central venous catheters in children: relative potential to perforate vessels. An in vitro study. J Clin Monit 13:75–79
Yanik GA, Levine JE, Matthay KK, Sisson JC, Shulkin BL, Shapiro B, Hubers D, Spalding S, Braun T, Ferrara JL, Hutchinson RJ (2002) Pilot study of iodine-131-metaiodobenzylguanidine in combination with myeloablative chemotherapy and autologous stem cell support for the treatment of neuroblastoma. J Clin Oncol 20:2142–2149
Yu J, Leisenring W, Bensinger WI, Holmberg LA, Rowley SD (1999) The predictive value of white cell or CD34+ cell count in the peripheral blood for timing apheresis and maximizing yield. Transfusion 39:442–450

11.7 Minimal Residual Disease Measurement

Irene Y. Cheung, Peter F. Ambros

11.7.1 Introduction

Patients with high-risk NB who are in clinical remission after completing induction chemotherapy are often left with minimal residual disease (MRD), i.e., the presence of microscopic levels of tumor cells not detectable by conventional clinicopathologic methods. MRD in high-risk patients is likely to contribute to the patient's eventual relapse and death. It stands to reason that accurate determination of MRD is crucial in the overall clinical management of NB patients. The bone marrow (BM), a frequent site of tumor recurrence, must be monitored for MRD. Peripheral blood (PB) is another reservoir of MRD, and sampling by venipuncture is less invasive and better tolerated by most patients.

The current multi-modality treatment for high-risk patients includes dose-intensive induction chemotherapy, tumor resection, local radiation, autologous stem cell harvest with or without purging, megatherapy with stem cell rescue, as well as biologic and/or differentiation therapy to eradicate MRD. Although methods to detect MRD are fully capable and useful for measuring large tumor loads, their clinical utility is most evident after the first three to five cycles of induction therapy, when residual NB are no longer detectable by conventional means. By serving as a surrogate end point, the "kinetics" of tumor response can be better defined by examining BM and PB during successive cycles of chemotherapy. MRD can also be used to evaluate the efficacy of various marrow/stem cell purging techniques, and to identify the optimal time to harvest stem cells. Despite positive selection of CD34+ cells from PB stem cells, substantial contaminating tumor cells remain (Moss et al. 1994; Lode et al. 1997). As therapy for NB becomes more effective, being able to quantify tumor cells during follow-up will help define the quality of remission. It is conceivable that patients in solid remission, without evidence of MRD, may be spared further cytotoxic therapy and treatment-related leukemia. Adjuvant therapy, be it mye-

Table 11.7.1 Techniques in the detection of minimal residual disease (MRD)

Method of detection	Sample source	Archived Samples	Turn-around time	Sensitivity
Cytology	BM Aspirate (BMA)	Yes	Hours	10^{-3}
Histology	BM Biopsy	Yes	2 days	10^{-3}
Immunocytology	BMA, PB	No	1 day	10^{-5}
Immunocytology/FISH	BMA, PB	No	2–3 days	10^{-5} to 10^{-6}
RT-PCR	BMA, PB	Yes	Hours to 1 day	10^{-6} to 10^{-7}

loablative therapy with autologous BM/stem cell rescue (Matthay et al. 1999; Pole et al. 1991; Ladenstein et al. 1998), or biologic therapy such as immunotherapy/differentiation therapy (Matthay et al. 1999; N.K. Cheung et al. 1998; Kushner et al. 2001; Yu et al. 1998), is typically applied at the time of clinical remission. An objective evaluation of the efficacy of these distinct adjuvant strategies is only possible when standardized protocols and quality-controlled detection techniques are used (Ambros and Ambros 2001). Ultimately, the rational choice of adjuvant therapies may become individualized depending on the MRD profile. To date, no treatment decision has been based solely on the detection of MRD.

11.7.2 Techniques in the Detection of Tumor Cells in the Hematopoietic System

11.7.2.1 Histology/Cytology

According to the International Neuroblastoma Staging System and International Neuroblastoma Response Criteria (Brodeur et al. 1993), BM studies evaluated by histologic or cytomorphologic examinations of biopsy specimens and of aspirates from bilateral anterior and bilateral posterior iliac crests are part of the extent-of-disease evaluation. It is also important to perform both biopsy and aspirate at different sites to achieve the highest detection sensitivity (Aronica et al. 1998); however, the sensitivity of tumor detection is relatively low, and thus the true prevalence of BM disease can be grossly underestimated (Cheung et al. 1997; Mehes et al. 2003). Nevertheless, histology and cytology are often used as the gold standard against which new detection techniques are measured (Cheung et al. 1998).

11.7.3 Detection Methods for MRD

Numerous diverse techniques have been developed to detect and in some assays to quantify MRD in NB, because there may be an advantage to know the amount of residual tumor cells over simply establishing its presence. Optimal MRD assays must have superior sensitivity and specificity. The sensitivity of MRD detection methods is influenced by the source of tissue being analyzed and is limited by the number of cells available to be assayed. Moreover, the heterogeneity of tumor cell populations can result in some residual disease escaping detection.

11.7.3.1 Immunocytology/Immunohistochemistry

In this cell surface antigen detection technique, mononuclear cells isolated from marrow aspirates and heparinized PB are incubated with a single or a panel of murine monoclonal antibodies directed against NB surface antigens. Monoclonal antibodies specific for the NB surface disialoganglioside GD2 are commonly used because this antigen is expressed homogeneously on NB cell surface in high density (Wu et al. 1986). The antibody of choice must have high affinity for tumor cells, with little or no cross reactivity to normal hematopoietic cells. Some examples of anti-GD2 monoclonal antibodies that have excellent specificity include 3F8 (Cheung et al. 1997; Faulkner et al. 1998), 14.18 (Mehes et al. 2001), 3A7 (Saarinen et al. 1996), and HSAN1.2 (Smith and Reynolds 1987). Its usual detection limit of 1 tumor cell in 10^5 normal hematopoietic cells may be improved to 1 in 10^6 or even lower by the use of a com-

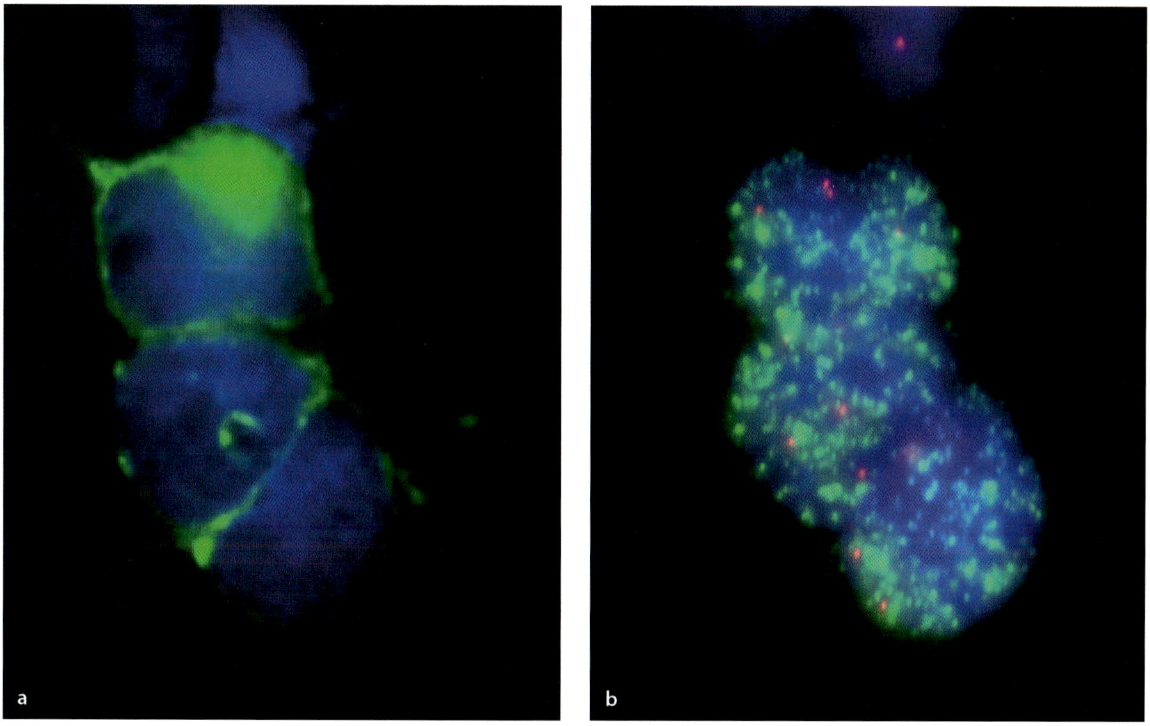

Figure 11.7.1 a,b

a Bone marrow cells from a neuroblastoma patient stained with FITC labeled GD2 antibody. **b** The same cells as in **a** were subsequently analyzed by fluorescence in situ hybridization using a *MYCN*-specific probe (FITC) and a chromosome-2 specific probe (TRITC). All three GD2 positive cells showed *MYCN* amplification.

bined immunofluorescence and genetic approach (Mehes et al. 2001) and to 1 in 10^7–10^8 by the use of immuno-magnetic sorting (Faulkner et al. 2000).

One important advantage of this method is the possibility to quantify the exact number of tumor cells in a specimen. It can exploit a mixture of monoclonal antibodies of different specificities (Moss et al. 1991). More importantly, it allows the genetic confirmation of malignant features of individual cells, and provides insights into the biologic make up of disseminated tumor cells (DTCs); however, this assay requires freshly collected samples which must be processed right away. The technique is also labor intensive because it requires counting and analyzing cells under the microscope.

11.7.3.2 Automatic Immunofluorescence Detection Techniques

The recent development of a fully automated microscopic device allows for the objective screening and quantitation of DTCs, as well as their immunologic and genetic analyses (Mehes et al. 2001a, 2003; Ambros et al. 2001; Ambros and Mehes 2002). The unequivocal identification of the true nature (malignant vs benign) of DTC can be achieved by a sequential fluorescence in situ hybridization (FISH) of the immunologically positive cells (Fig. 11.7.1). Furthermore, the visualization of different antibodies on the same cell can provide vital information on a tumor's aggressiveness. There is a fundamental difference between detecting a proliferative tumor cell vs an apoptotic cell (Mehes et al. 2001b).

11.7.3.3 Reverse Transcription-Polymerase Chain Reaction

In molecular methods to detect MRD, total RNA is first isolated from mononuclear cells. mRNA is reverse-transcribed to cDNA, then amplified by PCR using target gene-specific primers. In some assays, nested PCR is carried out, i.e., an aliquot of the PCR product is subjected to a second PCR reaction, although carryover contamination is a concern. The target gene is identified by the presence or absence of a band of the appropriate molecular size after separation by agarose gel electrophoresis of the PCR product. In some cases, the presence of a gene transcript is further verified using Southern blot, as well as DNA sequencing.

11.7.3.3.1 Real-Time Quantitative RT-PCR

The emergency of real-time quantitative PCR (qRT-PCR) technology permits not just the identification of a target gene, but also its transcript level (Heid et al. 1996; Gibson et al. 1996). Such a development has broadened the potentials in MRD monitoring. With a wide linear dynamic range, superior sensitivity and accuracy, real-time RT-PCR allows good intra-assay and inter-assay reproducibility. Additional attractions include high throughput capacity, speed, and elimination of lengthy post-PCR handling steps, preventing potential carryover contamination. Two major technical variables that need to be addressed are the selection of a reference gene against which the test samples can be normalized, and how to discriminate a positive from a negative result.

11.7.3.3.2 Molecular Targets

Several molecular targets have been studied extensively in the detection of residual NB cells in the BM and PB. Specificity is determined by the absence of gene expression when a series of normal BM and PB is evaluated. Sensitivity experiments are carried out by spiking varying concentration of tumor cells from a NB cell line to normal mononuclear cells, and assess the limit of detection. Depending on the specific gene expression of the cell line, sensitivity can reach as high as $1/10^7$. Tyrosine hydroxylase (TH, tyrosine 3-monoxygenase), being the first and rate-limiting enzyme in the biosynthesis of catecholamine, is a logical choice since most NBs secrete catecholamines. Detection of occult NB cells by RT-PCR of TH mRNA was first reported in BM by Naito et al. (1991), and by Burchill et al. (1994) in PB. Recently, several real-time RT-PCR assays for TH transcript have also been developed (Träger et al. 2003; Tchirkov et al. 2003).

Another useful molecular target is the transcript of GD2/GM2 synthase (β1,4-N-acetylgalactosaminyl-transferase). It is the key enzyme required for the synthesis of GD2 (Furukawa et al. 1996), an antigen ubiquitously expressed on NB. Its utility as a molecular marker in the detection of NB cells in the BM was first reported by Cheung et al. (Cheung and Cheung 2001; Lo Piccolo et al. 2001). A highly sensitive and specific quantitative RT-PCR assay which measures GD2 synthase mRNA was developed with transcript levels correlating well with the number of NB cells as measured by immunocytology (Cheung and Cheung 2001).

The cancer testis antigen *GAGE* belongs to a family of genes which encode distinct tumor-associated peptides recognizable by autologous cytolytic T lymphocytes when presented by HLA class-I molecules (Van den Eynde et al. 1995). It is expressed in human tumors of different histologic types including NB, but is silent in normal adult tissues except for placenta and testis (De Backer et al. 1999). *GAGE* was demonstrated to be a potentially useful MRD marker of NB (Cheung and Cheung 1997; Cheung et al. 2000) and melanoma (Cheung et al. 1999).

11.7.3.3.3 Perspectives on Molecular Detection

Molecular-based MRD assays can be hampered by the inherent pitfalls of DNA amplification. False-positive findings may result from "tumor-specific" genes which are occasionally transcribed even in normal tissues. Illegitimate transcription, i.e., the transcription of any gene in any cell type, and pseudogenes, which lack intronic sequences resulting in PCR products indistinguishable from those generated from the mRNA, also pose concerns. False-negative results in molecular assays can be due to degraded RNA, tumor cell heterogeneity, the presence of inhibitors, technical errors, sampling problem, as well as down-regulation of the target gene.

Table 11.7.2 MRD detection with prognostic significance in survival ($p<0.05$)

Study	Number of Patients	Sample	Time from diagnosis	Survival	Detection method	Reference
CCG-3891	242	BM	12 weeks from diagnosis (after three cycles of chemo)	PFS	Immunocytology	Seeger et al. (2000)
	195	BM	BM harvest	PFS	Immunocytology	Seeger et al. (2000)
France	22	BM	~3 months from diagnosis (after three cycles of chemo)	OS	TH qRT-PCR	Tchirkov et al. (2003)
	21	PBSC	PBSC harvest	OS	TH qRT-PCR	Tchirkov et al. (2003)
Japan	21	BM	4 months from diagnosis	PFS	TH RT-PCR	Fukuda et al. (2001)
MSKCC-N7	31	BM	Before 3F8[a] purging	OS	GD2 synthase qRT-PCR	Cheung et al. (2002)
Germany	24	PBSC	PBSC graft	PFS[c]	Immunocytology	Handgretinger et al. (2003)
MSKCC-N7	45	BM	Before ^{131}I-3F8 and 3F8[a]	PFS, OS	GD2 synthase qRT-PCR	Cheung et al. (2003a)
MSKCC-9418	74	BM	Before third cycle of 3F8[a]+GM-CSF (1.8 months from protocol entry)	PFS	GD2 synthase qRT-PCR	Cheung et al. (2003b)
UKCCSG-NB9305	112	PB	Off therapy in clinical remission[b]	PFS	TH RT-PCR	Burchill et al. (2001)
MSKCC-N6, N7	44	BM	24 months from diagnosis	PFS, OS	*GAGE* RT-PCR	Cheung et al. (2000)
MSKCC-N6, N7	44	BM	24 months from diagnosis	PFS, OS	GD2 synthase qRT-PCR	Cheung and Cheung (2001)

[a] 3F8 is a murine anti-GD2 monoclonal antibody
[b] Off therapy defined as after surgery and/or PBSC transplant
[c] Favorable survival with increased tumor cell contamination

11.7.4 Clinical Relevance of MRD

The ultimate utility of MRD detection is to determine the clinical significance of occult tumor cells in relations to patient relapse, survival, and even cure, using progression-free and overall survival as the clinical end points. Prognostic impact of MRD needs to factor in the genetic profile of the tumor. For example, NB patients with stage-4s disease are well known to have marrow disease, and yet they predictably have favorable outcome. This suggests that the presence of marrow disease may not necessarily be clinically relevant to all NB stages. In fact, a Children's Cancer Group study with 374 patients reported no statistically significant difference between stage-1 and stage-2 patients who had immunocytology-positive vs immunocytology-negative marrow disease at diagnosis (Perez et al. 2000). Interestingly, in a comparable patient group, a false-positive rate of >30% was found after genetic verification of the immunologically positive DTCs (Mehes et al. 2001). Indeed, an unambiguous identification and quantification of MRD must be a requisite for MRD monitoring. For patients with stage-4 NB undergoing multi-modality treatment, the clinical significance of MRD is highly dependent on when the sampling is being carried out.

Several research groups have reported that among stage-4 NB patients older than 1 year at diagnosis, MRD during and after therapy had a statistically significant impact on patient survival (Table 11.7.2). Some studies have further underscored the adverse effect of the presence of NB cells in BM and PB at diagnosis on clinical outcome (Seeger et al. 2000; Burchill et al. 2001). The implication of this conclusion is that emphasis must be placed on improved therapeutic strategies. It is not surprising to find the presence of MRD at the end of therapy to have prognostic importance, as demonstrated by the MSKCC and UKCCSG studies (Cheung and Cheung 2001; Cheung et al. 2000; Burchill et al. 2001). More relevant to the clinical management of NB is likely the impact of MRD during and after induction (Seeger et al. 2000; Fukuda et al. 2001). In BM/PBSC harvest, an adverse effect on survival was demonstrated with ≥100 tumor cells per 10^5 nucleated BM detected by immunocytology (Seeger et al. 2000), >500 TH transcripts in PBSC by qRT-PCR (Tchirkov et al. 2003), and >5 GD2 synthase transcript units in prepurged BM by qRT-PCR (Cheung et al. 2002). In contrast, Handgretinger et al. reported that patients with CD34+ PBSC grafts containing >2000 tumor cells as measured by immunocytology using chimeric anti-GD2 antibody ch14.18 had a lower risk of relapse than patients with fewer contaminating tumor cells (Handgretinger et al. 2003). It was suggested that a threshold number of tumor cells would elicit an anti-tumor immune response after autologous transplant, although false positivity remains a possibility. With the advent of novel post-induction therapies, MRD serves as a sensitive surrogate response marker in comparing the efficacy of different adjuvant therapies. The presence of positive GD2 synthase transcript in patients who did not achieve CR/VGPR before the onset of radioimmunotherapy had a higher risk of relapse and death (Cheung et al. 2003a). For patients undergoing another adjuvant therapy with a combination of anti-GD2 antibody 3F8 and GM-CSF, early molecular response was found to have prognostic impact on progression-free survival (Cheung et al. 2003b). The ability to identify a subset of patients who are unlikely to benefit from this adjuvant therapy and are at a great risk of relapse may provide the rationale for a more timely application of alternative treatment options.

11.7.5 Future Directions

Tumor heterogeneity as well as the occult nature of MRD often lead to failure in detection when only a single method is used; thus, optimal MRD surveillance should utilize multiple independent techniques, such as the inclusion of both immunologic and molecular based assays, as well as serial samplings over time. However, time, cost, and quality-control issues need to be considered. Potential NB targets identified by gene expression arrays will likely enhance detection sensitivity and specificity. The NB research thus far has implicated that, among selected groups of stage-4 NB patients, the presence of minimal residual tumor cells in the BM and PB at specific phases of the multi-modality treatment scheme is likely to portend an adverse survival outcome; however, to fully understand the role of MRD in the overall management of high-risk NB, a large multi-center prospective study with uniformly treated patients using quality-controlled detection techniques is warranted.

References

Ambros PF, Ambros IM (2001) Pathology and biology guidelines for resectable and unresectable neuroblastic tumors and bone marrow examination guidelines. Med Pediatr Oncol 37:492–504

Ambros PF, Mehes G (2003) Combined immunofluorescence and FISH: New prospects for tumor cell detection/identification. In: Robinson JP, Darzynkiewicz Z, Hyun W, Orfao A, Rabinovitch P (eds) Current protocols in cytometry. Wiley, New York, pp 8.13.1–8.13.10

Ambros PF, Mehes G, Hattinger C et al. (2001) Unequivocal identification of disseminated tumor cells in the bone marrow by combining immunological and genetic approaches: functional and prognostic information. Leukemia 15:275–277

Aronica PA, Pirrotta VT, Yunis EJ et al. (1998) Detection of neuroblastoma in the bone marrow: biopsy versus aspiration. J Pediatr Hematol Oncol 20:330–334

Brodeur G, Pritchard J, Berthold F et al. (1993) Revisions of the international criteria for neuroblastoma diagnosis, staging and response to treatment. J Clin Oncol 11:1466–1477

Burchill SA, Bradbury FM, Smith B et al. (1994) Neuroblastoma cell detection by reverse transcriptase-polymerase chain reaction (RT-PCR) for tyrosine hydroxylase mRNA. Int J Cancer 57:671–675

Burchill SA, Lewis IJ, Abrams KR et al. (2001) Circulating neuroblastoma cells detected by reverse transcriptase polymerase chain reaction for tyrosine hydroxylase mRNA are an independent poor prognostic indicator in stage 4 neuroblastoma in children over 1 year. J Clin Oncol 19:1795–1801

Cheung IY, Cheung NK (1997) Molecular detection of *GAGE* expression in peripheral blood and bone marrow: utility as a tumor marker for neuroblastoma. Clin Cancer Res 3:821–826

Cheung IY, Cheung NK (2001) Quantitation of marrow disease in neuroblastoma by real-time reverse transcription-PCR. Clin Cancer Res 7:1698–1705

Cheung IY, Barber D, Cheung NK (1998) Detection of microscopic neuroblastoma in marrow by histology, immunocytology, and reverse transcription-PCR of multiple molecular markers. Clin Cancer Res 4:2801–2805

Cheung IY, Cheung NKV, Ghossein RA et al. (1999) Association between molecular detection of *GAGE* and survival in patients with malignant melanoma: a retrospective cohort study. Clin Cancer Res 5:2042–2047

Cheung IY, Chi SN, Cheung NKV (2000) Prognostic significance of *GAGE* detection in bone marrows on survival of patients with metastatic neuroblastoma. Med Pediatr Oncol 35:632–634

Cheung IY, Lo Piccolo MS, Collins N et al. (2002) Quantitation of GD2 synthase mRNA by real-time reverse transcription-polymerase chain reaction: utility in bone marrow purging of neuroblastoma by anti-GD2 antibody 3F8. Cancer 94: 3042–3048

Cheung IY, Lo Piccolo MS, Kushner BH et al. (2003a) Quantitation of GD2 synthase mRNA by real-time reverse transcriptase polymerase chain reaction: clinical utility in evaluating adjuvant therapy in neuroblastoma. J Clin Oncol 21:1087–1093

Cheung IY, Lo Piccolo MS, Kushner BH et al. (2003b) Early molecular response of marrow disease to biologic therapy is highly prognostic in neuroblastoma. J Clin Oncol 21:3853–3858

Cheung NK, Heller G, Kushner BH et al. (1997) Detection of metastatic neuroblastoma in bone marrow: When is routine marrow histology insensitive? J Clin Oncol 15:2807–2817

Cheung NK, Kushner BH, Yeh SD et al. (1998) 3F8 monoclonal antibody treatment of patients with stage 4 neuroblastoma: a phase II study. Int J Oncol 12:1299–1306

De Backer O, Arden KC, Boretti M et al. (1999) Characterization of the *GAGE* genes that are expressed in various human cancers and in normal testis. Cancer Res 59:3157–3165

Faulkner LB, Tintori V, Tamburini A et al. (1998) High-sensitivity immunocytologic analysis of neuroblastoma cells in paired blood and marrow samples. J Hematother 7:361–366

Faulkner LB, Garaventa A, Paoli A et al. (2000) In vivo cytoreduction studies and cell sorting-enhanced tumor-cell detection in high-risk neuroblastoma patients: implications for leukapheresis strategies. J Clin Oncol 18:3829–3836

Fukuda M, Miyajima Y, Miyashita Y et al. (2001) Disease outcome may be predicted by molecular detection of minimal residual disease in bone marrow in advanced neuroblastoma: a pilot study. J Pediatr Hematol Oncol 23:10–13

Furukawa K, Soejima H, Niikawa N et al. (1996) Genomic organization and chromosomal assignment of the human β1,4-N-acetylgalactosaminyltransferase gene. J Biol Chem 271:20836–20844

Gibson UE, Heid CA, Williams PM (1996) A novel method for real time quantitative RT-PCR. Genome Res 6:995–1001

Handgretinger R, Leung W, Ihm K et al. (2003) Tumour cell contamination of autologous stem cells grafts in high-risk neuroblastoma: the good news? Br J Cancer 88:1874–1877

Heid CA, Stevens J, Livak KJ et al. (1996) Real time quantitative PCR. Genome Res 6:986–994

Kushner BH, Kramer K, Cheung NKV (2001) Phase II trial of the anti-G(D2) monoclonal antibody 3F8 and granulocyte-macrophage colony-stimulating factor for neuroblastoma. J Clin Oncol 19:4189–4194

Ladenstein R, Philip T, Lasset C et al. (1998) Multivariate analysis of risk factors in stage 4 neuroblastoma patients over the age of one year treated with megatherapy and stem cell transplantation: a report from the European Bone Marrow Transplantation Solid Tumor Registry. J Clin Oncol 16:953–965

Lo Piccolo MS, Cheung NK, Cheung IY (2001) GD2 synthase: a new molecular marker for detecting neuroblastoma. Cancer 92:924–931

Lode HN, Handgretinger R, Schuermann U et al. (1997) Detection of neuroblastoma cells in CD34+ selected peripheral peripheral stem cells using a combination of tyrosine hydroxylase nested RT-PCR and anti-ganglioside GD2 immunocytochemistry. Eur J Cancer 33:2024–2030

Matthay KK, Villablanca JG, Seeger RC et al. (1999) Treatment of high-risk neuroblastoma with intensive chemotherapy, radiotherapy, autologous bone marrow transplantation, and 13-cis-retinoic acid. Children's Cancer Group. N Engl J Med 341:1165–1173

Mehes G, Luegmayr A, Ambros IM et al. (2001a) Combined automatic immunological and molecular cytogenetic analysis allows exact identification and quantification of tumor cells in the bone marrow. Clin Cancer Res 7:1969–1975

Mehes G, Witt A, Kubista E et al. (2001b) Circulating breast cancer cells are frequently apoptotic. Am J Pathol 159:17–20

Mehes G, Luegmayr A, Kornmuller R et al. (2003) Detection of disseminated tumor cells in neuroblastoma: 3 log improvement in sensitivity by automatic immunofluorescence plus FISH (AIPF) analysis compared with classical bone marrow cytology. Am J Pathol 163:393–399

Moss TJ, Reynolds CP, Sather HN et al. (1991) Prognostic value of immunocytologic detection of bone marrow metastases in neuroblastoma. N Engl J Med 324:219–226

Moss TJ, Cairo M, Santana VM et al. (1994) Clonogenicity of circulating neuroblastoma cells: implications regarding peripheral blood stem cell transplantation. Blood 83:3085–3089

Naito H, Kuzumaki N, Uchino J et al. (1991) Detection of tyrosine hydroxylase mRNA and minimal neuroblastoma cells by the reverse transcription-polymerase chain reaction. Eur J Cancer 27:762–765

Perez CA, Matthay KK, Atkinson JB et al. (2000) Biologic variables in the outcome of stages I and II neuroblastoma treated with surgery as primary therapy: a Children's Cancer Group study. J Clin Oncol 18:18–26

Pole JG, Casper J, Elfenbein G et al. (1991) High-dose chemoradiotherapy supported by marrow infusions for advanced neuroblastoma: a Pediatric Oncology Group Study. J Clin Oncol 9:152–158

Saarinen U, Wikstrom S, Makipernaa A et al. (1996) In vivo purging of bone marrow in children with poor-risk neuroblastoma for marrow collection and autologous bone marrow transplantation. J Clin Oncol 14:2791–2802

Seeger RC, Reynolds CP, Gallego R et al. (2000) Quantitative tumor cell content of bone marrow and blood as a predictor of outcome in stage IV neuroblastoma: a Children's Cancer Group study. J Clin Oncol 18:4067–4076

Smith RG, Reynolds P (1987) Monoclonal antibody recognizing a human neuroblastoma-associated antigen. Diagn Clin Immunol 5:209–220

Tchirkov A, Paillard C, Halle P et al. (2003) Significance of molecular quantification of minimal residual disease in metastatic neuroblastoma. J Hematother Stem Cell Res 12:435–442

Träger C, Kogner P, Lindskog M et al. (2003) Quantitative analysis of tyrosine hydroxylase mRNA for sensitive detection of neuroblastoma cells in blood and bone marrow. Clin Chem 49:104–112

Van den Eynde B, Peeters O, De Backer O et al. (1995) A new family of genes coding for an antigen recognized by autologous cytolytic T lymphocytes on a human melanoma. J Exp Med 182:689–698

Wu Z, Schwartz E, Seeger RC et al. (1986) Expression of GD2 ganglioside by untreated primary human neuroblastomas. Cancer Res 46:440–443

Yu A, Uttenreuther-Fischer M, Huang C-S et al. (1998) Phase I trial of a human-mouse chimeric anti-disialoganglioside monoclonal antibody ch14.18 in patients with refractory neuroblastoma and osteosarcoma. J Clin Oncol 16:2169–2180

Treatment of Relapsed and Refractory Neuroblastoma

Katherine K. Matthay, Brian H. Kushner

Contents

12.1 Introduction

This chapter addresses the challenges of treating patients with high-risk neuroblastoma who have failed front-line therapy. Partially resected, incompletely responding, or locally recurrent low-risk neuroblastomas can usually be successful treated with little or no cytotoxic therapy (see Chap. 11.1). By contrast, despite aggressive multi-modality treatment, including dose-intensive and myeloablative chemotherapy, high-risk neuroblastoma eventually progresses and eventually proves lethal in more than 70% of cases (see Chap. 11.3). The prognosis of recurrent intermediate-risk disease is also guarded. This chapter focuses on resistant disease that portends a lethal outcome.

Relapse and recurrence are synonymous and refer to disease that re-emerges after complete or very good partial remission (CR/VGPR) has been achieved. Refractory disease indicates neuroblastoma that is stable or possibly reduced but still evident in macroscopic amounts after several months of adequate therapy, i.e., disease that responds incompletely to treatment. Resistant neuroblastoma encompasses both relapsed and refractory disease. In the International Neuroblastoma Response Criteria (INRC), refractory disease can be partial response, minor response, or no response, while relapsed/recurrent disease is progressive disease (PD). Persistence of metastases is particularly ominous after multiple cycles of intensive chemotherapy, whereas a partial response of the primary tumor may often be rendered CR or VGPR with surgery and radiotherapy. Progressive disease is also present when refractory disease spreads to a new site or when the volume of a refractory or residual lesion increases more than 25% (Brodeur et al. 1993).

If refractory disease could be detected at diagnosis or very early in induction, then such patients might be treated with novel approaches. Early detection of primary refractory disease is now possible via use of metaiodobenzylguanidine (MIBG) scintigraphy during the induction period as a semi-quantitative response measure (Matthay et al. 2003a; Ladenstein et al. 1998). Measurement of tumor cells in both blood and bone marrow by immunocytology and by the possibly more sensitive technique of reverse transcriptase-polymerase chain reaction may also be a means of early detection of refractory disease (Cheung et al. 2003; Burchill et al. 2001; Seeger et al. 2000) (see Chap. 11.7). In addition, genome-wide screening may lead to the identification of favorable vs unfavorable genetic patterns, which may, in the future, be used to distinguish resistant cases and stratify treatment at diagnosis (Keshelava et al. 2001; Takita et al. 2004; Hiyama et al. 2004).

Depending on the biology of the tumor, resistance to standard therapy is evident in 10–15% of children, resulting in disease that responds incompletely (primary refractory disease) to induction or initially responds but then recurs and progresses rapidly. More frequently, the typical patient with high-risk neuroblastoma will achieve remission, but suffer a relapse later, commonly within 2 years after myeloablative therapy with hematopoietic stem-cell support (Matthay et al. 1999). The approach to therapy of relapse in such patients should assume systemic dissemination. It is rare that even an isolated recurrence will be successfully treated with only local control measures. Bone and bone marrow are by far the most frequent sites of relapse (DuBois et al. 1999; Matthay et al. 1993b). Metastases in sites that are rarely involved at diagnosis, such as the central nervous system (CNS) and lungs, have been reported in up to 8% of relapsed patients (DuBois et al. 1999; Matthay et al. 2003b; Kramer et al. 2001). Regrowth of disease in the primary site has occurred in 10–20% of cases without and up to 50% of cases with distant disease. The incidence of local recurrence may decrease with dose-intensive chemotherapy, total resection, and adequate radiotherapy to the primary tumor bed plus regional nodal groups (Wolden et al. 2000; Haas-Kogan et al. 2002; Ikeda et al. 1992).

Mechanisms of tumor resistance are manifold, ranging from anatomic factors, such as sanctuary sites (CNS and testes), hypoxic conditions (bone or poorly perfused primary tumor), host factors (drug pharmacokinetics), and molecular features of the tumor cells. Examples of molecular changes include emergence of MRP1 and p-glycoprotein-mediated multi-drug resistance (Norris et al. 1996; Blanc et al. 2003; Manohar et al. 2004), altered DNA repair, decreased ability to undergo apoptosis because of p53 mutation (Keshelava et al. 2001; Tweddle et al. 2001, 2003), over-expression of Bcl-2 or Bcl-X_L Dole et al. 1994; Dole et al. 1995), and detoxification of alkylators via various enzymes that conjugate xenobiotics to glutathione (Tew 1994).

Relapse may also result from occult tumor cells admixed with autologous hematopoietic stem cells infused after myeloablative therapy. Support for this possibility comes from (a) the report that after infusion of unpurged autologous bone marrow marked with transduced neomycin-resistance gene, tumor cells in the recurrent neuroblastoma in all three cases showed the genetic marker (Rill et al. 1994), and (b) the occasional reports after autologous bone marrow transplantation of miliary metastases to the lung, a site at risk from infusion of tumor cells through a central venous catheter (Watts and Mroczek-Musulman 1996)and reports that circulating neuroblastoma cells in blood are clonogenic (Moss et al. 1994). The current Children's Oncology Group (COG) protocol for high-risk neuroblastoma is investigating the importance of tumor-free stem cells via a randomized study of ex vivo purging.

Herein we discuss the ever-expanding repertoire of cytotoxic agents (chemotherapy), tumor-targeted agents, and differentiating agents available for resistant neuroblastoma, and suggest how these therapies might best be integrated in an overall treatment plan for different subsets of resistant disease.

Table 12.1. Treatment approaches for different types of relapse (*MIBG* ^{131}I-metaiodobenzylguanidine, *MRD* multiply relapsed disease)

Disease status	Treatment approach
Primary refractory	Novel chemotherapy, MIBG+myeloablative therapy, MRD therapy
Early relapse	Novel chemotherapy, then targeted therapy, myeloablative therapy, MRD therapy
Late relapse	Standard combination chemotherapy, surgery, radiotherapy or MIBG, and novel MRD therapy
Multiple relapse	Low-toxicity oral chemotherapy or outpatient-targeted therapy

12.2 Treatment Strategies for Resistant Disease

The appropriate approach to the patient with recurrent or resistant neuroblastoma depends on the goals of the therapy. Although in previous studies the median survival for patients who relapsed after myeloablative therapy and bone marrow transplantation was only 3 months, with current multimodality approaches and judicious use of established as well as investigational agents, the survival can be prolonged for years (Kushner et al. 2002), and cure may be a possibility in some settings. Whether the goal is symptom palliation, prolongation of life, or complete remission depends on the timing and nature of the relapse, the prior therapy, and the tumor biology. General considerations in the choice of therapy include the use of agents with a different mechanism of action than those tried previously; tailoring therapy to sites of recurrence (e.g., agents with CNS penetration); the availability of stem cells for use with myelosuppressive or myeloablative agents (including ^{131}I-MIBG); and organ status (e.g., impaired renal function from prior cisplatin and/or ifosfamide; Table 12.1).

12.2.1 Primary Refractory Disease

Management of disease that responds incompletely to induction therapy has evolved considerably since the 1980s, which can be considered the beginning of the modern era of combination chemotherapy and myeloablative treatments for neuroblastoma. Early enthusiasm for use of myeloablative chemoradiotherapy for primary refractory neuroblastoma has waned due to the failure to achieve cure. In retrospect, the unsatisfactory results are not surprising, given the presence of a large residual tumor burden comprised of neuroblasts that have survived multiple cycles of combination chemotherapy, and given that the myeloablative regimens usually consist of agents identical to, or in the same drug categories as, those already used in the induction. The addition of total body irradiation does not appear to improve chances for cure, nor does the use of allogeneic stem cells. Myeloablative chemotherapy is ineffective against grossly visible residual soft tissue disease (incompletely resected primary tumor), and the same holds for local radiotherapy (Ladenstein et al. 1993, 1998).

Current treatment strategies for primary refractory disease can apply novel therapies that hold out the possibility of cure. These therapies include either prolongation of induction therapy with intensification of dose if there has been some response to treatment, or else adding chemotherapeutic agents that differ in their mechanism of action from those used in induction, biologic response modifiers, or targeted radiotherapy; thus, when standard induction regimens using alkylating agents (cyclophosphamide, ifosfamide), platinum compounds (cisplatin, carboplatin), and topoisomerase-II inhibitors (etoposide, doxorubicin) fail to achieve CR/VGPR, further cytoreduction is a good possibility by combining the topoisomerase-I inhibitor topotecan with one or two other agents. If there is a satisfactory response, then consideration can be given to myeloablative consolidation, followed by treatments for minimal residual disease such as local radiotherapy and the biologic response modifiers, 13-*cis*-retinoic acid and anti-GD2 antibodies. For morphologically detectable residual bone marrow disease, the use of 13-*cis*-retinoic acid and anti-GD2 antibodies can achieve CR/VGPR or even cure in a minority of patients, and some of the other biologic response modifiers may prove useful in the future (see Chaps. 14–17); however, for gross residual disease, approaches such as targeted radiotherapy with ^{131}I-MIBG or novel cytotoxic agents may be more appropriate for cytoreduction.

12.2.2 Early Relapse

The development of new disease during induction, although uncommon with the regimens currently in wide use, portends early death since a durable major response to different chemotherapy or to non-chemotherapeutic measures is unusual. The chance for cure is only slightly better when relapse occurs in the 6- to 12-month period after stem-cell rescue. In this situation, management is similar to that of primary refractory disease (see above), except that there is no role for (repeat) myeloablative therapy and organ toxicity may limit chemotherapeutic options. Poor bone marrow reserve post-transplant can be an obstacle to aggressive retrieval therapy, but this problem has lessened considerably with the excellent hematologic recovery that follows use of abundant peripheral blood stem cells (for the initial stem-cell rescue) or with the availability of previously collected stem cells for use with the retrieval program.

12.2.3 Late Relapse

Disease recurrence more than 1 year off therapy is usually responsive to retrieval chemotherapy. Thus, major disease regressions can be expected, even with use of the similar agents or regimens that comprised induction following the initial diagnosis; however, different consolidation measures are required to offer any chance for long-term control, which is still very limited in patients who have already received myeloablative therapy. For patients who achieve a second complete remission, there is a potential role for the same repertoire of treatments for minimal residual disease mentioned above, including retinoids, anti-GD2 antibodies, and local radiotherapy.

12.2.4 Multiply Relapsed Disease

Cure of multiply relapsed high-risk neuroblastoma is virtually unheard of; hence, quality of life becomes a predominant concern and toxic treatments should be avoided. Reasonable chemotherapeutic options include use of topotecan (i.v. or p.o.), irinotecan, etoposide (i.v. or p.o.), or temozolomide, singly or with other agents such as cyclophosphamide, carboplatin, temozolomide, and/or vincristine – all at relatively mild dosages. Widely available cytostatic agents that warrant consideration in this setting may include retinoids, Gleevec, and thalidomide. Phase-I therapies that have expected low toxicity and may be available on an outpatient basis may be reasonable. Local radiotherapy and low-dose ^{131}I-MIBG are useful for palliation of pain or for preventative treatment of heavily involved sites (especially skeletal) likely to become symptomatic.

12.3 Cytotoxic Chemotherapeutic Agents

Agents that may attack resistant neuroblastoma with novel mechanisms to overcome resistance may be divided into cytotoxic chemotherapeutic agents vs those that are targeted to either tumor-specific receptors or biochemical and genetic pathways that are relatively tumor specific. The cytotoxic agents may either be drugs already approved for other cancer indications, or else still under IND, which implies less certain future availability, depending on the overall marketability. In developing a new agent for use in a relatively rare tumor, such as neuroblastoma, it is important to establish efficacy using appropriate tumor models (Houghton et al. 2002). The section below discusses each of these approaches, both for agents that have undergone early clinical trials and those with preclinical data supporting ongoing trials (Table 12.2). In general, efficacy of these agents was based on small phase-I and phase-II clinical studies. Typically, there was substantial heterogeneity in the patient populations, including time from diagnosis and extent of relapse, as such response rates cannot be easily

Table 12.2. New agents with potential in neuroblastoma (*HDAC* histone deacetylase inhibitors)

Cytotoxic	Apoptotic pathway	Immunologic	Anti-angiogenic	Retinoids	Targeted radiotherapy
Topoisomerase inhibitors	HDAC inhibitors	Antibodies	Thalidomide	Fenretinide	^{131}I-MIBG
Alkylators	Demethylating agents	Cytokines	Antibodies	Other retinoids	^{131}I-anti-GD2
Cross-linkers	Tyrosine kinase inhibitors	Vaccines	Small molecules		

compared among these agents. Most would agree that cytotoxic therapy is necessary for large bulky recurrences, while cytostatic or biologic therapy may be most optimally applied when there is small tumor load.

12.3.1 Alkylating and DNA Cross-Linking Agents

12.3.1.1 Ifosfamide and Cyclophosphamide

Initial approaches to treatment of resistant or recurrent neuroblastoma in the previous decade concentrated on use of more intensive combination therapy or use of newer platinum or alkylating agents. Neuroblastoma was proven to be responsive to ifosfamide alone (Castleberry et al. 1994; Pratt 1992; Kellie et al. 1988), and then to combinations of ifosfamide with etoposide (Watts 1992; Kung et al. 1993) or with carboplatin with or without etoposide (Goorin et al. 1995; Alvarado et al. 1997) or with continuous infusion doxorubicin, cisplatin, and etoposide (Campbell et al. 1993; Fernandez et al. 2000). These studies resulted in the incorporation of ifosfamide subsequently into multiple induction regimens (Pinkerton et al. 1990; Olgun et al. 2003; Grupp et al. 2000). Since exposure to alkylating agents at high doses is now widely used in both induction and consolidation regimens for neuroblastoma, and since many patients may already have impairment of renal function due to surgery and prior cisplatin, ifosfamide may be currently less useful than cyclophosphamide as a treatment of relapse.

12.3.1.2 Melphalan Combined with Buthionine Sulfoximine

Since therapy for neuroblastoma relies heavily upon alkylating agents and acquired alkylator resistance likely contributes to recurrent disease, drugs that improve response to alkylating agents may be useful in resistant disease. Glutathione (GSH) is a ubiquitous, intracellular thiol containing tri-peptide that, along with its associated enzymes, plays a critical role in cell growth and metabolism, by maintaining the redox potential of the intracellular environment (Tew 1994; Stokes et al. 2000). Buthionine sulfoximine (BSO), a selective inhibitor of γ-glutamylcysteine synthetase (γ-GCS), the rate-limiting enzyme in GSH synthesis, can enhance alkylator anti-tumor efficacy in a variety of solid tumors. In vitro data have shown BSO to have significant single-agent cytotoxicity against neuroblastoma (Anderson et al. 1997, 1999). Pre-treatment of neuroblastoma cell lines with only 10 μM BSO for 24 h synergistically enhanced the cytotoxicity of 10 μM melphalan by 1–2 logs of cell kill (Anderson et al. 1997). Promising results have been found in adult trials for ovarian cancer, small cell lung cancer, and melanoma, using continuous infusion of BSO and non-myeloablative doses of melphalan, with myelosuppression as the main toxicity (Bailey et al. 1997; O'Dwyer et al. 1992; Yao et al. 1993).

A pilot study of BSO (3 g/m^2 bolus followed by a 72-h continuous infusion (CI) of 0.75–1.0 gm/m^2 h^{-1}) and L-PAM (15 mg/m^2 bolus at hour 48 of BSO infusion) was carried out in 32 patients with recurrent neuroblastoma (Anderson et al. 1998). Of 31 evaluable patients, there were 7 partial responses (PR), 2 minor responses (MR), 9 stable disease (SD), and 13 patients with progressive disease (PD). Nearly all patients experienced grade-3 leukopenia and thrombocytopenia, plus grade-2 nausea. There were two toxic deaths on study secondary to renal and CNS toxicity. At autopsy, both children had evidence of mid-brain edema and eosinophilic necrosis of the pons. Other patients on study showed no consistent pattern of impending renal/neurologic toxicity (Anderson et al. 1998). A phase-I study of BSO with melphalan is underway in the New Approaches to Neuroblastoma Therapy (NANT) consortium (N9902), which increases the melphalan to myeloablative doses with peripheral blood stem-cell support, while holding the BSO infusion constant, with close monitoring for possible renal or neurologic toxicity.

12.3.1.3 Platinum Compounds

Newer platinum derivatives with differing toxicity profiles have also been tested. Initially, carboplatin was tested in an attempt to reduce the nephrotoxicity of cisplatin and in the hope of non-cross-resistance. The drug showed excellent activity in phase-I and phase-II trials (Ettinger et al. 1994), in newly diagnosed patients in a phase-II window study (Castleberry et al. 1994), and in combination with etoposide (Frappaz et al. 1992). A recent phase-II trial combined cisplatin with carboplatin in relapsed patients, and showed a 42% response rate (Frappaz et al. 1998). Since myelosuppression is a prominent toxicity of carboplatin, several trials were then done incorporating high-dose carboplatin into regimens utilizing hematopoietic stem-cell infusion (Matthay et al. 1999; Kreissman et al. 1997; Park et al. 2000). Iproplatin produced a 67% response rate in newly diagnosed patients in a phase-II window (Castleberry et al. 1994). Current protocols are open to test oxaliplatin, a derivative with decreased nephrotoxicity, which showed activity in neuroblastoma in preclinical testing, and is apparently non-cross-resistant with cisplatin and carboplatin (Riccardi et al. 1999; Bleiberg 1998).

12.3.1.4 Temozolomide

Temozolomide, an imidazotetrazine prodrug, is an alkylating agent that mediates its cytotoxic effects via O(6)-methylguanine adducts in DNA and their recognition and processing by the post-replication mismatch repair system. Temozolomide is similar to dacarbazine (DTIC) in that they share the same active metabolite; however, activation of the parent drug is spontaneous with temozolomide and not dependent on enzymatic activity, as is the case with dacarbazine. Temozolomide has excellent oral bioavailability with a single-agent MTD of 200–215 mg/m^2 day^{-1} when given to pediatric patients on a 5-day schedule in 28-day cycles, with the dose-limiting toxicity being neutropenia and thrombocytopenia. Temozolomide readily crosses the blood-brain barrier, and has been proven to be active against a variety of brain tumors. Adult phase-II trials have shown response rates as high as 35–50% using temozolomide for recurrent high-grade glioma (Yung et al. 1999), leading to FDA approval for this indication. In addition to activity against brain tumors, temozolomide also appears to have modest activity against mouse models of non-CNS solid tumors, including neuroblastoma (Middlemas et al. 2000; Houghton et al. 2000). In a phase-II study recently reported in abstract form, 27 pediatric patients with refractory non-CNS solid tumors were treated with temozolomide 215 mg/m^2 day^{-1} in 5-day courses. Although no objective imaging responses were observed, two isolated bone marrow responses were noted in 13 evaluable neuroblastoma patients, of whom 10 (77%) had stable disease lasting a median of 7 months (Donfrancesco et al. 2004).

In addition to the single-agent activity, the combination of temozolomide and irinotecan is attractive because of non-overlapping toxicities and the significant therapeutic synergy demonstrated by Houghton et al. (2000) in preclinical experiments. The combination of sub-therapeutic doses of each drug resulted in complete responses in four different xenograft models of neuroblastoma. The proposed mechanism of synergy is temozolomide-induced methylation causing localization and enhancement of topoisomerase I-DNA cleavage complexes, allowing irinotecan to more effectively stabilize the DNA-enzyme complex and cause cytotoxicity after collision with the advancing replication fork (Pourquier et al. 2001). Interestingly, the synergy seen in the mouse models appeared to be partly independent of the DNA repair phenotype of tumor tissue, including *p53* status (Houghton et al. 2000). This observation is important in light of the frequency of acquired *p53* mutations in neuroblastoma cell lines established at the time of relapse (Keshelava et al. 2000a). A recent phase-I study of the combination of intravenous irinotecan and temozolomide in pediatric solid tumors established the MTD as temozolomide 100 mg/m^2 day^{-1} daily for 5 days the first week, with irinotecan, 10 mg/m^2 day^{-1} daily for 5 days $\times$ 2 consecutive weeks. Future studies may incorporate oral rather than intravenous irinotecan, and use an oral antibiotic to prevent the usual irinotecan-induced diarrhea (Takasuna et al. 1996; Cosetti et al. 2002; Furman et al. 2003).

12.3.1.5 Tirapazamine

Tirapazamine (TPZ), a benzotriazine di-*N*-oxide anti-cancer drug activated to a toxic free radical under hypoxic conditions, is the first drug of this class to enter clinical testing (Brown 1998). In preclinical models it has been shown to extend the activity of traditional cytotoxic chemotherapy, presumably by selective killing of the hypoxic fraction of tumor cells (Dorie and Brown 1993). It has been shown to be safe and effective when combined with cisplatin in adults with NSCLC, although patients receiving the combination experienced significantly more nausea and vomiting (Olgun et al. 2003). A pediatric phase-I trial of the tirapazamine/cyclophosphamide combination was just completed in POG (Yung et al. 1999). The MTD for tirapazamine when combined with 1.5 g/m^2 of cyclophosphamide was 325 mg/m^2. The DLT was reversible ototoxicity. There were 2 children who experienced grade-3 reversible ototoxicity at 420 mg/m^2. There were three responses (two in neuroblastoma and one in rhabdomyosarcoma; Aquino et al. 2004).

12.3.2 Topoisomerase Inhibitors

Topoisomerase-I and topoisomerase-II inhibitors were the next chemotherapy class to be investigated for treatment of relapsed and newly diagnosed neuroblastoma. Etoposide, a topoisomerase-II inhibitor, as detailed above, has been incorporated into relapse and primary treatment regimens for the past two decades, and is quite effective incorporated into regimens for newly diagnosed neuroblastoma (see Chap. 11). Unfortunately, a significant proportion of cell lines obtained from patients after relapse have demonstrated resistance to this agent, even when cell lines from the same patient obtained at diagnosis were sensitive. Furthermore, cross-resistance with other topoisomerase inhibitors, the camptothecins topotecan and irinotecan, was demonstrated in these cell lines (Keshelava et al. 2000b). Nonetheless, up to 10–15% of children with relapsed neuroblastoma could achieve disease stabilization or partial remission with chronic administration of oral etoposide (Davidson et al. 1997; Kushner et al. 1999; Ng et al. 2000; Schiavetti et al. 2001). Camptothecin is a naturally occurring cytotoxic alkaloid that targets topoisomerase I, a nuclear enzyme that reduces the torsional stress of supercoiled DNA during the replication, recombination, transcription, and repair of DNA. Topotecan and irinotecan are synthetic analogues developed for parenteral administration of the active lactone form of the compound (Garcia-Carbonero and Supko 2002).

12.3.2.1 Irinotecan

Other camptothecins under investigation include irinotecan, a prodrug that undergoes enzymatic conversion to the biologically active metabolite 7-ethyl-10-hydroxy-camptothecin (Garcia-Carbonero and Supko 2002). Irinotecan has shown efficacy in preclinical studies (Thompson et al. 1997; Komuro et al. 1994; Vassal et al. 1996; Shitara et al. 2003) and produced responses in refractory neuroblastoma (Shitara et al. 2003; Furman et al. 1999). Whereas the predominant toxicity of topotecan is myelosuppression, that of irinotecan is diarrhea (Furman et al. 1999; Rowinsky and Verweij 1997). It is usually administered intravenously, but trials of oral irinotecan are currently underway. As mentioned above, laboratory studies in neuroblastoma cell lines suggest that lines which are resistant to either etoposide or topotecan are also likely to be resistant to irinotecan (Keshelava et al. 2000b), although another study showed that irinotecan was effective in a xenograft model of neuroblastoma that was resistant to etoposide (Vassal et al. 1996). This drug has also been extensively studied in adult tumors, both alone and in combination with other chemotherapy. It has not yet been shown in human studies of neuroblastoma whether it is non-cross-resistant or in any way more advantageous than topotecan. Other camptothecin analogues are in various stages of clinical development, including 9-aminocamptothecin, 9-nitrocamptothecin, 7-(4-methylpiperazinomethylene)-10,11-ethylenedioxy-20(S)-camptothecin, exatecan mesylate, and karenitecin (Garcia-Carbonero and Supko 2002).

12.3.2.2 Topotecan

Multiple phase-I and phase-II single-agent studies have tested topotecan in neuroblastoma, using either a continuous 72-h infusion regimen (Pratt et al. 1994; Blaney et al. 1998) or a daily 1-h infusion for 5 days (Tubergen et al. 1996; Kretschmar et al. 1995; Nitschke et al. 1998; Langler et al. 2002). Responses were reported with both schedules in the phase-I studies, but in the phase-II studies there were no responses with the 72-h continuous infusion, though the response rate was significant in both relapsed patients (10–20%) and in a phase-II window using the 5-day schedule in newly diagnosed patients (37%). Oral topotecan has also been tested with some modest responses (Garcia-Carbonero and Supko 2002; Kramer et al. 2003; Zamboni et al. 1999). Topotecan in combination regimens with other agents active in neuroblastoma, such as cyclophosphamide, cisplatin, and etoposide, have been reported. A phase-I study of topotecan with cyclophosphamide showed that the maximum tolerated dose of topotecan was 0.75 $mg/m^2\ day^{-1}$ when given with a daily dose of 250 $mg/m^2\ day^{-1}$ of cyclophosphamide for 5 days (Saylors et al. 1998). A phase-II window study showed a significant response rate in newly diagnosed patients, and the results are pending for a recently completed randomized study (P9462) in the Children's Oncology Group in relapse patients, comparing topotecan alone at 2 $mg/m^2\ day^{-1}$ to the combined regimen of cyclophosphamide with topotecan (Frantz et al. 2004). Preclinical studies suggest that other cytotoxic agents, such as vincristine (Thompson et al. 1999) or MGI114 (iludin; Weitman et al. 2000), might provide synergistic cytotoxicity with topotecan. A few studies have investigated high-dose regimens incorporating topotecan with thiotepa and carboplatin using stem-cell support, but the dose of topotecan could not be substantially escalated in this regimen beyond standard dose due to mucositis (Park et al. 2000; Kushner et al. 2001). It is possible that further escalation of topotecan in combinations with other agents with less extra-hematopoietic toxicity, such as cyclophosphamide, may be possible with autologous stem-cell support.

12.3.2.3 Pyrazoloacridine

Pyrazoloacridine (PZA), a DNA intercalator, is a rationally synthesized acridine derivative that has been shown to have a broad spectrum of activity against tumor cells in vitro and in vivo (Jackson et al. 1990; LoRusso et al. 1990; Sebolt et al. 1987). Pyrazoloacridine binds nucleic acids (preferentially ribonucleic acid) and inhibits the activity of topoisomerase I and II, causing DNA fragmentation, and thus DNA strand breaks. It is effective against cells in a hypoxic environment as well as the normal oxygen environment, and it is equally effective in cycling and non-cycling cells (Cole 1990; Adjei et al. 1998). It has the further advantage of activity in cells that over-express P-glycoprotein or MRP, as well as in cells that have lost topoisomerase I or II (Cole 1990; Adjei et al. 1998; Sebolt et al. 1989). Preclinical data suggest that prolonged exposure to PZA may increase cytotoxicity (Grem et al. 1996). A recent in vitro study of resistant neuroblastoma cell lines showed that PZA effectively induced cytotoxicity in multi-drug-resistant neuroblastoma cell lines, as well as in drug-resistant p53 non-functional neuroblastoma cell lines. Pyrazoloacridine sensitivity could be shown even under hypoxic conditions, but only with PZA exposure times that exceeded those tested in previous clinical trials. The in vitro data demonstrated that PZA cytotoxicity is dose- and time dependent (Keshelava et al. 2003). Phase-I and phase-II clinical studies have been conducted, mostly using a short infusion schedule of <6 h, with hematologic toxicity as the main complication. Despite occasional reports of responses, the overall results in pediatric phase-II trials have been disappointing and failed to confirm the anti-cancer activity found in preclinical models (Berg et al. 2000). A possible explanation is that adequate PZA dose levels in humans were not achieved (Berg et al. 1998; LoRusso et al. 1995; Rowinsky et al. 1995). In children and young adults where 640 mg/m^2 of PZA was administered as a 1- or 24-h infusion (Berg et al. 1998), myelosuppression was the dose-limiting toxicity, in contrast to neurotoxicity in the adults.

12.3.2.4 Rebeccamycin

Indolocarbazoles are another group of topoisomerase-I inhibitors, of which rebeccamycin, a naturally occurring anti-tumor antibiotic, derived from an actinomycete. In addition to their action on DNA, rebeccamycin analogues may inhibit the SR kinase activity of topoisomerase I and therefore constitute a unique family of topoisomerase-I poisons quite different from the well-known camptothecins (Prudhomme 2000). In vitro studies support activity in neuroblastoma (Weitman et al. 1998; Marminon et al. 2003). Dose-limiting toxicity in both adults and children in phase-I studies was myelosuppression (Dowlati et al. 2001; Langevin et al. 2003). A phase-II study in pediatric solid tumors is currently ongoing at MSKCC and in the COG.

12.4 Tumor-Targeted Biologic Agents

12.4.1 Retinoids

For information on tumor-targeted biologic agents, including retinoids, see Chap. 15.

12.4.2 Tyrosine Kinase Inhibitors

c-kit has been shown to be expressed in some neuroblastoma cell lines, preferentially those with *MYCN* amplification, and therefore growth inhibitory activity of Gleevec has been demonstrated, both in vitro (Vitali et al. 2003) and in xenograft models (Beppu et al. 2004), leading to testing in pediatric phase-II studies. Another tyrosine kinase inhibitor in clinical testing is CEP-701, a selective inhibitor of several cell-surface receptor-linked tyrosine kinases, with highest affinity and specificity for the Trk receptors. The BDNF/TrkB signaling pathway is a key autocrine survival mechanism for neuroblastomas in patients with high-risk disease, where TrkB is over-expressed (Suzuki et al. 1993; Nakagawara et al. 1994). CEP-701 has high oral bioavailability and potently inhibits all three Trk tyrosine kinases with IC50 values of 3±1 nM (George et al. 1999). CEP-701 also inhibits VEGFR and PDGFR kinase activity, and inhibits the hematopoietic receptor, FLT-3, but has little inhibitory activity against other receptor tyrosine kinases (e.g., EGFR kinase). Targeted inhibition of this pathway has been proven efficacious in preclinical models of human neuroblastoma (Ho et al. 2002; Evans et al. 1999). Ongoing clinical trials of CEP-701 in adult patients with refractory acute myeloid leukemia have shown the drug to be relatively well tolerated, an MTD of 60 mg twice daily has been defined, and biologic and clinical activity has been shown (Smith et al. 2004). A phase-I trial in children with refractory neuroblastoma is ongoing in NANT.

12.4.3 Modulators of Apoptotic Pathway and Angiogenesis

Resistance of tumors to treatment with cytotoxic drugs, irradiation, or immunotherapy may be due to disrupted apoptosis programs.

12.4.3.1 Anti-Angiogenic Agents

Preclinical data have been published supporting the importance of angiogenesis and invasion in progression and prognosis of neuroblastoma (see Chap. 16). An initial report on 50 human tumor samples provided data that increased tumor vascularity correlated with a poorer prognosis (Meitar et al. 1996), though this was contradicted by a later Spanish report (Canete et al. 2000). High-risk neuroblastomas over-express the $\alpha_v\beta$ integrin, an endothelial transmembrane receptor for neovascular proliferation, which can be blocked with a monoclonal antibody, vitaxin, or an RGD peptide, resulting in increased ceramide production and endothelial cell death (Erdreich-Epstein et al. 2000). Phase-I trials of both the monoclonal antibody and the peptide, cilengitide, have shown promise in adult cancers (Eskens et al. 2003; Tucker 2003). Matrix metalloproteinases, MMP-2, and MMP-9, have a key role in invasion and metastasis, and are over-expressed in the stroma of high-risk neuroblastoma (Sugiura et al. 1998; Ara et al. 1998; Bjornland et al. 2001). In vivo xenograft studies in neuroblastoma have shown that inhibitors of MMPs can decrease angiogenesis and prolong survival (Chantrain et al. 2004). A number of inhibitors are currently in clinical testing, with a few positive results in adult cancers (Ramnath and Creaven 2004). Thalidomide is another agent with antiangiogenic actions in neuroblastoma (Kerbel et al. 2000; Kaicker et al. 2003) currently in clinical cancer trials (Fine et al. 2000, 2003). To date, no large-scale trial of anti-angiogenic or anti-invasion agents has been accomplished in neuroblastoma, although as some of these agents become available and have completed phase-I testing in adults, they will be appropriate for further trials in children.

12.4.3.2 Arsenic Trioxide

Multiple in vitro studies suggest activity of arsenic trioxide against neuroblastoma cell lines, through activation of apoptosis, and possible by differentiation and other mechanisms (Akao et al. 1999; Karlsson et al. 2004; Ora et al. 2000; Carre et al. 2002; Wang 2001). Clinical trials have shown good activity in acute promyelocytic leukemia, and are ongoing in neuroblastoma.

12.4.3.3 Demethylating Agents

Caspase-8 expression acts as a key determinant of sensitivity for apoptosis induced by death-inducing ligands or cytotoxic drugs. Caspase 8 has been shown to be preferentially silenced in neuroblastoma (Teitz et al. 2000). In tumor cell lines resistant to TRAIL, anti-CD95 or TNF-alpha, caspase-8 protein and mRNA expression was decreased or absent without caspase-8 gene loss. Methylation-specific PCR revealed hypermethylation of caspase-8 regulatory sequences in cells with impaired caspase-8 expression. Treatment with the demethylation agent 5-Aza-2'-deoxycytidine (decitabine) reversed hypermethylation of caspase-8 resulting in restoration of caspase-8 expression and recruitment and activation of caspase-8 for drug-induced apoptosis (Fulda et al. 2001; Eggert et al. 2001). The use of a demethylating agent in combination with chemotherapy is being tested in a phase-I trial in the COG.

12.4.3.4 Histone Deacetylase Inhibitors

A dynamic equilibrium of histone acetyltransferase and histone deacetylase (HDAC) controls the level of acetylated histones in nuclear chromatin. By inducing acetylation of the nuclear histones H3 and H4, HDAC inhibitors (HDACI) alter chromatin structure, affecting transcription of several genes, and resulting in growth arrest, differentiation, and apoptosis of tumor cells (Kuo and Allis 1998). Deregulation of histone acetylation has been implicated in the development of several types of cancer. Genes that encode HAT enzymes are translocated, amplified, over-expressed, and/or mutated in various cancers. Two closely related HATs, CBP and p300, are altered in some tumors by either mutation or translocation. A number of new compounds have been developed which inhibit HDAC activity. The best-known examples of this class of agents are the butyrates; however, the butyrates have a short plasma half-life and it is difficult to achieve therapeutic concentrations of butyrates in the plasma. Other compounds that have been developed more recently include depsipeptide (FK-228; Furumai et al. 2002), CBHA, suberoylanilide hydroxamic acid (SAHA), oxamflatin, depudecin, and MS-275 (Yoshida et al. 2001; Marks et al. 2004).

12.5 Immunologic Therapy

12.5.1 Anti-GD2

Multiple approaches are currently under investigation in phase-I, phase-II, and phase-III studies based on antibody targeting of the GD2 ganglioside expressed in >95% of neuroblastoma (see Chap. 14). Treatment with either murine or chimeric anti-GD2 antibody, with or without cytokines, or conjugated to iodine-131, has shown promise for minimal residual and bone marrow disease in refractory and newly diagnosed patients, with responses in phase-I and phase-II studies of 10–20% (Frost et al. 1997; Uttenreuther-Fischer et al. 1995; Handgretinger et al. 1995; Hank et al. 1994; Cheung et al. 1987, 1989; Saleh et al. 1992; Yu et al. 1997; Ozkaynak et al. 1998). A phase-III randomized trial is currently underway in the COG for treatment of minimal residual disease following myeloablative therapy. Current trials in refractory disease are testing the humanized anti-GD2, Hu14.18, covalently linked to interleukin-2 (IL-2; immunocytokine), or use with an immunologic enhancer such as glucan (Cheung and Modak 2002). An anti-idiotype vaccine to anti-GD2, using the monoclonal antibody 1A7 with adjuvant, has completed phase-I testing in neuroblastoma, with evidence of immunologic response.

12.5.2 Interleukins

Interleukin-2 is the most extensively investigated cytokine in clinical use at present. Interleukin-2 enhances the proliferation, cytokine production, and cytolytic activity of T and NK/LAK cell populations, various aspects of monocyte/macrophage function and global measures of immune responsiveness in vivo (Hladik et al. 1994; Foa et al. 1992; Higashi et al. 1991; Verstovsek et al. 1995; Nishimura et al. 1992; Cox et al. 1992). IL-2 has demonstrated anti-tumor activity in neuroblastoma (Lode et al. 1997) and may also have synergy when used in combination with IFN-γ to treat murine tumors, including neuroblastoma (Sigal et al. 1991). A total of 15 studies have reported on the use of IL-2 to treat pediatric patients with solid tumors, including over 100 patients with neuroblastoma (Frost et al. 1997; Negrier et al. 1991; Pardo et al. 1996; Valteau-Couanet et al. 1995; Bauer et al. 1995; Chien and Hsieh 1990; Nasr et al. 1989; Pais et al. 1992; Favrot et al. 1990; Truitt et al. 1992; Ribeiro et al. 1993; Roper et al. 1992; Toren et al. 2000; Pession et al. 1998). The majority of these early studies evaluated the use of chronic, intermittent dosing of IL-2 delivered as an intravenous bolus over periods ranging from 15 min to 2 h. Fever, vascular leak, and hypotension are common side effects, seen more frequently at the higher intravenous dosing schedules.

IL-2 alone has had little activity in relapsed bulky disease in any solid tumor other than renal cell carcinoma (Bauer et al. 1995), and has therefore been more extensively tested in the post-transplant setting. For relapsed disease, IL-2 may be more effective in combination with other immunotherapeutic agents, such as the anti-GD2 antibody or other cytokines. Recent preclinical evidence suggests that in combination, IL-12 with IL-2 may possess potent immunomodulatory and anti-tumor activity that exceeds the effect of either agent alone. IL-12 and IL-2 reciprocally upregulate the expression of their respective receptors (Bacon et al. 1995; Desai et al. 1992; Yanagida et al. 1994) and can greatly enhance T and/or NK cell proliferation, cytokine production, and cytolytic function. Systemic administration of IL-12 in combination with intermittent, weekly doses of IL-2 (pulse IL-2) is not only well tolerated, but can induce rapid and complete regression of established primary and/or metastatic tumor in several murine models (Wigginton et al. 1996, 2001a,b). Several reports have also demonstrated that IL-12 gene therapy administered alone or in conjunction with tumor-targeted IL-2 possesses anti-tumor activity in transplantable murine neuroblastoma tumor models (Lode et al. 1999; Davidoff et al. 1999). Based on preclinical data of the combination therapy in murine neuroblastoma models and the adult human trial data, a phase-I dose escalation trial of IL-12 combined with IL-2 is now underway in the NANT consortium.

12.5.3 Vaccines

Preclinical and clinical trials are in progress to try to further enhance the specificity and efficacy of cytokines by using autologous tumor cells transfected with cytokines such as IL-2 (Bowman et al. 1998a,b), IL-12, GM-CSF, interferon gamma (Bausero et al. 1996; Yoshida et al. 1999), or lymphotactin as vaccines to stimulate the host immune response to the neuroblastoma. Other vaccine approaches include the use of DNA vaccines (Pertl et al. 2003), or dendritic cell vaccines (Chen et al. 2003).

12.6 ^{131}I-Metaiodobenzylguanidine

^{131}I-Metaiodobenzylguanidine (MIBG) is a guanethidine derivative that is structurally similar to norepinephrine, and therefore concentrates in the neurosecretory granules of catecholamine-secreting cells. Radiolabeled MIBG provides very sensitive and specific visualization of primary and metastatic neuroblastoma by scintigraphy (Shulkin and Shapiro 1998). In an attempt to deliver higher doses of tumor-specific radiotherapy and avoid normal organ toxicity, iodine-131 MIBG therapy has been used in pilot trials since the mid 1980s, with more than 500 children reported in the literature. Initially, it was shown to induce 30–40% response rate in highly refractory relapsed patients, without significant non-hematologic toxicity (Klingebiel et al. 1991; Matthay et al. 1998; Voute et al. 1991). At low and moderate doses, up to 12 mCi/kg of ^{131}I-MIBG, the main toxicity has been thrombocytopenia, usually self-limited. Phase-I dose escalation studies showed that higher doses, up to 18 mCi/kg, could be administered with bone marrow or peripheral blood stem-cell support to mitigate the neutropenia and thrombocytopenia, but without clinical organ toxicity, excepting a 10–15% incidence of hypothyroidism due to uptake of some free iodide by the thyroid gland (Matthay et al. 1998; Lashford et al. 1992). There are a few reports of patients with secondary leukemia developing after MIBG therapy, but the estimated risk of this problem at 5 years post-therapy is only 4%, lower than with some chemotherapy regimens (Garaventa et al. 2003; Weiss et al. 2003). Despite a number of clinical studies worldwide, dose response to ^{131}I-MIBG has not been firmly established. Recent studies are investigating the use of low dose ^{131}I-MIBG at diagnosis prior to surgical resection (Troncone et al. 1995), or in combination with standard (Mastrangelo et al. 2001)or high-dose myeloablative chemotherapy (Yanik et al. 2002; Klingebiel et al. 1998). New phase-I studies are currently open in the NANT to test the use of double infusion of ^{131}I-MIBG with stem-cell support or further combination with myeloablative chemotherapy and stem cells. Further investigations are required to determine the optimal timing and use of this targeted approach.

12.7 Conclusion

Refractory and relapsed neuroblastoma is very difficult to eradicate, due to multiple mechanisms of drug resistance. Above all, compassion and consideration for quality of life must be incorporated into the therapeutic goals for the child with refractory neuroblastoma. Currently established therapies include only a few chemotherapeutic and targeted agents, and of these, only the chemotherapy agents are commercially available. Future success depends on rational preclinical in vitro and in vivo testing of new agents and combinations in panels of appropriate neuroblastoma cell lines and tumors, followed by careful clinical trials. Judicious selection of trials depending on the type of relapse, and willing cooperation of patients and parents after careful explanation of the goals of the study are essential to improve survival in this disease.

References

Adjei AA, Charron M, Rowinsky EK et al. (1998) Effect of pyrazoloacridine (NSC 366140) on DNA topoisomerases I and II. Clin Cancer Res 4:683–691

Akao Y, Nakagawa Y, Akiyama K (1999) Arsenic trioxide induces apoptosis in neuroblastoma cell lines through the activation of caspase 3 in vitro. FEBS Lett 455:59–62

Alvarado CS, Kretschmar C, Joshi VV et al. (1997) Chemotherapy for patients with recurrent or refractory neuroblastoma: a POG phase II study. J Pediatr Hematol Oncol 19:62–67

Anderson CP, Tsai JM, Chan WW et al. (1997) Buthionine sulfoximine (BSO) is cytotoxic and enhances the activity of melphalan for human neuroblastoma cell lines. Eur J Cancer 33:2016–2019

Anderson CP, Seeger RC, Matthay KK, Neglia JP, Bailey HH, Reynolds CP (1998) Pilot study of buthionine sulfoximine (BSO) and melphalan (L-PAM) in children with recurrent neuroblastoma. Proc Am Soc Clin Oncol 17:531a

Anderson CP, Tsai JM, Meek WE et al. (1999) Depletion of glutathione by buthionine sulfoxine is cytotoxic for human neuroblastoma cell lines via apoptosis. Exp Cell Res 246: 183–192

Aquino VM, Weitman SD, Winick NJ et al. (2004) Phase I trial of tirapazamine and cyclophosphamide in children with refractory solid tumors: a pediatric oncology group study. J Clin Oncol 22:1413–1419

Ara T, Fukuzawa M, Kusafuka T et al. (1998) Immunohistochemical expression of MMP-2, MMP-9, and TIMP-2 in neuroblastoma: association with tumor progression and clinical outcome. J Pediatr Surg 33:1272–1278

Bacon CM, McVicar DW, Ortaldo JR, Rees RC, O'Shea JJ, Johnston JA (1995) Interleukin 12 (IL-12) induces tyrosine phosphorylation of JAK2 and TYK2: differential use of Janus family tyrosine kinases by IL-2 and IL-12. J Exp Med 181: 399–404

Bailey HH, Ripple G, Tutsch KD et al. (1997) Phase I study of continuous-infusion L-S,R-buthionine sulfoximine with intravenous melphalan. J Natl Cancer Inst 89:1789–1796

Bauer M, Reaman GH, Hank JA et al. (1995) A phase II trial of human recombinant interleukin-2 administered as a 4-day continuous infusion for children with refractory neuroblastoma, non-Hodgkin's lymphoma, sarcoma, renal cell carcinoma, and malignant melanoma. A Childrens Cancer Group study. Cancer 75:2959–2965

Bausero MA, Panoskaltsis-Mortari A, Blazar BR, Katsanis E (1996) Effective immunization against neuroblastoma using double-transduced tumor cells secreting GM-CSF and interferon-gamma. J Immunother Emphasis Tumor Immunol 19:113–124

Beppu K, Jaboine J, Merchant MS, Mackall CL, Thiele CJ (2004) Effect of imatinib mesylate on neuroblastoma tumorigenesis and vascular endothelial growth factor expression. J Natl Cancer Inst 96:46–55

Berg SL, Blaney SM, Adamson PC et al. (1998) Phase I trial and pharmacokinetic study of pyrazoloacridine in children and young adults with refractory cancers. J Clin Oncol 16: 181–186

Berg SL, Blaney SM, Sullivan J, Bernstein M, Dubowy R, Harris MB (2000) Phase II trial of pyrazoloacridine in children with solid tumors: a Pediatric Oncology Group phase II study. J Pediatr Hematol Oncol 22:506–509

Bjornland K, Bratland A, Rugnes E et al. (2001) Expression of matrix metalloproteinases and the metastasis-associated gene S100A4 in human neuroblastoma and primitive neuroectodermal tumor cells. J Pediatr Surg 36:1040–1044

Blanc E, Goldschneider D, Ferrandis E, Barrois M, Le Roux G, Leonce S, Douc-Rasy S, Benard J, Raguenez G (2003) MYCN enhances P-gp/MDR1 gene expression in the human metastatic neuroblastoma IGR-N-91 model. Am J Pathol 163:321–331

Blaney SM, Needle MN, Gillespie A et al. (1998) Phase II trial of topotecan administered as 72-hour continuous infusion in children with refractory solid tumors: a collaborative Pediatric Branch, National Cancer Institute, and Children's Cancer Group Study. Clin Cancer Res 4:357–360

Bleiberg H (1998) Oxaliplatin (L-OHP): a new reality in colorectal cancer. Br J Cancer 77 (Suppl 4):1–3

Bowman L, Grossmann M, Rill D et al. (1998) IL-2 adenovector-transduced autologous tumor cells induce antitumor immune responses in patients with neuroblastoma. Blood 92:1941–1949

Bowman LC, Grossmann M, Rill D et al. (1998) Interleukin-2 gene-modified allogeneic tumor cells for treatment of relapsed neuroblastoma. Hum Gene Ther 9:1303–1311

Brodeur GM, Pritchard J, Berthold F et al. (1993) Revisions of the international criteria for neuroblastoma diagnosis, staging, and response to treatment (see comments). J Clin Oncol 11:1466–1477

Brown JM (1998) Exploiting tumour hypoxia and overcoming mutant p53 with tirapazamine. Br J Cancer 77 (Suppl 4): 12–14

Burchill SA, Lewis IJ, Abrams KR et al. (2001) Circulating neuroblastoma cells detected by reverse transcriptase polymerase chain reaction for tyrosine hydroxylase mRNA are an independent poor prognostic indicator in stage 4 neuroblastoma in children over 1 year. J Clin Oncol 19:1795–1801

Campbell LA, Seeger RC, Harris RE, Villablanca JG, Matthay KK (1993) Escalating dose of continuous infusion combination chemotherapy for refractory neuroblastoma. J Clin Oncol 11:623–629

Canete A, Navarro S, Bermudez J, Pellin A, Castel V, Llombart-Bosch A (2000) Angiogenesis in neuroblastoma: relationship to survival and other prognostic factors in a cohort of neuroblastoma patients. J Clin Oncol 18:27–34

Carre M, Carles G, Andre N et al. (2002) Involvement of microtubules and mitochondria in the antagonism of arsenic trioxide on paclitaxel-induced apoptosis. Biochem Pharmacol 63:1831–1842

Castleberry RP, Cantor AB, Green AA et al. (1994) Phase II investigational window using carboplatin, iproplatin, ifosfamide, and epirubicin in children with untreated disseminated neuroblastoma: a Pediatric Oncology Group study (see comments). J Clin Oncol 12:1616–1620

Chantrain CF, Shimada H, Jodele S et al. (2004) Stromal matrix metalloproteinase-9 regulates the vascular architecture in neuroblastoma by promoting pericyte recruitment. Cancer Res 64:1675–1686

Chen X, Doffek K, Sugg SL, Shilyansky J (2003) Neuroblastoma cells inhibit the immunostimulatory function of dendritic cells. J Pediatr Surg 38:901–905

Cheung IY, Lo Piccolo MS, Kushner BH, Kramer K, Cheung NK (2003) Quantitation of GD2 synthase mRNA by real-time reverse transcriptase polymerase chain reaction: clinical utility in evaluating adjuvant therapy in neuroblastoma. J Clin Oncol 21:1087–1093

Cheung NK, Modak S (2002) Oral (1->3),(1->4)-beta-D-glucan synergizes with antiganglioside GD2 monoclonal antibody 3F8 in the therapy of neuroblastoma. Clin Cancer Res 8:1217–1223

Cheung NK, Lazarus H, Miraldi FD et al. (1987) Ganglioside GD2 specific monoclonal antibody 3F8: a phase I study in patients with neuroblastoma and malignant melanoma (see comments). J Clin Oncol 5:1430–1440

Cheung NK, Munn D, Kushner BH, Usmani N, Yeh SD (1989) Targeted radiotherapy and immunotherapy of human neuroblastoma with GD2 specific monoclonal antibodies. Int J Rad Appl Instrum [B] 16:111–120

Chien CH, Hsieh KH (1990) Interleukin-2 immunotherapy in children. Pediatrics 86:937–943

Cole SP (1990) Patterns of cross-resistance in a multidrug-resistant small-cell lung carcinoma cell line. Cancer Chemother Pharmacol 26:250–256

Cosetti M, Wexler LH, Calleja E et al. (2002) Irinotecan for pediatric solid tumors: the Memorial Sloan-Kettering experience. J Pediatr Hematol Oncol 24:101–105

Cox GW, Melillo G, Chattopadhyay U, Mullet D, Fertel RH, Varesio L (1992) Tumor necrosis factor-alpha-dependent production of reactive nitrogen intermediates mediates IFN-gamma plus IL-2-induced murine macrophage tumoricidal activity. J Immunol 149:3290–3296

Davidoff AM, Kimbrough SA, Ng CY, Shochat SJ, Vanin EF (1999) Neuroblastoma regression and immunity induced by transgenic expression of interleukin-12. J Pediatr Surg 34:902–907

Davidson A, Gowing R, Lowis S et al. (1997) Phase II study of 21 day schedule oral etoposide in children. New Agents Group of the United Kingdom Children's Cancer Study Group UKCCSG. Eur J Cancer 33:1816–1822

Desai BB, Quinn PM, Wolitzky AG, Mongini PK, Chizzonite R, Gately MK (1992) IL-12 receptor. II. Distribution and regulation of receptor expression. J Immunol 148:3125–3132

Dole M, Nunez G, Merchant AK et al. (1994) Bcl-2 inhibits chemotherapy-induced apoptosis in neuroblastoma. Cancer Res 54:3253–3259

Dole MG, Jasty R, Cooper MJ, Thompson CB, Nunez G, Castle VP (1995) Bcl-xL is expressed in neuroblastoma cells and modulates chemotherapy-induced apoptosis. Cancer Res 55:2576–2582

Donfrancesco A, Jenkner A, Castellano A et al. (2004) Ifosfamide/carboplatin/etoposide (ICE) as front-line, topotecan/cyclophosphamide as second-line and oral temozolomide as third-line treatment for advanced neuroblastoma over one year of age. Acta Paediatr Suppl 93:6–11

Dorie MJ, Brown JM (1993) Tumor-specific, schedule-dependent interaction between tirapazamine (SR 4233) and cisplatin. Cancer Res 53:4633–4636

Dowlati A, Hoppel CL, Ingalls ST et al. (2001) Phase I clinical and pharmacokinetic study of rebeccamycin analog NSC 655649 given daily for five consecutive days. J Clin Oncol 19:2309–2318

DuBois SG, Kalika Y, Lukens JN et al. (1999) Metastatic sites in stage IV and IVS neuroblastoma correlate with age, tumor biology, and survival (see comments). J Pediatr Hematol Oncol 21:181–189

Eggert A, Grotzer MA, Zuzak TJ et al. (2001) Resistance to tumor necrosis factor-related apoptosis-inducing ligand (TRAIL)-induced apoptosis in neuroblastoma cells correlates with a loss of caspase-8 expression. Cancer Res 61:1314–1319

Erdreich-Epstein A, Shimada H, Groshen S et al. (2000) Integrins alpha(v)beta3 and alpha(v)beta5 are expressed by endothelium of high-risk neuroblastoma and their inhibition is associated with increased endogenous ceramide. Cancer Res 60:712–721

Eskens FA, Dumez H, Hoekstra R et al. (2003) Phase I and pharmacokinetic study of continuous twice weekly intravenous administration of Cilengitide (EMD 121974), a novel inhibitor of the integrins alphavbeta3 and alphavbeta5 in patients with advanced solid tumours. Eur J Cancer 39:917–926

Ettinger LJ, Gaynon PS, Krailo MD et al. (1994) A phase II study of carboplatin in children with recurrent or progressive solid tumors. A report from the Childrens Cancer Group. Cancer 73:1297–1301

Evans AE, Kisselbach KD, Yamashiro DJ et al. (1999) Antitumor activity of CEP-751 (KT-6587) on human neuroblastoma and medulloblastoma xenografts. Clin Cancer Res 5:3594–3602

Favrot MC, Michon J, Floret D et al. (1990) Interleukin 2 immunotherapy in children with neuroblastoma after high-dose chemotherapy and autologous bone marrow transplantation. Pediatr Hematol Oncol 7:275–284

Fernandez MC, Krailo MD, Gerbing RR, Matthay KK (2000) A phase I dose escalation of combination chemotherapy with granulocyte-macrophage-colony stimulating factor in patients with neuroblastoma. Cancer 88:2838–2844

Fine HA, Figg WD, Jaeckle K et al. (2000) Phase II trial of the antiangiogenic agent thalidomide in patients with recurrent high-grade gliomas. J Clin Oncol 18:708–715

Fine HA, Wen PY, Maher EA et al. (2003) Phase II trial of thalidomide and carmustine for patients with recurrent high-grade gliomas. J Clin Oncol 21:2299–2304
Foa R, Guarini A, Gansbacher B (1992) IL2 treatment for cancer: from biology to gene therapy. Br J Cancer 66:992–998
Frantz CN, London WB, Diller L, Seeger R, Sawyer K (2004) Recurrent neuroblastoma: Randomized treatment with topotecan+cyclophosphamide (T+C) vs. topotecan alone (T). A POG/CCG Intergroup Study. ASCO, abstract no. 8512
Frappaz D, Michon J, Hartmann O et al. (1992) Etoposide and carboplatin in neuroblastoma: a French Society of Pediatric Oncology phase II study. J Clin Oncol 10:1592–1601
Frappaz D, Bouffet E, Perel Y et al. (1998) Phase II study of cisplatinum and carboplatinum CACIS combination in advanced stage neuroblastomas. Med Pediatr Oncol 30:9–14
Frost JD, Hank JA, Reaman GH et al. (1997) A phase I/IB trial of murine monoclonal anti-GD2 antibody 14.G2a plus interleukin-2 in children with refractory neuroblastoma: a report of the Children's Cancer Group. Cancer 80:317–333
Fulda S, Kufer MU, Meyer E, van Valen F, Dockhorn-Dworniczak B, Debatin KM (2001) Sensitization for death receptor- or drug-induced apoptosis by re-expression of caspase-8 through demethylation or gene transfer. Oncogene 20:5865–5877
Furman WL, Stewart CF, Poquette CA et al. (1999) Direct translation of a protracted irinotecan schedule from a xenograft model to a phase I trial in children. J Clin Oncol 17: 1815–1824
Furman WL, Crews KR, Daw NC et al. (2003) Cefixime enables further dose-escalation of oral irinotecan in pediatric patients with refractory solid tumors. Proc Am Soc Clin Oncol 22:799
Furumai R, Matsuyama A, Kobashi N et al. (2002) FK228 (depsipeptide) as a natural prodrug that inhibits class I histone deacetylases. Cancer Res 62:4916–4921
Garaventa A, Gambini C, Villavecchia G et al. (2003) Second malignancies in children with neuroblastoma after combined treatment with 131I-metaiodobenzylguanidine. Cancer 97:1332–1338
Garcia-Carbonero R, Supko JG (2002) Current perspectives on the clinical experience, pharmacology, and continued development of the camptothecins. Clin Cancer Res 8:641–661
George DJ, Dionne CA, Jani J et al. (1999) Sustained in vivo regression of Dunning H rat prostate cancers treated with combinations of androgen ablation and Trk tyrosine kinase inhibitors, CEP-751 (KT-6587) or CEP-701 (KT-5555). Cancer Res 59:2395–2401
Goorin AM, Harris MB, Inoue S et al. (1995) Ifosfamide/carboplatin/etoposide (ICE) for recurrent malignant solid tumors of childhood: a Pediatric Oncology Group Phase I/II study. J Pediatr Hematol Oncol 17:265–269
Grem JL, Politi PM, Berg SL et al. (1996) Cytotoxicity and DNA damage associated with pyrazoloacridine in MCF-7 breast cancer cells. Biochem Pharmacol 51:1649–1659
Grupp SA, Stern JW, Bunin N et al. (2000) Tandem high-dose therapy in rapid sequence for children with high-risk neuroblastoma. J Clin Oncol 18:2567–2575
Haas-Kogan DA et al. (2002) Impact of radiotherapy for high risk neuroblastoma: a Children's Cancer Group study. J Clin Oncol 56:28–39
Handgretinger R, Anderson K, Lang P et al. (1995) A phase I study of human/mouse chimeric antiganglioside GD2 antibody ch14.18 in patients with neuroblastoma. Eur J Cancer 31A:261–267
Hank JA, Surfus J, Gan J et al. (1994) Treatment of neuroblastoma patients with antiganglioside GD2 antibody plus interleukin-2 induces antibody-dependent cellular cytotoxicity against neuroblastoma detected in vitro. J Immunother 15:29–37
Higashi N, Nishimura Y, Higuchi M, Osawa T (1991) Human monocytes in a long-term culture with interleukin-2 show high tumoricidal activity against various tumor cells. J Immunother 10:247–255
Hiyama E, Hiyama K, Yamaoka H, Sueda T, Reynolds CP, Yokoyama T (2004) Expression profiling of favorable and unfavorable neuroblastomas. Pediatr Surg Int 20:33–38
Hladik F, Tratkiewicz JA, Tilg H et al. (1994) Biologic activity of low dosage IL-2 treatment in vivo. Molecular assessment of cytokine network interaction. J Immunol 153:1449–1454
Ho R, Eggert A, Hishiki T et al. (2002) Resistance to chemotherapy mediated by TrkB in neuroblastomas. Cancer Res 62:6462–6466
Houghton PJ, Stewart CF, Cheshire PJ et al. (2000) Antitumor activity of temozolomide combined with irinotecan is partly independent of O6-methylguanine-DNA methyltransferase and mismatch repair phenotypes in xenograft models. Clin Cancer Res 6:4110–4118
Houghton PJ, Adamson PC, Blaney S et al. (2002) Testing of new agents in childhood cancer preclinical models: meeting summary. Clin Cancer Res 8:3646–3657
Ikeda H et al. (1992) Sites of relapse in patients with neuroblastoma following bone marrow transplantation in relation to preparatory "debulking" treatments. J Pediatr Surg 27:1438–1441
Jackson RC, Sebolt JS, Shillis JL, Leopold WR (1990) The pyrazoloacridines: approaches to the development of a carcinoma-selective cytotoxic agent. Cancer Invest 8:39–47
Kaicker S, McCrudden KW, Beck L et al. (2003) Thalidomide is anti-angiogenic in a xenograft model of neuroblastoma. Int J Oncol 23:1651–1655
Karlsson J, Ora I, Porn-Ares I, Pahlman S (2004) Arsenic trioxide-induced death of neuroblastoma cells involves activation of bax and does not require p53. Clin Cancer Res 10:3179–3188
Kellie SJ, de Kraker J, Lilleyman JS, Bowman A, Pritchard J (1988) Ifosfamide in previously untreated disseminated neuroblastoma. Results of study 3A of the European Neuroblastoma Study Group. Eur J Cancer Clin Oncol 24: 903–908

Kerbel RS, Viloria-Petit A, Klement G, Rak J (2000) 'Accidental' anti-angiogenic drugs. Anti-oncogene directed signal transduction inhibitors and conventional chemotherapeutic agents as examples. Eur J Cancer 36:1248–1257

Keshelava N, Zuo JJ, Waidyaratne NS, Triche TJ, Reynolds CP (2000a) p53 mutations and loss of p53 function confer multidrug resistance in neuroblastoma. Med Pediatr Oncol 35:563–568

Keshelava N, Groshen S, Reynolds CP (2000b) Cross-resistance of topoisomerase I and II inhibitors in neuroblastoma cell lines. Cancer Chemother Pharmacol 45:1–8

Keshelava N, Zuo JJ, Chen P et al. (2001) Loss of p53 function confers high-level multidrug resistance in neuroblastoma cell lines. Cancer Res 61:6185–6193

Keshelava N, Tsao-Wei D, Reynolds CP (2003) Pyrazoloacridine is active in multidrug-resistant neuroblastoma cell lines with nonfunctional p53. Clin Cancer Res 9:3492–3502

Klingebiel T, Bader P, Bares R et al. (1998) Treatment of neuroblastoma stage 4 with 131I-meta-iodo-benzylguanidine, high-dose chemotherapy and immunotherapy. A pilot study. Eur J Cancer 34:1398–1402

Klingebiel T, Berthold F, Treuner J et al. (1991) Metaiodobenzylguanidine (mIBG) in treatment of 47 patients with neuroblastoma: results of the German Neuroblastoma Trial. Med Pediatr Oncol 19:84–88

Komuro H, Li P, Tsuchida Y et al. (1994) Effects of CPT-11 (a unique DNA topoisomerase I inhibitor) on a highly malignant xeno-transplanted neuroblastoma. Med Pediatr Oncol 23:487–492

Kramer K, Kushner B, Heller G, Cheung NK (2001) Neuroblastoma metastatic to the central nervous system. The Memorial Sloan-kettering Cancer Center experience and a literature review. Cancer 91:1510–1519

Kramer K, Kushner BH, Cheung NK (2003) Oral topotecan for refractory and relapsed neuroblastoma: a retrospective analysis. J Pediatr Hematol Oncol 25:601–605

Kreissman SG, Rackoff W, Lee M, Breitfeld PP (1997) High dose cyclophosphamide with carboplatin: a tolerable regimen suitable for dose intensification in children with solid tumors. J Pediatr Hematol Oncol 19:309–312

Kretschmar CS, Kletzel K, Murray K, Smith EI, Marcus R, Castleberry R (1995) Phase II therapy with taxol and topotecan in untreated children (>365 days) with disseminated (INSS stage 4) neuroblastoma (NB). A POG study. Med Pediatr Oncol 24:243

Kung FH, Pratt CB, Vega RA et al. (1993) Ifosfamide/etoposide combination in the treatment of recurrent malignant solid tumors of childhood. A Pediatric Oncology Group Phase II study. Cancer 71:1898–1903

Kuo MH, Allis CD (1998) Roles of histone acetyltransferases and deacetylases in gene regulation. Bioessays 20:615–626

Kushner BH, Cheung NK, Kramer K, Dunkel IJ, Calleja E, Boulad F (2001) Topotecan combined with myeloablative doses of thiotepa and carboplatin for neuroblastoma, brain tumors, and other poor-risk solid tumors in children and young adults. Bone Marrow Transplant 28:551–556

Kushner BH, Kramer K, Cheung NK (2002) Chronic neuroblastoma. Cancer 95:1366–1375

Kushner BH, Kramer K, Cheung NK (1999) Oral etoposide for refractory and relapsed neuroblastoma. J Clin Oncol 17: 3221–3225

Ladenstein R, Lasset C, Hartmann O et al. (1993) Impact of megatherapy on survival after relapse from stage 4 neuroblastoma in patients over 1 year of age at diagnosis: a report from the European Group for Bone Marrow Transplantation. J Clin Oncol 11:2230–2341

Ladenstein R, Philip T, Lasset C et al. (1998) Multivariate analysis of risk factors in stage 4 neuroblastoma patients over the age of one year treated with megatherapy and stem-cell transplantation: a report from the European Bone Marrow Transplantation Solid Tumor Registry. J Clin Oncol 16: 953–965

Langevin AM, Weitman SD, Kuhn JG et al. (2003) Phase I trial of rebeccamycin analog (NSC #655649) in children with refractory solid tumors: a pediatric oncology group study. J Pediatr Hematol Oncol 25:526–533

Langler A, Christaras A, Abshagen K, Krauth K, Hero B, Berthold F (2002) Topotecan in the treatment of refractory neuroblastoma and other malignant tumors in childhood: a phase-II-study. Klin Padiatr 214:153–156

Lashford LS, Lewis IJ, Fielding SL et al. (1992) Phase I/II study of iodine 131 metaiodobenzylguanidine in chemoresistant neuroblastoma: a United Kingdom Children's Cancer Study Group investigation. J Clin Oncol 10:1889–1896

Lode HN, Xiang R, Varki NM, Dolman CS, Gillies SD, Reisfeld RA (1997) Targeted interleukin-2 therapy for spontaneous neuroblastoma metastases to bone marrow. J Natl Cancer Inst 89:1586–1594

Lode HN, Xiang R, Duncan SR, Theofilopoulos AN, Gillies SD, Reisfeld RA (1999) Tumor-targeted IL-2 amplifies T cell-mediated immune response induced by gene therapy with single-chain IL-12. Proc Natl Acad Sci USA 96:8591–8596

LoRusso P, Wozniak AJ, Polin L et al. (1990) Antitumor efficacy of PD115934 (NSC 366140) against solid tumors of mice. Cancer Res 50:4900–4905

LoRusso P, Foster BJ, Poplin E et al. (1995) Phase I clinical trial of pyrazoloacridine NSC366140 (PD115934). Clin Cancer Res 1:1487–1493

Manohar CF, Bray JA, Salwen HR, Madafiglio J, Cheng A, Flemming C, Marshall GM, Norris MD, Haber M, Cohn SL (2004) MYCN-mediated regulation of the MRP1 promoter in human neuroblastoma. Oncogene 23:753–762

Marks PA, Richon VM, Kelly WK, Chiao JH, Miller T (2004) Histone deacetylase inhibitors: development as cancer therapy. Novartis Found Symp 259:269–288

Marminon C, Pierre A, Pfeiffer B et al. (2003) Syntheses and antiproliferative activities of 7-azarebeccamycin analogues bearing one 7-azaindole moiety. J Med Chem 46:609–622

Mastrangelo S, Tornesello A, Diociaiuti L et al. (2001) Treatment of advanced neuroblastoma: feasibility and therapeutic potential of a novel approach combining 131-I-MIBG and multiple drug chemotherapy. Br J Cancer 84:460–464

Matthay KK, Atkinson JB, Stram DO, Selch M, Reynolds CP, Seeger RC (1993) Patterns of relapse after autologous purged bone marrow transplantation for neuroblastoma: a Childrens Cancer Group pilot study. J Clin Oncol 11:2226–2233
Matthay KK, DeSantes K, Hasegawa B et al. (1998) Phase I dose escalation of 131I-metaiodobenzylguanidine with autologous bone marrow support in refractory neuroblastoma. J Clin Oncol 16:229–236
Matthay KK, Villablanca JG, Seeger RC et al. (1999) Treatment of high-risk neuroblastoma with intensive chemotherapy, radiotherapy, autologous bone marrow transplantation, and 13-cis- retinoic acid. Children's Cancer Group. N Engl J Med 341:1165–1173
Matthay KK, Edeline V, Lumbroso J et al. (2003a) Correlation of early metastatic response by 123I-metaiodobenzylguanidine scintigraphy with overall response and event-free survival in stage IV neuroblastoma. J Clin Oncol 21:2486–2491
Matthay KK, Brisse H, Couanet D et al. (2003b) Central nervous system metastases in neuroblastoma: radiologic, clinical, and biologic features in 23 patients. Cancer 98:155–165
Meitar D, Crawford SE, Rademaker AW, Cohn SL (1996) Tumor angiogenesis correlates with metastatic disease, N-myc amplification, and poor outcome in human neuroblastoma. J Clin Oncol 14:405–414
Middlemas DS, Stewart CF, Kirstein MN et al. (2000) Biochemical correlates of temozolomide sensitivity in pediatric solid tumor xenograft models. Clin Cancer Res 6:998–1007
Moss TJ, Cairo M, Santana VM, Weinthal J, Hurvitz C, Bostrom B (1994) Clonogenicity of circulating neuroblastoma cells: implications regarding peripheral blood stem cell transplantation. Blood 83:3085–3089
Nakagawara A, Azar CG, Scavarda NJ, Brodeur GM (1994) Expression and function of TRK-B and BDNF in human neuroblastomas. Mol Cell Biol 14:759–767
Nasr S, McKolanis J, Pais R et al. (1989) A phase I study of interleukin-2 in children with cancer and evaluation of clinical and immunologic status during therapy. A Pediatric Oncology Group Study. Cancer 64:783–788
Negrier S, Michon J, Floret D et al. (1991) Interleukin-2 and lymphokine-activated killer cells in 15 children with advanced metastatic neuroblastoma (published erratum appears in J Clin Oncol 1992, 6:1026). J Clin Oncol 9:1363–1370
Ng A, Taylor GM, Eden OB (2000) Secondary leukemia in a child with neuroblastoma while on oral etoposide: What is the cause? Pediatr Hematol Oncol 17:273–279
Nishimura Y, Higashi N, Tsuji T, Higuchi M, Osawa T (1992) Activation of human monocytes by interleukin-2 and various cytokines. J Immunother 12:90–97
Nitschke R, Parkhurst J, Sullivan J, Harris MB, Bernstein M, Pratt C (1998) Topotecan in pediatric patients with recurrent and progressive solid tumors: a Pediatric Oncology Group phase II study. J Pediatr Hematol Oncol 20:315–318
Norris MD, Bordow SB, Marshall GM, Haber PS, Cohn SL, Haber M (1996) Expression of the gene for multidrug-resistance-associated protein and outcome in patients with neuroblastoma. N Engl J Med 334:231–238
O'Dwyer PJ, Hamilton TC, Young RC et al. (1992) Depletion of glutathione in normal and malignant human cells in vivo by buthionine sulfoximine: clinical and biochemical results. J Natl Cancer Inst 84:264–267
Olgun N, Kansoy S, Aksoylar S et al. (2003) Experience of the Izmir Pediatric Oncology Group on Neuroblastoma: IPOG-NBL-92 Protocol. Pediatr Hematol Oncol 20:211–218
Ora I, Bondesson L, Jonsson C et al. (2000) Arsenic trioxide inhibits neuroblastoma growth in vivo and promotes apoptotic cell death in vitro. Biochem Biophys Res Commun 277:179–185
Ozkaynak MF, Seeger RC, Krailo M, Sondel P, Matthay K, Reaman G (1998) Phase I study of chimeric human/murine anti-GD2 monoclonal antibody (ch14.18) with GM-CSF in children with neuroblastoma immediately post hematopoietic stem cell transplantation (HSCT): a Children's Cancer Group study. Proc Am Soc Clin Oncol 17:532a
Pais RC, Abdel-Mageed A, Ghim TT et al. (1992) Phase I study of recombinant human interleukin-2 for pediatric malignancies: feasibility of outpatient therapy. A Pediatric Oncology Group Study. J Immunother 12:138–146
Pardo N, Marti F, Fraga G et al. (1996) High-dose systemic interleukin-2 therapy in stage IV neuroblastoma for one year after autologous bone marrow transplantation: pilot study. Med Pediatr Oncol 27:534–539
Park JR, Slattery J, Gooley T et al. (2000) Phase I topotecan preparative regimen for high-risk neuroblastoma, high-grade glioma, and refractory/recurrent pediatric solid tumors. Med Pediatr Oncol 35:719–723
Pertl U, Wodrich H, Ruehlmann JM, Gillies SD, Lode HN, Reisfeld RA (2003) Immunotherapy with a posttranscriptionally modified DNA vaccine induces complete protection against metastatic neuroblastoma. Blood 101:649–654
Pession A, Prete A, Locatelli F et al. (1998) Immunotherapy with low-dose recombinant interleukin 2 after high-dose chemotherapy and autologous stem cell transplantation in neuroblastoma. Br J Cancer 78:528–533
Pinkerton CR, Zucker JM, Hartmann O et al. (1990) Short duration, high dose, alternating chemotherapy in metastatic neuroblastoma. (ENSG 3C induction regimen). The European Neuroblastoma Study Group. Br J Cancer 62:319–323
Pourquier P, Waltman JL, Urasaki Y et al. (2001) Topoisomerase I-mediated cytotoxicity of N-methyl-N'-nitro-N-nitrosoguanidine: trapping of topoisomerase I by the O6-methylguanine. Cancer Res 61:53–58
Pratt CB (1992) Current studies of ifosfamide for pediatric solid tumors and leukemia in the United States. Semin Oncol 19:43–49
Pratt CB, Stewart C, Santana VM et al. (1994) Phase I study of topotecan for pediatric patients with malignant solid tumors. J Clin Oncol 12:539–543
Prudhomme M (2000) Recent developments of rebeccamycin analogues as topoisomerase I inhibitors and antitumor agents. Curr Med Chem 7:1189–1212

Ramnath N, Creaven PJ (2004) Matrix metalloproteinase inhibitors. Curr Oncol Rep 6:96–102

Ribeiro RC, Rill D, Roberson PK et al. (1993) Continuous infusion of interleukin-2 in children with refractory malignancies. Cancer 72:623–628

Riccardi A, Ferlini C, Meco D, Mastrangelo R, Scambia G, Riccardi R (1999) Antitumour activity of oxaliplatin in neuroblastoma cell lines. Eur J Cancer 35:86–90

Rill DR, Santana VM, Roberts WM et al. (1994) Direct demonstration that autologous bone marrow transplantation for solid tumors can return a multiplicity of tumorigenic cells. Blood 84:380–383

Roper M, Smith MA, Sondel PM et al. (1992) A phase I study of interleukin-2 in children with cancer. Am J Pediatr Hematol Oncol 14:305–311

Rowinsky EK, Verweij J (1997) Review of phase I clinical studies with topotecan. Semin Oncol 24:S20-3–S20-10

Rowinsky EK, Noe DA, Grochow LB et al. (1995) Phase I and pharmacologic studies of pyrazoloacridine, a novel DNA intercalating agent, on single-dosing and multiple-dosing schedules. J Clin Oncol 13:1975–1984

Saleh MN, Khazaeli MB, Wheeler RH et al. (1992) Phase I trial of the chimeric anti-GD2 monoclonal antibody ch14.18 in patients with malignant melanoma. Hum Antibodies Hybridomas 3:19–24

Saylors RL III, Stewart CF, Zamboni WC et al. (1998) Phase I study of topotecan in combination with cyclophosphamide in pediatric patients with malignant solid tumors: a Pediatric Oncology Group Study. J Clin Oncol 16:945–952

Schiavetti A, Varrasso G, Maurizi P, Castello MA (2001) Two secondary leukemias among 15 children given oral etoposide. Med Pediatr Oncol 37:148–149

Sebolt JS, Scavone SV, Pinter CD, Hamelehle KL, Hoff DD von, Jackson RC (1987) Pyrazoloacridines, a new class of anticancer agents with selectivity against solid tumors in vitro. Cancer Res 47:4299–4304

Sebolt J, Havlick M, Hamelehle K, Nelson J, Leopold W, Jackson R (1989) Activity of the pyrazoloacridines against multidrug-resistant tumor cells. Cancer Chemother Pharmacol 24:219–224

Seeger RC, Reynolds CP, Gallego R, Stram DO, Gerbing RB, Matthay KK (2000) Quantitative tumor cell content of bone marrow and blood as a predictor of outcome in stage IV neuroblastoma: a Children's Cancer Group Study. J Clin Oncol 18:4067–4076

Shitara T, Shimada A, Tsuchida Y, Suzuki N, Toki F, Kuroiwa M (2003) Successful clinical response to irinotecan in relapsed neuroblastoma. Med Pediatr Oncol 40:126–128

Shulkin BL, Shapiro B (1998) Current concepts on the diagnostic use of MIBG in children. J Nucl Med 39:679–688

Sigal RK, Lieberman MD, Reynolds JV, Shou J, Ziegler MM, Daly JM (1991) Low-dose interferon gamma renders neuroblastoma more susceptible to interleukin-2 immunotherapy. J Pediatr Surg 26:389–396

Smith BD, Levis M, Beran M et al. (2004) Single agent CEP-701, a novel FLT3 inhibitor, shows biologic and clinical activity in patients with relapsed or refractory acute myeloid leukemia CEP-701 and CEP-751 inhibit constitutively activated RET tyrosine kinase activity and block medullary thyroid carcinoma cell growth. Blood 63:5559–5563

Smith MA, Parkinson DR, Cheson BD, Friedman MA (1992) Retinoids in cancer therapy. J Clin Oncol 10:839–864

Stokes AH, Lewis DY, Lash LH et al. (2000) Dopamine toxicity in neuroblastoma cells: role of glutathione depletion by L-BSO and apoptosis. Brain Res 858:1–8

Sugiura Y, Shimada H, Seeger RC, Laug WE, DeClerck YA (1998) Matrix metalloproteinases-2 and -9 are expressed in human neuroblastoma: contribution of stromal cells to their production and correlation with metastasis. Cancer Res 58:2209–2216

Suzuki T, Bogenmann E, Shimada H, Stram D, Seeger RC (1993) Lack of high-affinity nerve growth factor receptors in aggressive neuroblastomas (see comments). J Natl Cancer Inst 85:377–384

Takasuna K, Hagiwara T, Hirohashi M et al. (1996) Involvement of beta-glucuronidase in intestinal microflora in the intestinal toxicity of the antitumor camptothecin derivative irinotecan hydrochloride (CPT-11) in rats. Cancer Res 56:3752–3757

Takita J, Ishii M, Tsutsumi S et al. (2004) Gene expression profiling and identification of novel prognostic marker genes in neuroblastoma. Genes Chromosomes Cancer 40:120–132

Teitz T, Wei T, Valentine MB et al. (2000) Caspase 8 is deleted or silenced preferentially in childhood neuroblastomas with amplification of MYCN (see comments). Nat Med 6:529–535

Tew KD (1994) Glutathione-associated enzymes in anticancer drug resistance. Cancer Res 54:4313–4320

Thompson J, Zamboni WC, Cheshire PJ et al. (1997) Efficacy of oral irinotecan against neuroblastoma xenografts. Anticancer Drugs 8:313–322

Thompson J, George EO, Poquette CA et al. (1999) Synergy of topotecan in combination with vincristine for treatment of pediatric solid tumor xenografts. Clin Cancer Res 5:3617–3631

Toren A, Nagler A, Rozenfeld-Granot G et al. (2000) Amplification of immunological functions by subcutaneous injection of intermediate-high dose interleukin-2 for 2 years after autologous stem cell transplantation in children with stage IV neuroblastoma. Transplantation 70:1100–1104

Troncone L, Rufini V, Luzi S, Mastrangelo R, Riccardi R (1995) The treatment of neuroblastoma with [131I]MIBG at diagnosis. Q J Nucl Med 39:65–68

Truitt RL, Piaskowski V, Kirchner P, McOlash L, Camitta BM, Casper JT (1992) Immunological evaluation of pediatric cancer patients receiving recombinant interleukin-2 in a phase I trial. J Immunother 11:274–285

Tubergen DG, Stewart CF, Pratt CB et al. (1996) Phase I trial and pharmacokinetic (PK) and pharmacodynamics (PD) study of topotecan using a five-day course in children with refractory solid tumors: a pediatric oncology group study. J Pediatr Hematol Oncol 18:352–361

Tucker GC (2003) Alpha v integrin inhibitors and cancer therapy. Curr Opin Invest Drugs 4:722–731

Tweddle DA, Malcolm AJ, Bown N, Pearson AD, Lunec J (2001) Evidence for the development of p53 mutations after cytotoxic therapy in a neuroblastoma cell line. Cancer Res 61:8–13

Tweddle DA, Pearson AD, Haber M et al. (2003) The p53 pathway and its inactivation in neuroblastoma. Cancer Lett 197:93–98

Uttenreuther-Fischer MM, Huang CS, Reisfeld RA, Yu AL (1995) Pharmacokinetics of anti-ganglioside GD2 mAb 14G2a in a phase I trial in pediatric cancer patients. Cancer Immunol Immunother 41:29–36

Valteau-Couanet D, Rubie H, Meresse V, Farace F, Brandely M, Hartmann O (1995) Phase I-II study of interleukin-2 after high-dose chemotherapy and autologous bone marrow transplantation in poorly responding neuroblastoma. Bone Marrow Transplant 16:515–520

Vassal G, Terrier-Lacombe MJ, Bissery MC et al. (1996) Therapeutic activity of CPT-11, a DNA-topoisomerase I inhibitor, against peripheral primitive neuroectodermal tumour and neuroblastoma xenografts. Br J Cancer 74:537–545

Verstovsek S, Eppolito C, Ujhazy P, Maccubbin DL, Ehrke MJ, Mihich E (1995) Murine splenic macrophage tumoricidal activation by cytokines. Exp Hematol 23:519–528

Vitali R, Cesi V, Nicotra MR, McDowell HP, Donfrancesco A, Mannarino O, Natali PG, Raschella G, Dominici C (2003) c-Kit is preferentially expressed in MYCN-amplified neuroblastoma and its effect on cell proliferation is inhibited in vitro by STI-571. Int J Cancer 106:147–152

Voute PA, Hoefnagel CA, de Kraker J, Valdes Olmos R, Bakker DJ, van de Kleij AJ (1991) Results of treatment with ^{131}I-metaiodobenzylguanidine 131 I-MIBG in patients with neuroblastoma. Future prospects of zetotherapy. Prog Clin Biol Res 366:439–445

Wang ZY (2001) Arsenic compounds as anticancer agents. Cancer Chemother Pharmacol 48 (Suppl 1):S72–S76

Watts RG (1992) Combination chemotherapy with ifosfamide and etoposide is effective in the treatment of central nervous system metastasis of childhood neuroblastoma. Cancer 69:3012–3014

Watts RG, Mroczek-Musulman E (1996) Pulmonary interstitial disease mimicking idiopathic pneumonia syndrome as the initial site of relapse of neuroblastoma following autologous bone-marrow transplantation: a case report. Am J Hematol 53:137–140

Weiss B, Vora A, Huberty J, Hawkins RA, Matthay KK (2003) Secondary myelodysplastic syndrome and leukemia following 131I-metaiodobenzylguanidine therapy for relapsed neuroblastoma. J Pediatr Hematol Oncol 25:543–547

Weitman S, Moore R, Barrera H, Cheung NK, Izbicka E, Hoff DD von (1998) In vitro antitumor activity of rebeccamycin analog (NSC# 655649) against pediatric solid tumors. J Pediatr Hematol Oncol 20:136–139

Weitman S, Barrera H, Moore R et al. (2000) MGI 114: augmentation of antitumor activity when combined with topotecan. J Pediatr Hematol Oncol 22:306–314

Wigginton JM, Komschlies KL, Back TC, Franco JL, Brunda MJ, Wiltrout RH (1996) Administration of interleukin 12 with pulse interleukin 2 and the rapid and complete eradication of murine renal carcinoma. J Natl Cancer Inst 88:38–43

Wigginton JM, Park JW, Gruys ME et al. (2001a) Complete regression of established spontaneous mammary carcinoma and the therapeutic prevention of genetically programmed neoplastic transition by IL-12/pulse IL-2: induction of local T cell infiltration, Fas/Fas ligand gene expression, and mammary epithelial apoptosis. J Immunol 166:1156–1168

Wigginton JM, Gruys E, Geiselhart L et al. (2001b) IFN-gamma and Fas/FasL are required for the antitumor and antiangiogenic effects of IL-12/pulse IL-2 therapy. J Clin Invest 108: 51–62

Wolden SL, Gollamudi SV, Kushner BH, LaQuaglia M, Kramer K, Rosen N, Abramson S, Cheung NV et al. (2000) Local control with multimodality therapy for Stage 4 neuroblastoma. Int J Radiat Oncol Biol Phys 46:969–974

Yanagida T, Kato T, Igarashi O, Inoue T, Nariuchi H (1994) Second signal activity of IL-12 on the proliferation and IL-2R expression of T helper cell-1 clone. J Immunol 152:4919–4928

Yanik GA, Levine JE, Matthay KK et al. (2002) Pilot study of iodine-131-metaiodobenzylguanidine in combination with myeloablative chemotherapy and autologous stem-cell support for the treatment of neuroblastoma. J Clin Oncol 20:2142–2149

Yao K, Godwin AK, Ozols RF, Hamilton TC, O'Dwyer PJ (1993) Variable baseline gamma-glutamylcysteine synthetase messenger RNA expression in peripheral mononuclear cells of cancer patients, and its induction by buthionine sulfoximine treatment. Cancer Res 53:3662–3666

Yoshida H, Tanabe M, Miyauchi M et al. (1999) Induced immunity by expression of interleukin-2 or GM-CSF gene in murine neuroblastoma cells can generate antitumor response to established tumors. Cancer Gene Ther 6:395–401

Yoshida M, Furumai R, Nishiyama M, Komatsu Y, Nishino N, Horinouchi S (2001) Histone deacetylase as a new target for cancer chemotherapy. Cancer Chemother Pharmacol 48 Suppl 1:S20–S26

Yu AL, Batova A, Alvarado C, Rao VJ, Castleberry RP (1997) Usefulness of a chimeric anti-GD2 (ch14.18) and GM-CSF for refractory neuroblastoma: a POG Phase II study. Proc Am Soc Clin Oncol 16:513a

Yung WK, Prados MD, Yaya-Tur R et al. (1999) Multicenter phase II trial of temozolomide in patients with anaplastic astrocytoma or anaplastic oligoastrocytoma at first relapse. Temodal Brain Tumor Group. J Clin Oncol 17:2762–2771

Zamboni WC, Bowman LC, Tan M et al. (1999) Interpatient variability in bioavailability of the intravenous formulation of topotecan given orally to children with recurrent solid tumors. Cancer Chemother Pharmacol 43:454–460

the greatest efficacy when immunotherapy is applied at the time of small tumor load; thus, application of immunotherapeutic interventions for patients with high-risk NB is likely to be most effective if utilized at the time of minimal residual disease.

14.2 The Immunobiology of Neuroblastoma

To recognize human NB, antibodies, T-cell receptors, and receptors of the innate immune system (e.g., NK, NKT, and γ/δ+T cells) (Jameson et al. 2003) have been explored. Antigens recognized by antibodies on NB are summarized in Table 14.1. Several antigen systems recognized by cytotoxic T lymphocytes (CTLS) have also been demonstrated in NB; these include cancer–testes antigens [*MAGE* (Ishida et al. 1996; Cheung et al. 1998),[5] *GAGE* (Cheung and Cheung 1997), NY-Eso-1 (Soling et al. 1999)], *MYCN* oncogene (Sarkar and Nuchtern 2000), kinase (ALK; Passoni et al. 2002), and others. The activation of antigen-specific T lymphocytes is a multi-step process requiring antigen-specific triggering of the T-cell receptor (TCR) complex on the T cell, and additional signaling via the costimulatory molecules CD28 that interact with CD80 (B7–1/BB1) and CD86 (B7–2/B70)

Table 14.1. Neuroblastoma antigens recognized by antibodies

Antigen	Biochemical nature Target antigen	Antibody forms		Immunoconjugates
GD2	Ganglioside	Human:	OFA-1-2 (Tai et al. 1984)	
		Humanized:	KM8138 (Nakamura et al. 2001)	
		Chimeric:	ch14.18 (Yu et al. 1998)	IL-2 (Hank et al. 1996)
			KM1138 (Nakamura et al. 2001)	GM-CSF (Batova et al. 1999)
		Mouse:	3F8 (Cheung et al. 1987)	^{131}I (Cheung et al. 1986, 2001b)
			14.G2a (Yu et al. 1997)	^{124}I (Larson et al. 1991)
			BW625 (Berthold et al. 1989)	^{225}Ac (Miederer et al. 2004)
			AI (Kawashima et al. 1988)	
		ScFv (Moutel et al. 1997; Tur et al. 2001a)		scFv-CIR (Krause et al. 1998; Rossig et al. 2001; Cheung et al. 2003c) scFv-PE-toxin (Tur et al. 2001b)
GD3	Ganglioside	Humanized:	KM8871 (Nakamura et al. 2001)	
		Chimeric:	KM871 (Nakamura et al. 2001; Scott et al. 2001)	I-131 (Scott et al. 2001)
		Mouse:	R24 (Houghton et al. 1985)	
GM2	Ganglioside	Humanized:	KM8969 (Nakamura et al. 2001)	
		Chimeric:	KM966 (Nakamura et al. 2001)	
NCAM (CD56)	Glycoprotein	Humanized:	HuN901 (Roguska et al. 1996)	Maytansinoid (Tassone et al. 2004)
		Mouse:	UJ13A (Lashford et al. 1987),	I-131 (Goldman et al. 1984)
			N901 (McGarry et al. 1988)	blocked-Ricin (Lynch et al. 1997)
				CC-1065 (Chari et al. 1995)
L1-CAM	Glycoprotein	Chimeric:	chCE7 (Amstutz et al. 1993)	I-131 (Hoefnagel et al. 2003) Cu-64 (Novak-Hofer et al. 2003) Cu-67 (Carrel et al. 1997)
		Mouse:	CE7 (Schonmann et al. 1986)	
		ScFv (Carrel et a. 1997)		
GP58	Glycoprotein	Mouse:	8H9 (Modak et al. 2001)	scFv-Fc (Cheung et al. 2002) scFc-CIR (Cheung et al. 2003c)
GP95	Glycoprotein	Mouse:	BW575 (Berthold et al. 1989)	
NB-p260	Protein	Natural IgM (Ollert et al. 1996)		

ligands on the APCs, plus CD40-CD154 (CD40L) interactions. Adhesion molecules, such as leukocyte function antigen (LFA)-1, LFA-3, and intercellular adhesion molecule (ICAM)-1, are also important in the initial binding of CTLs to APC and to tumor targets. The CTLs must receive the appropriate help before expansion can occur. Antigen-specific T-helper cells with T-helper 1 (TH1) activity must be coactivated by the APCs. Th1 cells release Th1 cytokines, such as interferon (IFN)-γ and interleukin (IL)-12, which are also necessary for CTL activation, and interleukin-2 (IL-2), which is necessary for CTL expansion (Cheung and Rooney 2002). A tumor cell that induces the secretion of T-helper 2 (TH2) cytokines, such as IL-4 and IL-10, may promote antibody instead of CTL responses.

Because of the propensity for NB to undergo "spontaneous regression," many have implicated an endogenous anti-NB immune response. The recent discovery of a natural IgM anti-NB antibody in children suggests that innate immunity may have a potential role in surveillance against this tumor (Ollert et al. 1996). Besides IgM, lymphocytes of the innate immune system (NK, NKT, γ/δ-T cells) (Jameson et al. 2003) interact with tumors through unique activation and inhibitory receptors. The NK cells can lyse human NB in vitro and inhibit xenograft growth (Colucci et al. 2003; Cheung and Modak 2002). Specific ligands on tumor cells trigger activating or inhibitory receptors on NK cells (Schilbach et al. 2000). The NKT cells bear NK markers (CD161, CD122) and are thymus dependent, expressing CD3 plus TCR (Kronenberg and Gapin 2002). They recognize α-galactosyl-ceramide as well as ganglioside GD3 presented on CD1d, a nonclassical major histocompatibility (MHC) molecule (Wu et al. 2003). These NKT cells are effective anti-tumor vehicles in preclinical cellular targeting strategies (Metelitsa et al. 2001; Smyth et al. 2002). Human γδT cells isolated from PBL and expanded with IL-2 in vitro also mediate effective cytotoxicity against NB cells (Schilbach et al. 2000; Carding and Egan 2002).

14.3 How Neuroblastoma Escapes the Innate and Adaptive Immune Systems

Neuroblastoma employs a variety of tactics to evade the immune system (Table 14.2). It downregulates "immune-activating" while overexpressing "immune-inhibitory" receptors. By repressing the expression of class-I and class-II MHC (Lampson et al. 1983) as well as CD1d (Metelitsa et al. 2001), they interfere with both the afferent and efferent arms of adaptive immune response. In addition, NB cells can avoid immune recognition and destruction by releas-

Table 14.2. Neuroblastoma can evade the immune system

Immune function	Modulated Ags	Escape mechanism used by NB
Adaptive immunity		
T cells	↓MHC Class I	↓β2m, ↓TAP1, ↓TAP2, ↓LMP2, ↓LMP7*
	↓Adhesion	↓ICAM2, ↓ICAM3, ↓LFA3
Innate immunity		
NK cells	↓Activation	↓MICA (cytoplasmic), ↓MICB (cytoplasmic) (Raffaghello et al. 2004)
	↑*Inhibition*	Soluble MICA (Doubrovina et al. 2003; Raffaghello et al. 2004)
NKT cells	↓Activation	↓CD1d
Complement	↑Inhibition	CD46, ↑CD59
	↓Inhibition	↓CD55
Inhibition of immune cells		
Lymphocytes	↑Apoptosis	↑GD1a, ↑FasL, ↑GD2
APC	↓Function	↑GD2

* N.K. Cheung and W. Gerald, microarray gene expression analysis of human NB, unpublished results
LMP low molecular weight protein, *TAP* transporter-associated protein

ing the ganglioside GD1a which is directly toxic to human lymphocytes while uncoupling cell signaling through the NFκB pathway (Shen and Ladisch 2002), as well as disialoganglioside GD2 which interferes with T-cell (Li et al. 1995) and APC functions (Shurin et al. 2001; Heitger and Ladisch 1996). Furthermore, some NB cells have been shown to express FAS-ligand (Fas-L) (Shurin et al. 1998), which may act as a death signal causing apoptosis of effector cells, such as T cells or NK cells, which themselves express the surface Fas death receptor (Takamizawa et al. 2000; Li et al. 2002). On the other hand, when confronted with antibodies, despite their low levels of CD55 (decay accelerating factor), some neuroblastomas cells have increased CD59 (homologous restriction factor) and sufficient CD46 (membrane cofactor protein) expression to render them resistant to terminal complement pathways (see 14.4.1). Effective in vivo immunotherapy must circumvent these protective mechanisms of NB in order to ultimately maximize clinical benefit.

14.4 Humoral Immunotherapy

With the introduction of the hybridoma technique in 1975 by Koehler and Milstein (Koehler and Milstein 1975), and the more recent emergence of recombinant technology, monoclonal antibodies have transformed the original "serum therapy" concept of Emil Behring and Shibasaburo Kitasato into a pharmaceutical industry. Monoclonal antibodies (MAb) have generated excitement on many frontiers and will likely play an important role in the future of cancer medicine.

14.4.1 Effector Mechanisms of MAb

Anti-tumor MAb can carry out highly effective tumoricidal functions both in vitro and in vivo; these include signaling through receptor binding, antibody-dependent cell-mediated cytotoxicity (ADCC), and complement-mediated cytotoxicity (CMC) (Cheung 2004). MAb vary in their ability to induce downstream effects. For example, MAb 3F8 is unique among anti-GD2 antibodies in its ability to induce apoptosis among EL4 murine lymphoma cells (Tomlinson et al., unpublished results). MAb can also block receptor functions (e.g., EGF-R) (Mendelsohn 2003), and vascular endothelial growth factor receptor (VEGF-R) (Prewett et al. 1999) by interfering with binding of the natural ligands.

There are three types of IgG Fc receptors (FcγR): FcγRI (CD64); FcγRII (CD32); and low-affinity FcγRIII (CD16; Ravetch and Bolland 2001). Most FcγRs are of the activating type except for the inhibitory receptor FcγRIIB. Recent correlation of FcγRIIIA polymorphism with clinical response to rituximab suggests that IgG affinity for Fc receptor can influence anti-tumor response in patients (Cartron et al. 2002; Kimberly et al. 2002). Neuroblastoma cells are effectively killed by NK lymphocytes, granulocytes, and activated monocytes in vitro in the presence of specific MAb. Chimeric hIgG1 specific for GD2 (ch14.18) fused to GM-CSF depends on FcγRII in neutrophil ADCC (Metelitsa et al. 2002). In contrast, 3F8 (murine IgG3 specific for GD2) utilizes both FcγRII and FcγRIII for ADCC (Kushner and Cheung 1992). In addition to FcR, adhesion molecules including CR3 (CD11b/Cd18) (Metelitsa et al. 2002; Kushner and Cheung 1992; Ottonello et al. 1999) and CD66b (Ottonello et al. 1999) for neutrophils, and LFA-1 (CD11a/CD18) for lymphocytes (Edwards et al. 1992), are important in modulating tumor cytotoxicity. When their expression is increased by granulocyte macrophage colony stimulating factor (GM-CSF) or IFN-γ, granulocyte ADCC can be enhanced (Metelitsa et al. 2002; Kushner and Cheung 1989; Vaickus et al. 1990; Masucci et al. 1990). Similarly, IL-2 can increase lymphocyte ADCC (Munn and Cheung 1987; Sondel and Hank 1997). Furthermore, since both GM-CSF and IL-2 expand the effector cell pools, they have potential clinical benefits in tumor therapy when combined with MAb (Fig. 14.1).

Most NB cell lines are sensitive to CMC; however, some are resistant to complement because of anti-complement surface proteins, including CD55 (Cheung et al. 1988; Gorter and Meri 1999), CD59 (Gorter and Meri 1999; Cheng et al. 2000b) and CD46 (Gorter and Meri 1999). The effect of complement activation extends beyond direct tumor lysis. C3b deposited on tumor cells is rapidly cleaved by plasma protease factor I to iC3b. Through CR3 (Mac-1

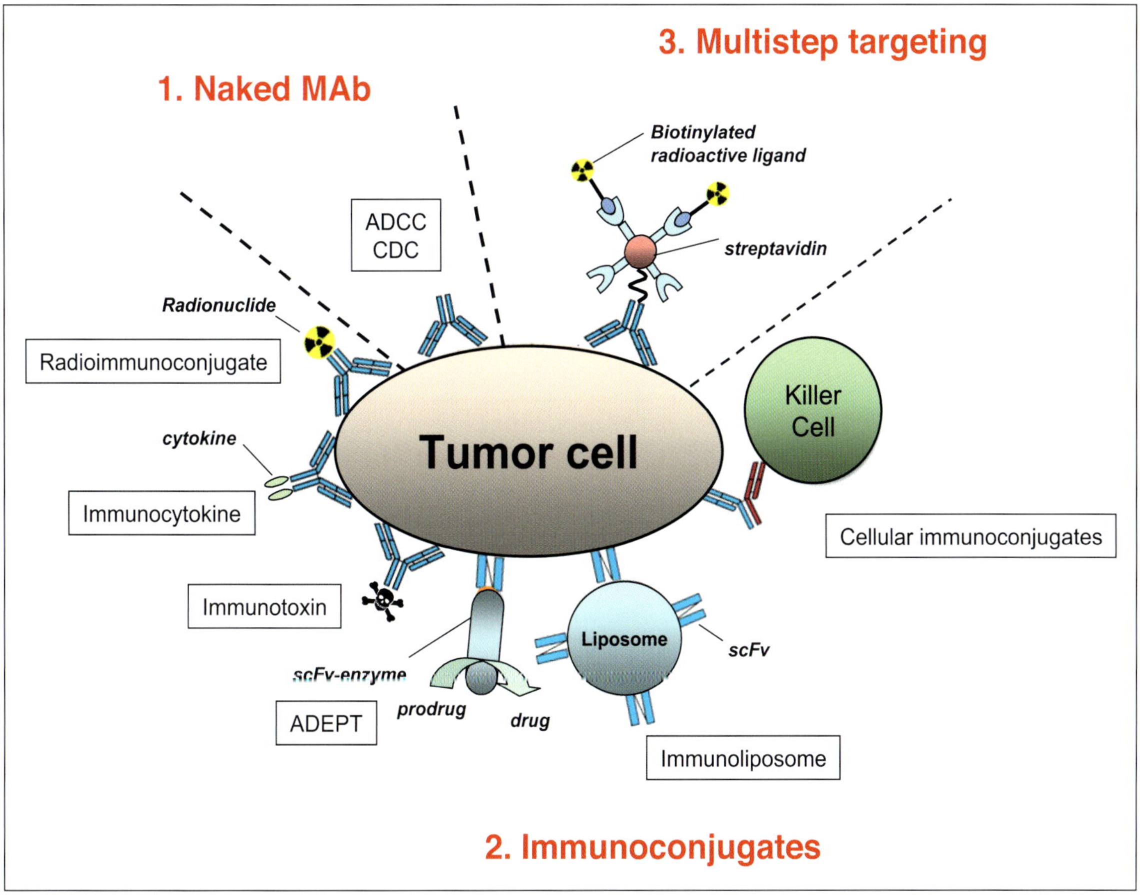

Figure 14.1

Effector mechanisms of monoclonal antibodies. *ADEPT* antibody directed enzyme prodrug therapy; *ADCC* antibody-dependent cell-mediated cytotoxicity, *CMC* complement mediated cytotoxicity, *MAb* monoclonal antibody, *scFv* single-chain Fv fragment. (From Cheung 2004; Carter 2001).

or alpha$_M$beta$_2$-integrin), and CR4 (CD11c/CD18, alpha$_X$beta$_2$-integrin) receptors on leukocytes, tumor cells are opsonized (Ross et al. 1999). C3a and C5a, byproducts of complement activation, are potent mediators of inflammation (Hugli 1978) and are chemotactic for phagocytic leukocytes, drawing them to the tumor sites. C5a can also induce secondary cytokines to increase vascular permeability for both MAb and effector cells.

14.4.2 Clinical Application of MAb

14.4.2.1 Naked MAb

Among the ganglioside antigens, GD2 is particularly relevant for the treatment of NB. Neuroblastoma cells express GD2 at high density, with relatively little heterogeneity within tumors or among patients (Schulz et al. 1984; Kramer et al. 1998). GD2 is not lost from the cell surface when bound to antibodies. In normal serum, GD2 is found in low concentrations typically bound to lipoproteins. This may explain why circu-

Table 14.3. Use of MAb for clinical diagnosis and therapy of neuroblastoma[a]

Radiolabeled antibody for imaging	Sensitivity
^{131}I-UJ13A[a] (Goldman et al. 1984)	89%
^{131}I-3F8 (Miraldi et al. 1986; Yeh et al. 1991)	90%
^{131}I-14.G2a (Podoloff et al. 1991)	85%
^{99m}Tc-BW575 (Smolarz et al. 1989)	90%
^{131}I-CE7 (Carrel et al. 1997)	–

Radiolabeled antibody for therapy	Overall response[b]	BM CR[b]
^{131}I-UJ13A (Kemshead et al. 1985)	–	1/4
^{131}I-3F8 (Larson et al. 2000)	2/10	2/10
^{131}I-3F8 (IT) (Kramer et al. 2000b)	–[c]	–

Naked antibody for therapy[d]	Cytokine	Total dose mg/m^2	Overall Response			BM CR	Bone CR/PR	Masses CR/PR
			N	CR/VGPR	PR			
Phase I								
3F8 (Cheung et al. 1987)	–	5–100	8	0	1	1/8[e]	1/8	0/4
14.G2a (Huang et al. 1992)	–	25–200	15	1	0	2/8	0/12	0/11
14.G2a (Handgretinger et al. 1992)	–	100–400	6	2	2	–	–	–
14.G2a (Murray et al. 1994)	–	50–200	5	0	2	–	–	–
ch14.18 (Yu et al. 1998)	–	10–200	9	0	1	3/7	0/9	1/8
ch14.18 (Handgretinger et al. 1995)	–	150–250	9	2	2	–	–	–
14.G2a (Frost et al. 1997)	IL-2 +/– GMCSF	10–100	31	0	1	–	–	1/1
Phase II								
3F8 (Cheung et al. 1998c)	–	50	16	1	0	3/8	2/7	0/8
3F8 (Kushner et al. 2001)	GM-CSF	100[f]	43[g]	11	–	31/42	–	–
ch14.18 (Simon et al. 2004)	–	100	166	–	–	↓marrow relapse, ↑survival, but no effect on event-free survival		
ch14.18 (Yu et al. 1997)	GM-CSF	200	27	1	3	5/13	0/9	0/7

[a] Antibodies were injected intravenously unless otherwise stated. *IT* = intrathecal
[b] BM CR was proportion of patients clearing marrow disease. Overall response = CR + PR, unless otherwise stated
[c] 1 radiographic and 2 CSF cytologic responses from the first 12 patients
[d] I=phase I, II=phase II
[e] No. of responses/no. of evaluable patients with neuroblastoma
[f] Patients without HAMA after 400 mg/m^2 (4 cycles of 10 days/cycle, 10 mg/m^2 day) were treated q1–2 months (100 mg/m^2/cycle) until 24 months from the first day of enrollment on the protocol
[g] Only patients with evaluable disease (primary resistance to induction or secondary resistance to retrieval therapy) were included in this analysis

lating GD2 in most patients has not interfered with antibody targeting which typically achieved high percent injected dose per gram (%ID/g) with high tumor-to-normal-tissue ratio, and unusually low liver and spleen uptake in patient studies (Yeh et al. 1991; Larson et al. 2000).

Clinical Trials

The first IgG anti-GD2 MAb to undergo clinical testing was 3F8 (murine IgG3; Table 14.3; Cheung et al. 1987, 1998a), followed subsequently by 14.G2a (murine IgG2a; Handgretinger et al. 1992; Frost et al. 1997). and a chimeric form ch14.18 (Yu et al. 1998). In clinical trials (Yu et al. 1998; Handgretinger et al. 1995; Ozkaynak et al. 2000), ch14.18 had a more prolonged serum half-life and lower immunogenicity compared with its mouse counterpart. Most of the responses noted in phase I and II clinical trials of unconjugated anti-GD2 MAbs involved metastatic disease in bone marrow, with less certain effects on bulky tumors. The predominant toxicity was pain, attributed to cross-reactivity of antibodies with peripheral pain fibers (Lammie et al. 1993; Xiao et al. 1997; Yuki et al. 1997). Other side effects included tachycardia, hypotension, fever, anaphylactoid reactions, nausea, vomiting, diarrhea, and transient neuropathy. Most side effects were dose dependent, rarely noted at dosages of $<10\ mg/m^2$ (14G.2a or ch14.18) or $<1\ mg/m^2$ (3F8), and compatible with outpatient treatment. Over a 15-year period, more than 350 patients with NB have been treated with >10,000 infusions of 3F8 at Memorial Sloan-Kettering Cancer Center. There was no treatment-associated mortality. Similarly, the COG (and its component organizations) have been administering 14.G2a or ch14.18 anti-GD2 MAb since 1989 with good safety record. Patients have been followed for up to 15 years. No long-term neurological complications have been noted. The clinical development of anti-GD2 MAb was partly hindered by its pain side effects which have precluded dose escalation.

Although the anti-tumor effect of anti-GD2 MAb was modest, response of microscopic marrow disease was more consistent (Cheung et al. 1998b, 2001a, 2003a,b; Kushner et al. 2001). An association of human anti-mouse antibody (HAMA) response and favorable patient outcome, plus the induction of anti-idiotypic Ab2 and anti-idiotypic Ab3/antibodies through the idiotype network, implicate the potential role of the host immune response in maintaining clinical remission (Cheung et al. 1994, 2000). In a recent update of 98 patients with stage-4 NB newly diagnosed after 18 month of age, who received anti-GD2 MAb 3F8 as part of their combined modality therapy at MSKCC, the induction of a HAMA response and a lower number of tumor cells in the diagnostic bone marrow were the most significant independent prognostic variables for both progression-free and overall survival (N.-K.V. Cheung et al., unpublished results).

14.4.2.2 Antibody in Combination with Cytokines

While cytokines can induce proliferation and activation of effector cells, in the absence of cytophilic MAb, they lack tumor selectivity. Antibody-dependent cellular cytotoxicity (ADCC) is greatly augmented in vitro by cytokines (Kushner and Cheung 1989; Munn and Cheung 1987; Hank et al. 1990; Barker and Reisfeld 1993). Clinical trials of anti-NB antibody combined with GM-CSF (Ozkaynak et al. 2000; Kushner et al. 2001) or combined with IL-2 (Sondel and Hank 1997; Frost et al. 1997) have shown modest anti-tumor effects. While large tumor masses rarely responded to these combinations, microscopic marrow disease showed consistent response in over 50% of patients whether measured by conventional histology (Kushner et al. 2001) or by RT-PCR (Cheung et al. 2003b). In addition, response may translate into improved survival (Cheung et al. 1998a, 2003b). To prospectively evaluate the clinical efficacy of antibody in combination with cytokine therapy, ch14.18 is being tested in combination with GM-CSF and IL-2 following autologous stem-cell transplant in a phase-III U.S. Children's Oncology Group (COG) randomized trial (A. Yu et al., unpublished results).

14.4.2.3 Antibody Immunoconjugates

The clinical utility of naked MAb has been limited by both host (number and activity of effector cells, FcR polymorphism, and interference by inhibitory FcR) and tumor factors (antigen heterogeneity and com-

Holzer U, Bethge W, Krull F et al. (1995) Superantigen-staphylococcal-enterotoxin-A-dependent and antibody-targeted lysis of GD2-positive neuroblastoma cells. Cancer Immunol Immunother 41:129–136

Houghton AN, Mintzer D, Cordon-Cardo C et al. (1985) Mouse monoclonal IgG3 antibody detecting GD3 ganglioside: a phase I trial in patients with malignant melanoma. Proc Natl Acad Sci USA 82:1242–1246

Huang CS, Utterreuther M, Reisfeld RA (1992) Immunotherapy of GD2+ tumors with a murine monoclonal antibody (MAB) 14G2a; a phase I study. Proc ASCO 11:364

Hugli TE, Muller-Eberhard HJ (1978Anaphylatoxins: C3a and C5a. Adv Immunol 26:1–53

Ishida H, Matsumura T, Salgaller ML et al. (1996) MAGE-1 and MAGE-3 or -6 expression in neuroblastoma-related pediatric solid tumors. Int J Cancer 69:375–380

Jameson J, Witherden D, Havran WL (2003) T-cell effector mechanisms: gammadelta and CD1d-restricted subsets. Curr Opin Immunol 15:349–353

Janeway CA, Travers P, Walport M et al. (2001) Immunobiology-5: the immune system in health and disease, 5th edn. Garland Publishing, Taylor and Francis Group, New York

Juhl H, Petrella EC, Cheung NK et al. (1997) Additive cytotoxicity of different monoclonal antibody-cobra venom factor conjugates for human neuroblastoma cells. Immunobiology 197:444–459

Jurcic JG, Larson SM, Sgouros G et al. (2002) Targeted alpha particle immunotherapy for myeloid leukemia. Blood 100:1233–1239

Kawashima I, Tada N, Ikegami S et al. (1988) Mouse monoclonal antibodies detecting disialogangliosides on mouse and human T lymphomas. Int J Cancer 41:267–274

Kemshead JT, Goldman A, Jones D et al. (1985) Therapeutic application of radiolabelled monoclonal antibody UJ13A in children with disseminated neuroblastoma-a phase I study. In: Evans AE, D'Angio GJ, Seeger RC (eds) Advances in neuroblastoma research. Prog Clin Biol Res. Liss, New York, pp 533–544

Kennedy RC, Zhou EM, Lanford RE et al. (1987) Possible role of anti-idiotypic antibodies in the induction of tumor immunity. J Clin Invest 80:1217–1224

Kimberly RP, Wu J, Gibson AW et al. (2002) Diversity and duplicity: human FCgamma receptors in host defense and autoimmunity. Immunol Res 26:177–189

King D, Albertini M, Schalch H et al. (2002) Phase I/II trial of the immunocytokine hu14.18-IL2 in patients with metastatic melanoma. Proc Am Soc Clin Oncol 21:16a

Koehler G, Milstein C (1975) Continuous culture of fused cells secreting antibody of pre-defined specificity. Nature 256: 495–496

Koehne G, Guo HF, Trivedi RY et al. (2003) Redirecting NK-cell cytolytic activity to solid tumors using chimeric scFv receptor gene-modified adoptive immunotherapy. Proc Am Soc Clin Oncol 22:175

Kramer K, Gerald WL, Kushner BH et al. (1998) Disialoganglioside G(D2) loss following monoclonal antibody therapy is rare in neuroblastoma. Clin Cancer Res 4:2135–2139

Kramer K, Cheung NK, Humm JL et al. (2000) Targeted radioimmunotherapy for leptomeningeal cancer using (131)I-3F8. Med Pediatr Oncol 35:716–718

Krause A, Guo HF, Latouche JB et al. (1998) Antigen-dependent CD28 signaling electively enhances survival and proliferation in genetically modified activated human primary T lymphocytes. J Exp Med 188:619–626

Kronenberg M, Gapin L (2002) The unconventional lifestyle of NKT cells. Nat Rev Immunol 2:557–568

Kushner BH, Cheung NK (1989) GM-CSF enhances 3F8 monoclonal antibody-dependent cellular cytotoxicity against human melanoma and neuroblastoma. Blood 73:1936–1941

Kushner BH, Cheung NK (1992) Absolute requirement of CD11/CD18 adhesion molecules, FcRII and the phosphatidylinositol-linked FcRIII for monoclonal antibody-mediated neutrophil antihuman tumor cytotoxicity. Blood 79:1484–1490

Kushner BH, Kramer K, Cheung NKV (2001) Phase II trial of the anti-G(D2) monoclonal antibody 3F8 and granulocyte-macrophage colony-stimulating factor for neuroblastoma. J Clin Oncol 19:4189–4194

Lammie GA, Cheung NKV, Gerald W et al. (1993) Ganglioside GD2 expression in the human nervous system and in neuroblastomas: an immunohistochemical study. Int J Oncol 3:909–915

Lampson LA, Fisher CA, Whelan JP (1983) Striking paucity of HLA-A, B, C and B2-microglobulin on human neuroblastoma cell lines. J Immunol 130:2471–2478

Larson SM, Pentlow KS, Volkow ND et al. (1991) PET scanning of 124I-3F8 as a novel method of tumor dosimetry during treatment planning for radioimmunotherapy in a child with neuroblastoma. Antibody Immunoconjug Radiopharmaceut 4:34

Larson SM, Divgi C, Sgouros G et al. (2000) Monoclonal antibodies: basic principles – radioisotope conjugates. In: DeVita VT, Hellman S, Rosenberg SA (eds) Biologic therapy of cancer: principles and practice. Lippincott, Philadelphia, pp 396–412

Lashford L, Jones D, Pritchard J et al. (1987) Therapeutic application of radiolabeled monoclonal antibody UJ13A in children with disseminated neuroblastoma. NCI Monogr 3:53–57

Lashford LS, Davies AG, Richardson RB et al. (1988) A pilot study of 131I monoclonal antibodies in the therapy of leptomeningeal tumors. Cancer 61:857–868

Li JH, Rosen D, Sondel P et al. (2002) Immune privilege and FasL: two ways to inactivate effector cytotoxic T lymphocytes by FasL-expressing cells. Immunology 105:267–277

Li R, Villacreses N, Ladisch S (1995) Human tumor gangliosides inhibit murine immune responses in vivo. Cancer Res 55:211–214

Lode HN, Reisfeld RA (2000) Targeted cytokines for cancer immunotherapy. Immunol Res 21:279–288

Lode HN, Xiang R, Varki NM et al. (1997) Targeted interleukin-2 therapy for spontaneous neuroblastoma metastases to bone marrow. J Natl Cancer Inst 89:1586–1594

Lode HN, Moehler T, Xiang R et al. (1999) Synergy between an antiangiogenic integrin alphav antagonist and an antibody-cytokine fusion protein eradicates spontaneous tumor metastases. Proc Natl Acad Sci USA 96:1591–1596

Lynch TJ Jr, Lambert JM, Coral F et al. (1997) Immunotoxin therapy of small-cell lung cancer: a phase I study of N901-blocked ricin. J Clin Oncol 15:723–734

Manzke O, Russello O, Leenen C et al. (2001) Immunotherapeutic strategies in neuroblastoma: antitumoral activity of deglycosylated Ricin A conjugated anti-GD2 antibodies and anti-CD3xanti-GD2 bispecific antibodies. Med Pediatr Oncol 36:185–189

Marti F, Pardo N, Peiro M et al. (1995) Progression of natural immunity during one-year treatment of residual disease in neuroblastoma patients with high doses of interleukin-2 after autologous bone marrow transplantation. Exp Hematol 23:1445–1452

Masucci G, Ragnhammar P, Wersall P et al. (1990) Granulocyte-monocyte colony-stimulating-factor augments the interleukin-2-induced cytotoxic activity of human lymphocytes in the absence and presence of mouse or chimeric monoclonal antibodies (mAb 17–1A). Cancer Immunol Immunother 31:231–235

Matthay KK, Seeger RC, Reynolds CP et al. (1994) Allogeneic versus autologous purged bone marrow transplantation for neuroblastoma: a report from the Childrens Cancer Group. J Clin Oncol 12:2382–2389

McDevitt MR, Sgouros G, Finn RD et al. (1998) Radioimmunotherapy with alpha-emitting nuclides. Eur J Nucl Med 25:1341–1351

McGarry RC, Pinto A, Hammersley-Straw DR et al. (1988) Expression of markers shared between human natural killer cells and neuroblastoma lines. Cancer Immunol Immunother 27:47–52

Mendelsohn J (2003) Antibody-mediated EGF receptor blockade as an anticancer therapy: from the laboratory to the clinic. Cancer Immunol Immunother 52:342–346

Metelitsa LS, Gillies SD, Super M et al. (2002) Antidisialoganglioside/granulocyte macrophage-colony-stimulating factor fusion protein facilitates neutrophil antibody-dependent cellular cytotoxicity and depends on FcgammaRII (CD32) and Mac-1 (CD11b/CD18) for enhanced effector cell adhesion and azurophil granule exocytosis. Blood 99:4166–4173

Metelitsa LS, Naidenko OV, Kant A et al. (2001) Human NKT cells mediate antitumor cytotoxicity directly by recognizing target cell CD1d with bound ligand or indirectly by producing IL-2 to activate NK cells. J Immunol 167:3114–3122

Michon J, Moutel S, Barbet J et al. (1995a) In vitro killing of neuroblastoma cells by neutrophils derived from granulocyte colony-stimulating factor-treated cancer patients using an anti-disialoganglioside/anti-Fc gamma RI bispecific antibody. Blood 86:1124–1130

Michon J, Perdereau B, Brixy F et al. (1995b) In vivo targeting of human neuroblastoma xenograft by anti-GD2/anti-Fc gamma RI (CD64) bispecific antibody. Eur J Cancer 31A: 631–636

Miraldi FD, Nelson AD, Kraly C et al. (1986) Diagnostic imaging of human neuroblastoma with radiolabeled antibody. Radiology 161:413–418

Modak S, Kramer K, Gultekin SH et al. (2001) Monoclonal antibody 8H9 targets a novel cell surface antigen expressed by a wide spectrum of human solid tumors. Cancer Res 61:4048–4054

Moutel S, Birkle S, Laurence V et al. (1997) Generation and characterization of a mouse single-chain antibody fragment specific for disialoganglioside (GD2). Hybridoma 16: 335–346

Mujoo K, Reisfeld RA, Cheung L et al. (1991) A potent and specific immunotoxin for tumor cells expressing disialoganglioside GD2. Cancer Immunol Immunother 34:198–204

Munn DH, Cheung NK (1987) Interleukin-2 enhancement of monoclonal antibody-mediated cellular cytotoxicity (ADCC) against human melanoma. Cancer Res 47:6600–6605

Murray JL, Cunningham JE, Brewer H et al. (1994) Phase I trial of murine monoclonal antibody 14G2a administered by prolonged intravenous infusion in patients with neuroectodermal tumors. J Clin Oncol 12:184–193

Nakamura K, Tanaka Y, Shitara K et al. (2001) Construction of humanized anti-ganglioside monoclonal antibodies with potent immune effector functions. Cancer Immunol Immunother 50:275–284

Neal ZC, Imboden M, Rakhmilevich AL et al. (2003) Recurrent murine neuroblastomas increase or decrease MHC class I expression to escape NK- or T cell dependent immune destruction. Cancer Immunol Immunother 53:41–52

Novak-Hofer I, Honer M, Ametamey S et al. (2003) Imaging of renal carcinoma xenografts with (64)Cu-labelled anti-L1-CAM antibody chCE7. Eur J Nucl Med Mol Imaging 30:1066

Ohta S, Igarashi S, Honda A et al. (1993) Cytotoxicity of adriamycin-containing immunoliposomes targeted with anti-ganglioside monoclonal antibodies. Anticancer Res 13:331–336

Ollert MW, David K, Schmitt C et al. (1996) Normal human serum contains a natural IgM antibody cytotoxic for human neuroblastoma cells. Proc Natl Acad Sci USA 93:4498–4503

Ottonello L, Epstein AL, Dapino P et al. (1999) Monoclonal Lym-1 antibody-dependent cytolysis by neutrophils exposed to granulocyte-macrophage colony-stimulating factor: intervention of FcgammaRII (CD32), CD11b-CD18 integrins, and CD66b glycoproteins. Blood 93:3505–3511

Ozkaynak MF, Sondel PM, Krailo MD et al. (2000) Phase I study of chimeric human/murine antiganglioside GD2 monoclonal antibody (ch14.18) with granulocyte-macrophage colony-stimulating factor in children with neuroblastoma inmmediately after hematopoietic stem-cell transplantation: a Children's Cancer Group Study. J Clin Oncol 18:4077–4085

Paganelli G, Bartolomei M, Ferrari M et al. (2001) Pre-targeted locoregional radioimmunotherapy with 90Y-biotin in glioma patients: phase I study and preliminary therapeutic results. Cancer Biother Radiopharm 16:227–235

Passoni L, Scardino A, Bertazzoli C et al. (2002) ALK as a novel lymphoma-associated tumor antigen: identification of 2 HLA-A2.1-restricted CD8+ T-cell epitopes. Blood 99:2100–2106

Pastan I (2003) Immunotoxins containing *Pseudomonas* exotoxin A: a short history. Cancer Immunol Immunother 52:338–341

Pertl U, Luster AD, Varki NM et al. (2001) IFN-gamma-inducible protein-10 is essential for the generation of a protective tumor-specific CD8 T cell response induced by single-chain IL-12 gene therapy. J Immunol 166:6944–6951

Pertl U, Wodrich H, Ruehlmann JM et al. (2003) Immunotherapy with a posttranscriptionally modified DNA vaccine induces complete protection against metastatic neuroblastoma. Blood 101:649–654

Pession A, Prete A, Locatelli F et al. (1998) Immunotherapy with low-dose recombinant interleukin 2 after high-dose chemotherapy and autologous stem cell transplantation in neuroblastoma. Br J Cancer 78:528–533

Philip T, Ladenstein R, Lasset C et al. (1997) 1070 myeloablative megatherapy procedures followed by stem cell rescue for neuroblastoma: 17 years of European experience and conclusions. European Group for Blood and Marrow Transplant Registry Solid Tumour Working Party. Eur J Cancer 33:2130–2135

Podoloff JL, Murray JL, Bhadkamkar VA et al. (1991) Radioimmunolocalization (RIL) of an anti-ganglioside antibody directed against GD2 ganglioside: imaging considerations. J Nucl Med 32:970

Posey JA, Ng TC, Yang B et al. (2003) A phase I study of anti-kinase insert domain-containing receptor antibody, IMC-1C11, in patients with liver metastases from colorectal carcinoma. Clin Cancer Res 9:1323–1332

Presta LG, Chen H, O'Connor SJ et al. (1997) Humanization of an anti-vascular endothelial growth factor monoclonal antibody for the therapy of solid tumors and other disorders. Cancer Res 57:4593–4599

Prewett M, Huber J, Li Y et al. (1999) Antivascular endothelial growth factor receptor (fetal liver kinase 1) monoclonal antibody inhibits tumor angiogenesis and growth of several mouse and human tumors. Cancer Res 59:5209–5218

Raffaghello L, Pagnan G, Pastorino F et al. (2003) In vitro and in vivo antitumor activity of liposomal Fenretinide targeted to human neuroblastoma. Int J Cancer 104:559–567

Raffaghello L, Airoldi I, Prigione I et al. (2004) Functional expression and release of ligands for the activating immunoreceptor NKG2D in human neuroblastoma. Adv Neuroblast Res 11th abstract #202.1

Ragupathi G, Livingston P, Hood C et al. (2003) Immunogenicity of GD2 lactone (GD2L)-KLH conjugate plus immunological adjuvant QS-21 vaccine in patients wtih melanoma. Clin Cancer Res 9:5214–5220

Ravetch JV, Bolland S (2001) IgG Fc receptors. Annu Rev Immunol 19:275–290

Reiter Y (2001) Recombinant immunotoxins in targeted cancer cell therapy. Adv Cancer Res 81:93–124

Roguska MA, Pedersen JT, Henry AH et al. (1996) A comparison of two murine monoclonal antibodies humanized by CDR-grafting and variable domain resurfacing. Protein Eng 9:895–904

Ross GD, Vetvicka V, Yan J et al. (1999) Therapeutic intervention with complement and beta-glucan in cancer. Immunopharmacology 42:61–74

Rossig C, Bollard CM, Nuchtern JG et al. (2001) Targeting of G(D2)-positive tumor cells by human T lymphocytes engineered to express chimeric T-cell receptor genes. Int J Cancer 94:228–236

Rousseau RF, Haight AE, Hirschmann-Jax C et al. (2003) Local and systemic effects of an allogeneic tumor cell vaccine combining transgenic human lymphotactin with interleukin-2 in patients with advanced or refractory neuroblastoma. Blood 101:1718–1726

Sandler AD, Chihara H, Kobayashi G et al. (2003) CpG oligonucleotides enhance the tumor antigen-specific immune response of a granulocyte macrophage colony-stimulating factor-based vaccine strategy in neuroblastoma. Cancer Res 63:394–399

Sarkar AK, Nuchtern JG (2000) Lysis of MYCN-amplified neuroblastoma cells by *MYCN* peptide-specific cytotoxic T lymphocytes. Cancer Res 60:1908–1913

Satoh J, Kurohara K, Yukitake M et al. (1998) Interleukin-15, a T-cell growth factor, is expressed in human neural cell lines and tissues. J Neurol Sci 155:170–177

Scanlan MJ, Gure AO, Jungbluth AA et al. (2002) Cancer/testis antigens: an expanding family of targets for cancer immunotherapy. Immunol Rev 188:22–32

Scheffold C, Kornacker M, Scheffold YC et al. (2002) Visualization of effective tumor targeting by CD8+ natural killer T cells redirected with bispecific antibody F(ab')(2) HER2xCD3. Cancer Res 62:5785–5791

Schilbach KE, Geiselhart A, Wessels JT et al. (2000) Human gammadelta T lymphocytes exert natural and IL-2-induced cytotoxicity to neuroblastoma cells. J Immunother 23:536–548

Schonmann SM, Iyer J, Laeng H et al. (1986) Production and characterization of monoclonal antibodies against human neuroblastoma. Int J Cancer 37:255–262

Schulz G, Cheresh DA, Varki NM et al. (1984) Detection of ganglioside GD2 in tumor tissues and sera of neuroblastoma patients. Cancer Res 44:5914–5920

Scott AM, Lee FT, Hopkins W et al. (2001) Specific targeting, biodistribution, and lack of immunogenicity of chimeric anti-GD3 monoclonal antibody KM871 in patients with metastatic melanoma: results of a phase I trial. J Clin Oncol 19:3976–3987

Sen G, Chakraborty M, Foon KA et al. (1998) Induction of IgG antibodies by an anti-idiotype antibody mimicking disialoganglioside GD2. J Immunother 21:75–83

Shen W, Ladisch S (2002) Ganglioside GD1a impedes lipopolysaccharide-induced maturation of human dendritic cells. Cell Immunol 220:125–133

Shimizu M, Fontana A, Takeda Y et al. (1999) Induction of antitumor immunity with Fas/APO-1 ligand (CD95L)-transfected neuroblastoma neuro-2a cells. J Immunol 162:7350–7357

Shimizu T, Berhanu A, Redlinger RE Jr et al. (2001) Interleukin-12 transduced dendritic cells induce regression of established murine neuroblastoma. J Pediatr Surg 36:1285–1292

Shurin GV, Gerein V, Lotze MT et al. (1998) Apoptosis induced in T cells by human neuroblastoma cells: role of Fas ligand. Nat Immun 16:263–274

Shurin GV, Shurin MR, Bykovskaia S et al. (2001) Neuroblastoma-derived gangliosides inhibit dendritic cell generation and function. Cancer Res 61:363–369

Siapati KE, Barker S, Kinnon C et al. (2003) Improved antitumour immunity in murine neuroblastoma using a combination of IL-2 and IL-12. Br J Cancer 88:1641–1648

Smolarz K, Waters W, Sieverts H et al. (1989) Immunoscintigraphy with Tc-99m-labeled monoclonal antibody BW575 compared with I-123 MIBG scintigraphy in neuroblastoma. Radiology 173:152–153

Smyth MJ, Crowe NY, Hayakawa Y et al. (2002) NKT cells: conductors of tumor immunity? Curr Opin Immunol 14:165–171

Soling A, Schurr P, Berthold F (1999) Expression and clinical relevance of NY-ESO-1, MAGE-1 and MAGE-3 in neuroblastoma. Anticancer Res 19:2205–2209

Sondel PM, Hank JA (1997) Combination therapy with interleukin-2 and antitumor monoclonal antibodies. Cancer J Sci Am 3 (Suppl 1):S121–S127

Tai T, Cahan LD, Paulson JC et al. (1984) Human monoclonal antibody against ganglioside GD2: use in development of enzyme-linked immunosorbent assay for the monitoring of anti-GD2 in cancer patients. J Natl Cancer Inst 73:627–633

Takamizawa S, Okamoto S, Wen J et al. (2000) Overexpression of Fas-ligand by neuroblastoma: a novel mechanism of tumor-cell killing. J Pediatr Surg 35:375–379

Thomas PB, Delatte SJ, Sutphin A et al. (2002) Effective targeted cytotoxicity of neuroblastoma cells. J Pediatr Surg 37: 539–544

Todo T, Martuza RL, Dallman MJ et al. (2001) In situ expression of soluble B7-1 in the context of oncolytic herpes simplex virus induces potent antitumor immunity. Cancer Res 61:153–161

Toren A, Nagler A, Rozenfeld-Granot G et al. (2000) Amplification of immunological functions by subcutaneous injection of intermediate-high dose interleukin-2 for 2 years after autologous stem cell transplantation in children with stage IV neuroblastoma. Transplantation 70:1100–1104

Tsao CY, Lou W, Wang S et al. (2002) Identification of GD2 ganglioside peptide mimics by using phage display peptide libraries. Proc Am Assoc Cancer Res 43:280

Tur MK, Sasse S, Stocker M et al. (2001a) An anti-GD2 single chain Fv selected by phage display and fused to Pseudomonas exotoxin A develops specific cytotoxic activity against neuroblastoma derived cell lines. Int J Mol Med 8:579–584

Tur MK, Huhn M, Sasse S et al. (2001b) Selection of scFv phages on intact cells under low pH conditions leads to a significant loss of insert-free phages. Biotechniques 30:404–408, 410, 412–413

Turner JG, Rakhmilevich AL, Burdelya L et al. (2001) Anti-CD40 antibody induces antitumor and antimetastatic effects: the role of NK cells. J Immunol 166:89–94

Vaickus L, Biddle W, Cemerlic D et al. (1990) Interferon gamma augments Lym-1-dependent, granulocyte-mediated tumor cell lysis. Blood 75:2408–2416

Valteau-Couanet D, Leboulaire C, Maincent K et al. (2002) Dendritic cells for NK/LAK activation: rationale for multicellular immunotherapy in neuroblastoma patients. Blood 100:2554–2561

Van der Bruggen P, Zhang Y, Chaux P et al. (2002) Tumor-specific shared antigenic peptides recognized by human T cells. Immunol Rev 188:51–64

Van Spriel AB, van Ojik HH, van de Winkel JG (2000) Immunotherapeutic perspective for bispecific antibodies. Immunol Today 21:391–397

Vlk V, Eckschlager T, Kavan P et al. (2000) Clinical ineffectiveness of IL-2 and/or IFN alpha administration after autologous PBSC transplantation in pediatric oncological patients. Pediatr Hematol Oncol 17:31–44

Wargalla UC, Reisfeld RA (1989) Rate of internalization of an immunotoxin correlates with cytotoxic activity against human tumor cells. Proc Natl Acad Sci USA 86:5146–5150

Wigginton JM, Wiltrout RH (2002) IL-12/IL-2 combination cytokine therapy for solid tumours: translation from bench to bedside. Exp Opin Biol Ther 2:513–524

Wu DY, Segal NH, Sidobre S et al. (2003) Cross-presentation of Disialoganglioside GD3 to Natural Killer T Cells. J Exp Med 198:173–181

Xiao W-h, Yu A, Sorkin LS (1997) Electrophysiological characteristics of primary afferent fibers after systemic administration of anti-GD2 ganglioside antibody. Pain 69:145–151

Yeh SD, Larson SM, Burch L et al. (1991) Radioimmunodetection of neuroblastoma with iodine-131-3F8: correlation with biopsy, iodine-131-metaiodobenzylguanidine (MIBG) and standard diagnostic modalities. J Nucl Med 32:769–776
Yoshida H, Tanabe M, Miyauchi M et al. (1999) Induced immunity by expression of interleukin-2 or GM-CSF gene in murine neuroblastoma cells can generate antitumor response to established tumors. Cancer Gene Ther 6:395–401
Yu AL, Batova A, Alvarado C, Rao VJ, Castelberry RP (1997) Usefulness of a chimeric anti-GD2 (ch.14.18) and GM-CSF for refractory neuroblastoma: a POG phase II study. Proc ASCO 16:1846
Yu A, Uttenreuther-Fischer M, Huang C-S et al. (1998) Phase I trial of a human-mouse chimeric anti-disialoganglioside monoclonal antibody ch14.18 in patients with refractory neuroblastoma and osteosarcoma. J Clin Oncol 16:2169–2180
Yuki N, Yamada M, Tagawa Y et al. (1997) Pathogenesis of the neurotoxicity caused by anti-GD2 antibody therapy. J Neurol Sci 149:127–130
Zalutsky MR, Vaidyanathan G (2000) Astatine-211-labeled radiotherapeutics: an emerging approach to targeted alpha-particle radiotherapy. Curr Pharm Des 6:1433–1455
Zeytin HE, Tripathi PK, Bhattacharya-Chatterjee M et al. (2000) Construction and characterization of DNA vaccines encoding the single-chain variable fragment of the anti-idiotype antibody 1A7 mimicking the tumor-associated antigen disialoganglioside GD2. Cancer Gene Therapy 7:1426–1436
Zhu Z, Hattori K, Zhang H et al. (2003) Inhibition of human leukemia in an animal model with human antibodies directed against vascular endothelial growth factor receptor 2. Correlation between antibody affinity and biological activity. Leukemia 17:604–611

Differentiation and Retinoids

Carol J. Thiele, C. Patrick Reynolds

Contents

15.1 Introduction

The clinical behavior as well as the associated histopathologic features of neuroblastomas (NB) have long suggested that tumorigenesis of this pediatric cancer is, at least in part, related to defects in the process of cellular differentiation. Primary and metastatic NBs consist of different cell types, and the cells commonly have different stages of differentiation. The histologically more mature forms of NB, ganglioneuroblastoma and ganglioneuroma, correspond to the normal differentiation patterns seen in the developing sympathetic nervous system. Moreover, the histologic classification of NB into subsets based on the extent of differentiation, the presence of stroma or Schwannian tissue, and the degree of mitotic/karyorrhectic cells when combined with age is highly predictive of outcome (Shimada et al. 1984).

15.1.1 Neural Crest Development

The neural crest is a transient embryonal structure that arises at the interface between the non-neural and neural ectoderm or neural plate. As the neural plate invaginates and the folds approximate to form the neural tube, inductive influences from the underlying mesoderm and the overlying non-neural ectoderm stimulate the dorsal aspect of the developing neural tube to form the neural crest cells. Cells migrate laterally from the neural tube to form or contribute to a variety of cell types including:

1. Neuronal cells; the sensory ganglia of several cranial nerves, spinal ganglia and ganglion of the autonomic nervous system

2. Supportive cells of the nervous system; glial, of the peripheral ganglion; Schwann cells of the peripheral nerves, and meninges of the anterior brain
3. Pigmented cells; except pigmented retina
4. Endocrine and paraedocrine cells; adrenomedullary cells, calcitonin-producing cells and type-I cells of the carotid body
5. Mesectodermal derivatives; visceral and facial skeleton; walls of the large arteries derived from the aortic arches, connective tissue of thymus and parathyroid glands, and dermis of the neck and facial regions (Le Dourain and Kalcheim 1999)

The fate or specialization of neural crest cells depends on their rostro-caudal location along the neural tube; however, in vitro and in vivo studies indicate that neural crest cells retain a high degree of plasticity even after they migrate from the neural tube. Interestingly, these are also features that mark highly malignant NB cells.

15.1.2 NB as a Neural Crest Derivative

Neuroblastomas frequently express both tyrosine hydroxylase (TH) and dopamine-β-hydroxylase (DβH), enzymes involved in the synthesis of the catecholamines. Not only are catecholamines characteristic of sympathetic neurons, but migrating neural crest cells are also catecholaminergic (Smith and Fauquet 1984). Tyrosine hydroxylase and DβH provided the earliest molecular markers that distinguished NB from other small round blue cell tumors such as Askin's tumor, Ewing's sarcomas, and peripheral neuroectodermal tumors, which express high levels of choline acetyltransferase (Thiele et al. 1988). Tyrosine hydroxylase and DβH expression are associated with the secretion of catecholamines and their metabolites (VMH and HVA) into the urine, providing diagnostic (Lopez-Ibor and Schwartz 1985) and screening markers (see Chap. 2) for NB.

Clinically, NBs present in a number of different anatomic locations most frequently reflecting the sites of sympathetic nervous system tissues. These sites include postganglionic neuronal precursors that are found in paravertebral ganglia of the sympathetic trunk, pre-aortic ganglia in the plexus around the branches of the abdominal aorta, and in the medullary and/or ganglionic cells of the adrenal gland (Jaffe 1976). During fetal development, sites of sympathetic nervous system tissue also include neuroendocrine structures with rests of neuroblasts in the adrenal gland and paraganglia adjacent to the sympathetic ganglia.

15.1.3 NB and Adrenal Medullary Development

During development of human adrenal medullary chromaffin tissue, cells express TH, chromogranin A (CgA), and neuropeptide Y (NPY) within the first 10 weeks of gestation (Cooper et al. 1990). By 26 weeks of gestation, cells co-express delta (a ligand for the notch receptor) but lose NPY expression until after birth when they express β2-microglobulin, the light chain receptor of the major histocompatibility complex, and re-express NPY. A second population of fetal ganglionic neuroblasts develops in the medullary region that expresses HNK-1 but not TH, CgA, or delta (Cooper et al. 1990). The NB cell lines also express these patterns of gene expression indicating that some NB tumors may arise from tumorigenic events occurring at different stages of adrenal medullary cell development (Cooper et al. 1990). Furthermore, NB tumor tissue express patterns of chromaffin-related genes that correlate with the patterns of gene expression observed during maturation of adrenal medullary chromaffin tissues (Cohen et al. 1990; Cooper et al. 1992).

In vitro studies showed that NB cell lines treated with compounds that raised intracellular cAMP levels stimulated a more neuroendocrine pattern of gene expression, while signal transduction pathways regulated by retinoid receptors stimulated more neuronal gene expression patterns (Gaetano et al. 1991). Oxygen deprivation, as would occur in a necrotic area may cause a hypoxic response and induction of the transcription factor HIF1α. In vitro, the induction of HIF1α leads to decreased expression of more mature neuronal and neuroendocrine markers such as NPY, CgA, and TH, and increased expression of growth factors such as VEGF, IGF-2, and a bHLH transcription factor inhibitor of differentiation, Id-2. These genes are more highly expressed in immature neural crest cells (Jogi et al. 2002), and VEGF (Eggert et al. 2000) is expressed in more immature and aggressive NBs, suggesting that the underlying biologic features of tumor cells are influenced not only by genetic events involved in tumorigenesis but also by their environment.

15.1.4 Neural Crest Gene Expression During Development

More recently in animal studies, a number of genes, including *slug, AP-2, HNK-1, and Krox-20,* distinguish the earliest neural crest cells from other neighboring epithelial and mesoderm derivatives in normal or genetically modified chicks, frogs, zebrafish, and mice. Many of these genes encode proteins that are thought to regulate gene transcription and neural crest cell determination. These genes are regulated in part by signals induced by bone morphogenic protein (BMP2/4) or Wnts. The BMPs are members of the TGFβ signaling path that utilize serine/threonine kinase receptors to transmit extracellular signals to the cytoplasm where a series of intracellular signaling intermediaries (SMADs) relay signals to the nucleus and regulate gene expression. Activation of the Wnt signal transduction path stabilizes the cytoplasmic protein β-catenin enabling its translocation into the nucleus and activation of neural crest markers (Wu et al. 2003). The BMP alone and in combination with retinoids have been found to induce differentiation of NB tumor cells and control their growth (Y. Nakamura et al. 2003; Sumantran et al. 2003).

15.1.5 *MYCN* in Neural Crest Development

As described in Chap. 4, *MYCN* amplification contributes to the clinically aggressive behavior of NB tumors (Seeger et al. 1985). *MYCN* has also been shown to play an important role in the development of sympathetic neurons. Deletion of the *MYCN* gene in animal models leads to a reduction in the number of mature neurons in the dorsal root and sympathetic ganglia (Sawai et al. 1993; Stanton et al. 1992). In addition, *MYCN* can stimulate post-mitotic sympathetic neurons to re-enter the cell cycle and enhance their survival (Wartiovaara et al. 2002). In avian embryos, migrating neural crest cells express *MYCN*. After cessation of the major wave of neural crest cell migration, *MYCN* expression is heterogeneous in the dorsal root and sympathetic ganglia, being more highly expressed in the nucleus of neuronal cells and decreased in Schwann and glial cells. In explants of neural crest cells in vitro, expression of *MYCN* stimulates an increase in differentiated neural crest cells without affecting proliferation. Implantation of *MYCN*-transduced neural crest cells in vivo leads to a massive migration of cells into the sympathetic ganglia and an increase in differentiated cells; thus, *MYCN* functions at an early phase of neural crest development increasing their migratory potential and a later phase promoting their neural differentiation (Wakamatsu et al. 1997).

15.2 Neurotrophins in Neural Crest Development

Neurogenesis in the sympathetic ganglia is governed by precursor proliferation, followed by a period of apoptosis as neuroblasts that fail to innervate their target tissues die, while others complete functional maturation. Upon innervation of their target tissues, neuroblast survival is mediated by growth/survival factors called neurotrophins (NTs). Neurotrophins exist as precursor proteins (proNTs) that are processed to mature NT proteins. The NT family of secreted growth factors include nerve growth factor (NGF), brain-derived neurotrophic factor (BDNF), NT-3, and NT-4/5 that bind to their cognate tyrosine kinase receptors TrkA, TrkB, and TrkC (Fig. 15.1). Neurotrophins bind and facilitate dimerization of Trk receptors, activating their intrinsic tyrosine kinase activities that initiate a kinase cascade that transmits signals to the nucleus to regulate genes important in neural survival and growth (Teng and Hempstead 2004). Both proNTs and mature NTs bind to the p75 receptor, which has limited homology to death receptor transmembrane proteins (Fig. 15.1). Recent evidence indicates that proNT interacts solely with p75 and in association with an accessory receptor, sortilin, is a potent death signal (Nykjaer et al.

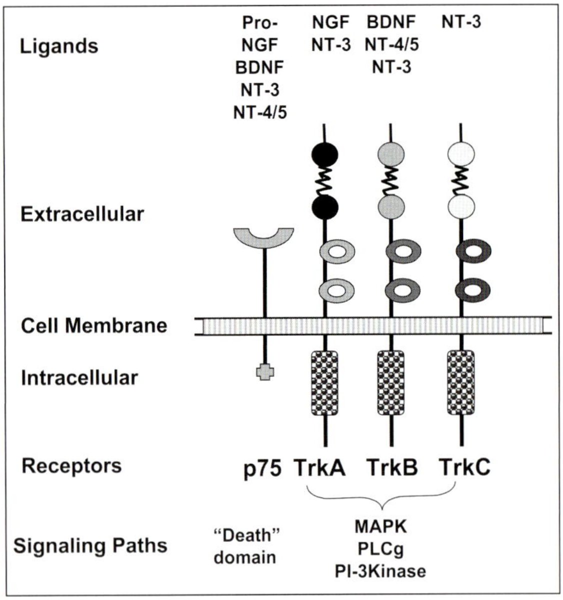

Figure 15.1

The cognate receptors for neurotrophins (NGF, BDNF, NT-3, and NT4/5). The p75 or nerve growth factor receptor (NGFR) binds all pre-processed (i.e., pro-NGF) and processed neurotrophins with equal affinity. p75 shares homology with the death receptor family of signaling receptors and this receptor may transmit either death-inducing or survival signals depending on cell type and context. Different neurotrophins interact selectively with distinct members of the Trk family of tyrosine kinase receptors. The structure of the Trk receptors contains several distinct protein motifs. The *filled circles* represent cysteine-rich regions separated by a fibronectin type-III repeat. The *open circles* to the right of the line contain Ig-like loops and the *sphere-filled rectangle* on the intracellular portion of the receptor contains the catalytic tyrosine kinase domain which is activated upon interaction of the extracellular portion of the receptor with the cognate ligand. Activation of the tyrosine kinase leads to activation of other signaling paths including the MAPK path, the PLCγ path, and the PI-3 kinase paths that ultimately transmit signals to the nucleus regulating gene transcription and ultimately affecting cell survival, growth, and differentiation.

2004). The NT/Trk (Kaplan and Miller 2000), p75 and the membrane bound kinase receptors of glial-derived neurotrophic factors (GDNF/RET), play important roles in the development of the peripheral nervous system.

The majority of migrating neural crest cells express TrkC and p75 and may be mitotically active or post-mitotic. A fraction of these also co-express TrkA. In the adrenal gland. The BDNF is expressed in the adrenal cortex during embryogenesis but is restricted to the interface of the adrenal cortex and medulla in the adult. Another TrkB ligand, NT-4, is highly expressed in the adrenal medulla. The majority of neuronal cells in the medulla express TrkA and p75 but not TrkB, although TrkB is restricted to a small number of ganglion cells. Under certain conditions NT-4 activates TrkA and may serve as a physiologic ligand for TrkA expressing chromaffin cells; however the neurons of the intermediolateral column of the spinal cord express TrkB and BDNF and innervate adrenal medullary chromaffin cells (Schober et al. 1999).

15.2.1 TrkA and NB

In NBs the expression of the neurotrophin receptors, Trks, have prognostic significance (see Chap. 5). TrkA and/or TrkC are more highly expressed in primary NBs tumors from patients who have a good prognosis (Nakagawara et al. 1993; Yamashiro et al. 1997), while expression of $p145^{TrkB}$ and its ligand BDNF is more highly expressed in primary NBs from patients with an unfavorable prognosis (Nakagawara et al. 1994). In NB cell lines engineered to express high levels of TrkA, activation with nerve growth factor (NGF) can decrease MYCN levels (Matsushima and Bogenmann 1993; Woo et al. 2004) by mediating signals transduced through the MAP kinase pathway (Woo et al. 2004). In NB cell lines, interferon gamma (Lucarelli et al. 1995), and to a lesser extent retinoids (Kaplan and Miller 2000), induce TrkA, suggesting that the levels of TrkA may be amenable to regulation in clinically aggressive NBs.

15.2.2 TrkB and NB

Activation of TrkB by its ligand BDNF has been shown to promote survival, alter sensitivity to chemotherapeutic drugs, and stimulate invasiveness – all properties of highly malignant tumors cells (Matsumoto et al. 1995) (see Chap. 5). An interesting aspect of the clinical behavior of poor prognosis NBs is that even though they are initially sensitive to chemotherapeutic agents, they often ultimately become resistant. The basis of this chemoresistance is probably multi-factorial being influenced by traditional chemoresistance factors such as the level of expression of drug efflux pumps such as MRP (Norris et al. 1996) and mutations in *TP53* (Keshelava et al. 2001; Tweddle et al. 2001). In addition, the level of expression of BDNF and its receptor TrkB may also contribute to the escape of NB cells from the effects of cytotoxic chemotherapy. Drug-resistant NB cell lines have increased levels of expression of BDNF and the levels of BDNF increase as the cells become progressively resistant to higher concentrations of cytotoxic drugs (Scala et al. 1996). Additionally, both the concentration of BDNF and the level of expression of TrkB have been shown to diminish the sensitivity of cells to drugs typically used in the therapy of NB (Jaboin et al. 2002). Recent studies have identified two targets of the TrkB pathway amenable to drug development. A drug targeting Trk tyrosine kinases (CEP-701) is in clinical trials and has shown preclinical efficacy against NB mouse xenografts (Evans et al. 1999). Furthermore, a number of compounds targeting the PI-3-kinase pathway and its downstream targets are in pre-clinical development. Such agents may enhance the toxicity of chemotherapeutic agents against aggressive NB.

15.3 Differentiation

Neuroblastoma cell lines are comprised of at least three morphologically distinct phenotypes: neuroblastic cells (N-type); non-neuronal substrate-adherent cells (S-type), and cells with an intermediate phenotype (I type), with distinct morphologic, biochemical, and tumorigenic properties (see Chap. 8). I-type cells can be induced to differentiate into N-type or S-type cells under selective culture conditions. Cytotoxic chemotherapeutic regimens can also induce NB maturation (McLaughlin and Urich 1977; Raaf et al. 1982). These observations led to subsequent studies aimed at evaluating induction of differentiation as a therapeutic strategy. A variety of chemicals and biologic response modifiers, including retinoids, histone-deacetylase inhibitors, agents that raise intracellular calcium levels, activators of protein kinase C, neurotrophins, and cytokines, have been shown to suppress tumorigenicity, control growth, and induce NB differentiation of NB cell lines.

15.3.1 Retinoids

Vitamin A or retinol primarily from the diet plays a critical role in normal neural crest development. The metabolism and storage of retinol is mediated by a number of binding proteins and enzymes. Intracellular retinol is metabolized to all-trans retinoic acid (ATRA). All-trans retinoic acid is a major mediator of the effects of vitamin A via activation of a number of RAR and RXR nuclear receptors that heterodimerize and regulate gene transcription (see below). Exposure of human neuroblastoma cell lines to supraphysiologic doses (micromolar) of ATRA caused a reduction of cell growth and induction of neurite extension and differentiation that was ultrastructurally, biochemically, and electro-physiologically similar to normal neural cells (Fig. 15.2; Sidell 1982; Abemayor and Sidell 1989).

The ATRA treatment of NB cells was accompanied by a decrease in the expression (Thiele et al. 1985) and transcription (Thiele and Israel 1988) of the *MYCN* gene. The decrease in *MYCN* expression preceded the ATRA-induced G1 arrest and evidence of morphologic differentiation (Thiele et al. 1985), and the *MYCN* over-expression blocked differentiation (Peverali et al. 1996). All-trans retinoic acid induced decreases in *MYCN* levels and increases in the cyclin-dependent kinase inhibitor p27 which may mediate the G1 arrest of NB cell cycle (Matsuo and Thiele 1998; M. Nakamura et al. 2003). Pulse therapy with retinoic acid showed a sustained arrest of tu-

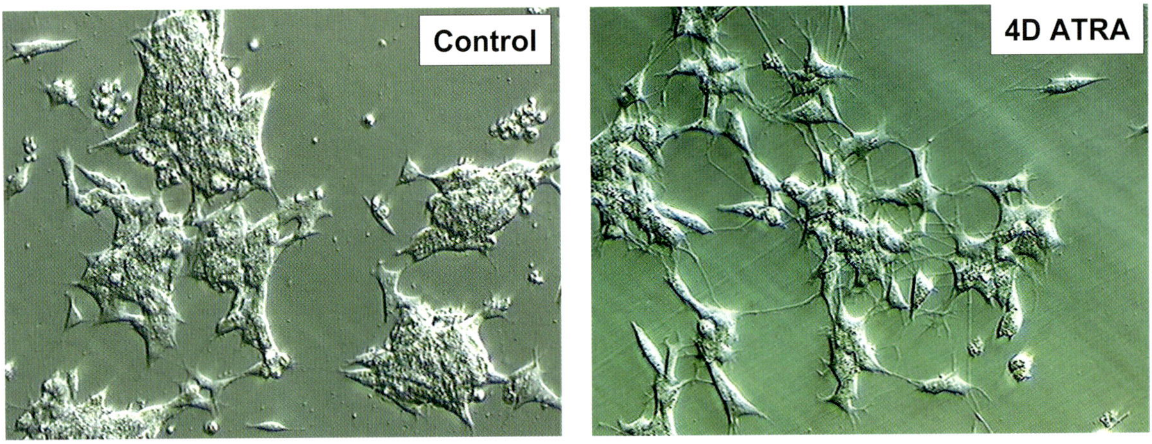

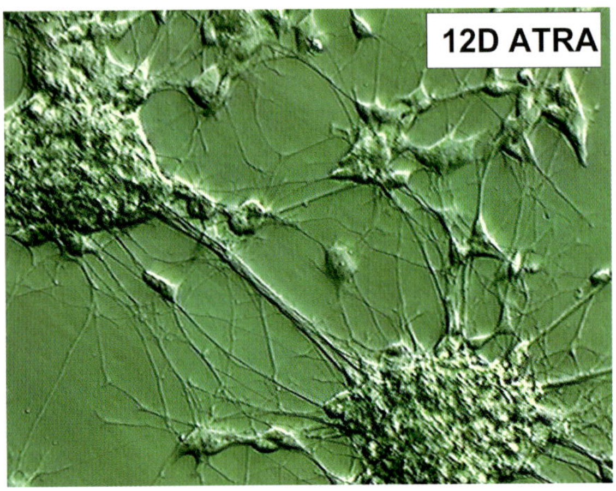

Figure 15.2

Morphologic appearance of SMS-KCNR cells cultured in control solvent or 5-µM all-trans retinoic acid for indicated days

mor cell proliferation in NB cell lines, suggesting that high-dose pulse retinoid therapy (as opposed to the more traditional low-dose continuous retinoid therapy) might be effective in vivo (Reynolds et al. 1991).

15.3.2 Retinoic Acid Receptors

The differentiation and growth arrest of malignant cells produced by retinoic acid are likely mediated by one or more of the two families of retinoic acid receptors (RAR or RXR): RAR α, β, γ; and RXR α, β, γ (Linney 1992); all belong to the steroid/thyroid hormone family of transcription factors and possess discrete DNA-binding and retinoic acid-binding domains. As depicted in Fig. 15.3, retinoic acid binds to the RA receptors, causing conformational changes that promote binding to specific cis-acting DNA sequences, which regulate transcription of certain target genes (Reynolds and Lemons 2001). A study of the RAR and RXR families of RA receptors in NB showed that they were expressed in most NB cell lines and primary tumors (Li et al. 1994). While RAR β was only expressed in 4 of 14 *MYCN* amplified cell lines, it could be induced by ATRA in most of these cell lines (Li et al. 1994). There was no correlation between resistance to ATRA and the level of RAR or RXR expression; however, higher expression of RARβ has been associated with good outcome in NB and RARβ over-expression by transfection in-

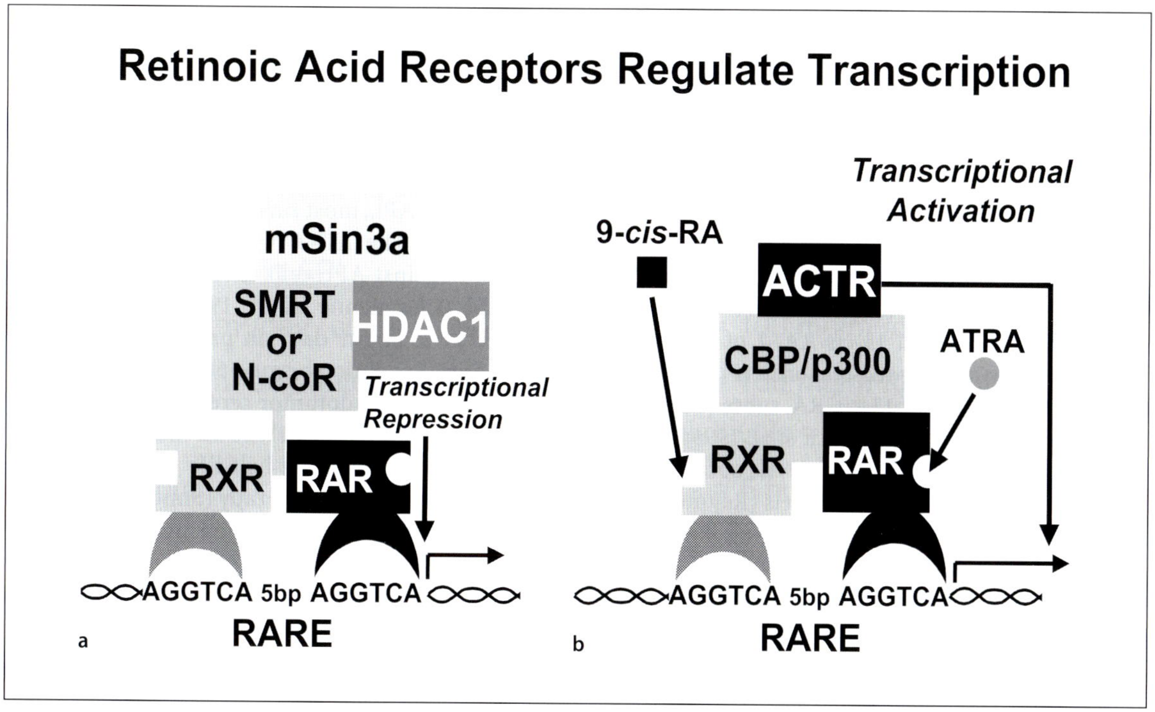

Figure 15.3 a,b

The mechanism of action of retinoids is mediated via zinc-finger transcriptional regulators which function as heterodimers to regulate promoter activity of certain target genes. The RAR and RXR proteins bind to specific direct repeat DNA sequences (AGGTCA are separated by either two or five nucleotides) in gene promoters, known as retinoic acid response elements, or RARE. **a** In the absence of ligand, the RAR/RXR heterodimers interact with nuclear co-repressors including N-CoR and SMRT, which in turn bind to a common adapter protein mSin3 which complexes to proteins with histone deacetylase activity to repress transcription. **b** Retinoic acid binds to the RAR portion of the complex causing a conformational change in the RAR and RXR proteins which releases the co-repressor complex and facilitates binding of 9-cis-RA to the RXR protein (the latter enhances the activation response). The transcriptional co-regulator CBP/p300 then binds to the receptor complex and recruits the coactivator protein ACTR, which contains histone acetyltransferase activity, and promotes transcription (Reynolds and Lemons 2001)

creases the responsiveness of some NB cell lines to RA (Cheung et al. 1998). Furthermore, RARβ selective agonists mediate growth inhibitory signals in NB cell lines (Giannini et al. 1997); thus, while alterations in RAR or RXR do not appear to be a major resistance mechanism, higher levels of expression of these receptors may enhance sensitivity to retinoids.

15.4 13-cis-Retinoic Acid

In the mid-1980s the only retinoid available for clinical use was 13-cis-retinoic acid (13-cis-RA), which induced differentiation in promyelocytic leukemia, and produced objective clinical responses in promyelocytic leukemia, myelodysplastic syndrome, cutaneous T-cell lymphoma (mycosis fungoides), and advanced squamous carcinoma of the skin (Reynolds and Lemons 2001). Although 13-cis-RA has limited

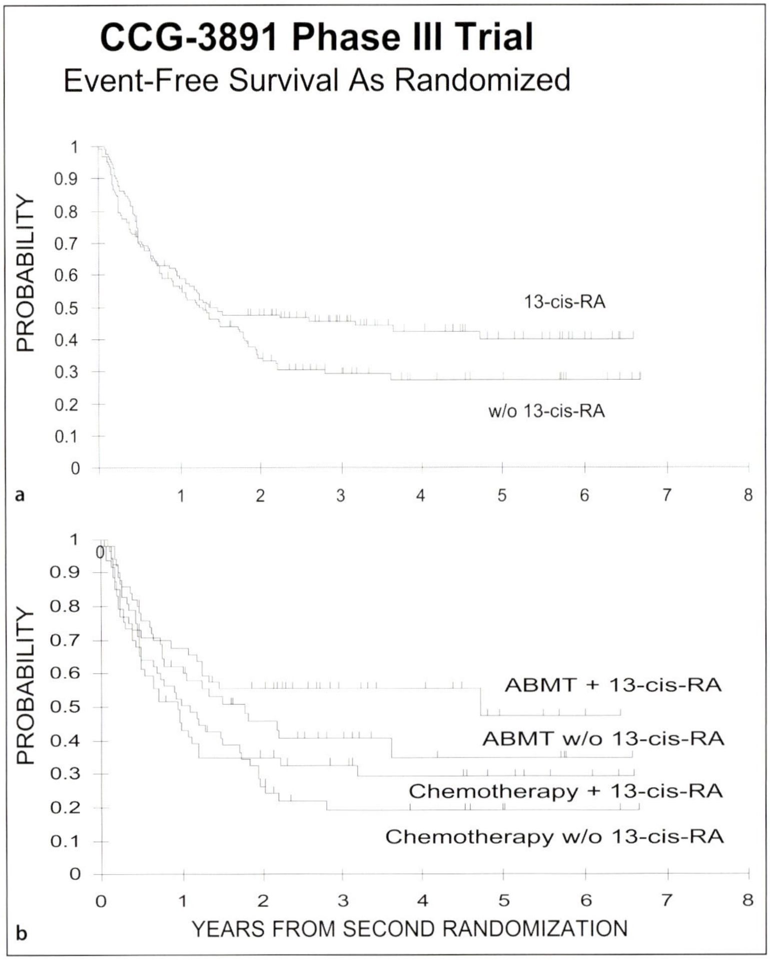

Figure 15.5 a,b

Event-free survival for CCG-3891 showing the second randomization between13-cis-RA vs no further therapy (**a**), and the four groups created by the quasi-factorial design (**b**). The latter curves are limited to only those patients completing both randomizations. All curves are shown from time of randomization (Matthay et al. 1999)

for patients who received either ABMT or non-myeloablative chemotherapy. As shown in Fig. 15.5b, there appeared to be a higher 3-year EFS from time of second randomization in patients undergoing both randomizations for those randomized to both ABMT and 13-cis-RA (55±10%), compared with ABMT alone (41±10%; P=0.28). The 3-year EFS for chemotherapy and 13-cis-RA was 33±7%, compared with chemotherapy alone (19±7%; P=0.17).

In 1989 the European NB Study Group (ENSG) initiated a randomized trial of 13-cis-RA vs no further therapy in children with advanced NB who achieved remission after high-dose therapy (Kohler et al. 2000). Patients randomized to 13-cis-RA on the ENSG study were given a single daily dose of 0.75 mg/kg (22.5 mg/m^2 day^{-1} continuously for 4 years or until relapse). Approximately 175 children were entered into the study with 88 patients randomized to receive 13-cis-RA (3-year event-free survival=37%) and 87 patients randomized to placebo (3-year event-free survival=42%); thus, in contrast to the CCG study, no advantage in event-free survival was shown in this trial for children randomized to receive low-dose, continuous 13-cis-RA. These results emphasize the importance of utilizing adequate dose levels and optimal dosing schedules to achieve pharmacologically efficacious drug levels when employing retinoids as anti-cancer agents.

15.5 Fenretinide

N-(4-hydroxyphenyl) retinamide or fenretinide (4-HPR is a synthetic retinoid; Fig. 15.6) inhibits NB growth in vitro at 1–10 µM (Ponzoni et al. 1995) and was highly active against retinoic-acid resistant NB lines at 5–10 µM (Reynolds et al. 2000). In contrast to 13-cis-RA and ATRA, 4-HPR does not induce maturational changes, but is cytotoxic, causing both apoptosis and necrosis (Maurer et al. 1999). Toxicity of 4-HPR in chemoprevention clinical trials has been minimal. The major clinical toxicity of 4-HPR is decreased night vision, due to decreased plasma retinol levels. No hematologic toxicity has been reported (Reynolds and Lemons 2001). In pediatrics, fenretinide has been well tolerated (Garaventa et al. 2003), and the MTD of oral 4-HPR given for 7 days every 3 weeks is 2475 mg/m^2 day^{-1}, which achieved 4-HPR plasma levels of 6–10 µM (Villablanca et al. 2002).

4-HPR has been shown to achieve multi-log cytotoxicity in NB cell lines resistant to ATRA and 13-cis-RA (Reynolds et al. 2000). Resistance to 13-cis-RA in NB cell lines appears to involve selection for increased expression of *MYCN* or c-*myc*, and such retinoic acid-resistant NB cell lines are collaterally hypersensitive to 4-HPR; thus, pre-clinical data suggest that sequential use of 13-cis-RA, followed by 4-HPR, could be an effective approach to treating minimal residual disease in NB patients after myeloablative therapy.

The mechanisms by which 4-HPR achieves anti-tumor cytotoxicity are not completely understood. One mechanism by which 4-HPR stimulates apoptosis is the induction of reactive oxygen species in NB cells (Maurer et al. 1999; Lovat et al. 2003a). Other possible mechanisms include induction of lipo-oxygenase, the stress-induced transcription factor GADD153 (Lovat et al. 2002; Corazzari et al. 2003), and Bak, a pro-apoptotic member of the bcl-2 family (Lovat et al. 2003b).

A major portion of fenretinide cytotoxicity for NB cell lines at high concentrations (~ 5–10 µM) is via non-apoptotic mechanisms (Maurer et al. 1999). Fenretinide stimulated large increases of ceramide in NB cell lines, which may account for its non-apoptotic cytotoxicity (Reynolds et al. 2004). Agents that modulate ceramide metabolism can increase the anti-tumor activity of 4-HPR. Drugs that inhibit glucosylceramide synthase/1-O-acylceramide synthase or sphingosine kinase, or safingol (L-threo-dihydrosphingosine), which modulate ceramide metabolism and/or action, can significantly increase 4-HPR anti-tumor activity with minimal toxicity to normal fibroblasts or bone marrow myeloid progenitors (CFU-GM; Maurer et al. 2000). Fenretinide has also been shown to inhibit NB-induced angiogenesis (Ribatti et al. 2001), and the anti-angiogenic activity of 4-HPR may be in part mediated via ceramide (Erdreich-Epstein et al. 2002). The latter data suggest that 4-HPR alone or in combination with ceramide mod-

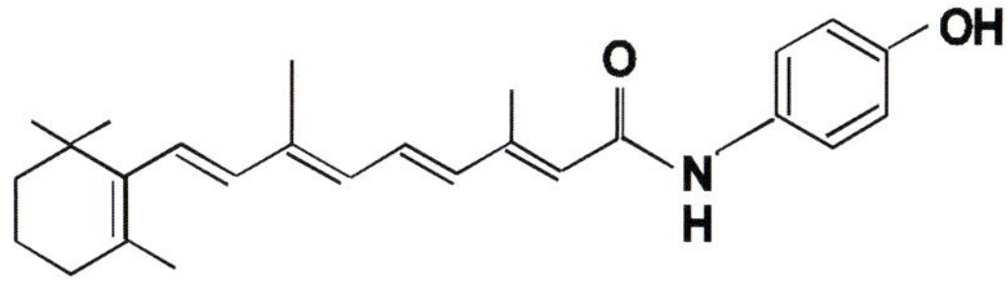

fenretinide (4-HPR)

Synthetic retinoid

Active against retinoic acid-resistant neuroblastoma cell lines

Cytotoxic for tumor cells via reactive oxygen species and increasing ceramide

Phase I therapeutic trials in pediatrics showed minimal systemic toxicity

Figure 15.6

Structure of the cytotoxic retinoid N-(4-hydroxyphenyl) retinamide=fenretinide (4-HPR) and a summary of its properties ulators may achieve anti-tumor activity in vivo by both direct effects against tumor and anti-angiogenesis.

One limitation with fenretinide is the need for large administered doses to achieve effective drug levels. Although the currently available oral capsular dose form of 4-HPR is poorly bioavailable and difficult to administer to small children, a phase-II study of the 4-HPR oral capsule formulation in recurrent NB is ongoing in the Children's Oncology Group (COG). Pre-clinical studies have been reported with a liposome formulation of 4-HPR targeted to NB via an anti-GD2 monoclonal antibody looks promising (Raffaghello et al. 2003). New oral and intravenous formulations of fenretinide have been developed via the NCI RAID program and these are entering clinical trials in 2004 (www.nant.org). These new formulations are likely more bioavailable, and will enable the administration of 4-HPR to small children.

15.6 Conclusions

Neuroblastoma tumorigenesis is related in part to defects in cellular differentiation. A number of agents, including 13-cis-RA, are capable of inducing NB differentiation in vitro, and a phase-III trial has definitively shown the clinical benefit of high-dose pulse 13-cis-RA following consolidation therapy; however, there are still tumors that do not respond to 13-cis-RA, even at the time of minimal residual disease, and additional therapies in the post-myeloablative period are clearly needed. Pre-clinical studies have shown that cytotoxic retinoid fenretinide (4-HPR) can achieve multi-log cell kills against NB cell lines resistant to 13-cis-RA, especially when combined with modulators of ceramide metabolism. A challenge with 4-HPR is that the current oral (capsule) formulation is poorly bioavailable and is not suitable for administration to young children. New formulations are currently in development. Randomized clinical trials are needed to determine if incorporating new approaches to treating minimal residual disease in high-risk NB patients, such as use of 4-HPR±ceramide modulators, can improve event-free survival.

Acknowledgements. The authors thank D.R. Reed for outstanding editorial assistance. This work was supported in part by the Neil Bogart Memorial Laboratories of the T.J. Martell Foundation for Leukemia, Cancer, and AIDS Research and by National Cancer Institute Grant CA81403.

References

Abemayor E, Sidell N (1989) Human neuroblastoma cell lines as models for the in vitro study of neoplastic and neuronal cell differentiation. Environ Health Perspect 80:3–15

Cheung B, Hocker JE, Smith SA, Norris MD, Haber M, Marshall GM (1998) Favorable prognostic significance of high-level retinoic acid receptor beta expression in neuroblastoma mediated by effects on cell cycle regulation. Oncogene 17:751–759

Chomienne C et al (1990) All-trans retinoic acid in acute promyelocytic leukemias. II. In vitro studies: structure-function relationship. Blood 76:1710–1717

Cohen PS, Cooper MJ, Helman LJ, Thiele CJ, Seeger RC, Israel MA (1990) Neuropeptide Y expression in the developing adrenal gland and in childhood neuroblastoma tumors. Cancer Res 50:6055–6061

Cooper MJ, Hutchins GM, Cohen PS, Helman LJ, Mennie RJ, Israel MA (1990) Human neuroblastoma tumor cell lines correspond to the arrested differentiation of chromaffin adrenal medullary neuroblasts. Cell Growth Differ 1:149–159

Cooper MJ, Steinberg SM, Chatten J, Evans AE, Israel MA (1992) Plasticity of neuroblastoma tumor cells to differentiate along a fetal adrenal ganglionic lineage predicts for improved patient survival. J Clin Invest 90:2402–2408

Corazzari M, Lovat PE, Oliverio S, Pearson AD, Piacentini M, Redfern CP (2003) Growth and DNA damage-inducible transcription factor 153 mediates apoptosis in response to fenretinide but not synergy between fenretinide and chemotherapeutic drugs in neuroblastoma. Mol Pharmacol 64:1370–1378

Eggert A, Ikegaki N, Kwiatkowski J, Zhao H, Brodeur GM, Himelstein BP (2000) High-level expression of angiogenic factors is associated with advanced tumor stage in human neuroblastomas. Clin Cancer Res 6:1900–1908

Erdreich-Epstein A et al. (2002) Ceramide signaling in fenretinide-induced endothelial cell apoptosis. J Biol Chem 277:49531–49537

Evans AE et al. (1999) Antitumor activity of CEP-751 (KT-6587) on human neuroblastoma and medulloblastoma xenografts. Clin Cancer Res 5:3594–3602

Finklestein JZ et al. (1992) 13-cis-retinoic acid (NSC 122758) in the treatment of children with metastatic neuroblastoma unresponsive to conventional chemotherapy: report from the Childrens Cancer Study Group. Med Pediatr Oncol 20:307–311

Gaetano C, Matsumoto K, Thiele CJ (1991) Retinoic acid negatively regulates p34cdc2 expression during human neuroblastoma differentiation. Cell Growth Differ 2:487–493

Garaventa A et al. (2003) Phase I trial and pharmacokinetics of fenretinide in children with neuroblastoma. Clin Cancer Res 9:2032–2039

Giannini G, Dawson MI, Zhang X, Thiele CJ (1997) Activation of three distinct RXR/RAR heterodimers induces growth arrest and differentiation of neuroblastoma cells. J Biol Chem 272:26693–26701

Jaboin J, Kim CJ, Kaplan DR, Thiele CJ (2002) Brain-derived neurotrophic factor activation of TrkB protects neuroblastoma cells from chemotherapy-induced apoptosis via phosphatidylinositol 3'-kinase pathway. Cancer Res 62:6756–6763

Jaffe N (1976) neuroblastoma: review of the literature and an examination of factors contributing to its enigmatic character. Cancer Treat Rev 3:61–82

Jogi A et al. (2002) Hypoxia alters gene expression in human neuroblastoma cells toward an immature and neural crest-like phenotype. Proc Natl Acad Sci USA 99:7021–7026

Kaplan DR, Miller FD (2000) Neurotrophin signal transduction in the nervous system. Curr Opin Neurobiol 10:381–391

Keshelava N et al. (2001) Loss of p53 function confers high-level multidrug resistance in neuroblastoma cell lines. Cancer Res 61:6185–6193

Khan AA, Villablanca JG, Reynolds CP, Avramis VI (1996) Pharmacokinetic studies of 13-cis-retinoic acid in pediatric patients with neuroblastoma following bone marrow transplantation. Cancer Chemother Pharmacol 39:34–41

Kohler JA, Imeson J, Ellershaw C, Lie SO (2000) A randomized trial of 13-cis retinoic acid in children with advanced neuroblastoma after high-dose therapy. Br J Cancer 83:1124–1127

Le Dourain N, Kalcheim C (1999) The neural crest, 2nd edn. Cambridge University Press, New York

Li C, Einhorn PA, Reynolds CP (1994) Expression of retinoic acid receptors alpha, beta, and gamma in human neuroblastoma cell lines. Prog Clin Biol Res 385:221–227

Linney E (1992) Retinoic acid receptors: transcription factors modulating gene regulation, development, and differentiation. Curr Top Dev Biol 27:309–350

Lopez-Ibor B, Schwartz AD (1985) Neuroblastoma. Pediatr Clin North Am 32:755–778

Lovat PE et al. (2002) GADD153 and 12-lipoxygenase mediate fenretinide-induced apoptosis of neuroblastoma. Cancer Res 62:5158–5167

Lovat PE et al. (2003a) Bak: a downstream mediator of fenretinide-induced apoptosis of SH-SY5Y neuroblastoma cells. Cancer Res 63:7310–7313

Lovat PE et al. (2003b) Mechanisms of free-radical induction in relation to fenretinide-induced apoptosis of neuroblastoma. J Cell Biochem 89:698–708

Lucarelli E, Kaplan DR, Thiele CJ (1995) Selective regulation of TrkA and TrkB receptors by retinoic acid and interferon-gamma in human neuroblastoma cell lines. J Biol Chem 270:24725–24731

Matsumoto K, Wada RK, Yamashiro JM, Kaplan DR, Thiele CJ (1995) Expression of brain-derived neurotrophic factor and p145TrkB affects survival, differentiation, and invasiveness of human neuroblastoma cells. Cancer Res 55:1798–1806

Matsuo T, Thiele CJ (1998) p27Kip1: a key mediator of retinoic acid induced growth arrest in the SMS-KCNR human neuroblastoma cell line. Oncogene 16:3337–3343

Matsushima H, Bogenmann E (1993) Expression of trkA cDNA in neuroblastomas mediates differentiation in vitro and in vivo. Mol Cell Biol 13:7447–7456

Matthay K et al. (1999) Treatment of high risk neuroblastoma with intensive chemotherapy, radiotherapy, autologous bone marrow transplantation, and 13-cis-retinoic acid. N Engl J Med 341:1165–1173

Maurer BJ, Metelitsa LS, Seeger RC, Cabot MC, Reynolds CP (1999) N-(4-hydroxyphenyl)retinamide increases ceramide and reactive oxygen species and induces mixed apoptosis/necrosis in neuroblastoma cell lines. J Natl Cancer Inst 91:1138–1146

Maurer BJ, Melton L, Billups C, Cabot MC, Reynolds CP (2000) Synergistic cytotoxicity in solid tumor cell lines between N-(4-hydroxyphenyl)retinamide and modulators of ceramide metabolism. J Natl Cancer Inst 92:1897

McLaughlin JE, Urich H (1977) Maturing neuroblastoma and ganglioneuroblastoma: a study of four cases with long survival. J Pathol 121:19–26

Nakagawara A, Arima Nakagawara M, Scavarda NJ, Azar CG, Cantor AB, Brodeur GM (1993) Association between high levels of expression of the TRK gene and favorable outcome in human neuroblastoma. N Engl J Med 328:847–854

Nakagawara A, Azar CG, Scavarda NJ, Brodeur GM (1994) Expression and function of TRK-B and BDNF in human neuroblastomas. Mol Cell Biol 14:759–767

Nakamura M, Matsuo T, Stauffer J, Neckers L, Thiele CJ (2003) Retinoic acid decreases targeting of p27 for degradation via an N-myc-dependent decrease in p27 phosphorylation and an N-myc-independent decrease in Skp2. Cell Death Differ 10:230–239

Nakamura Y, Ozaki T, Koseki H, Nakagawara A, Sakiyama S (2003) Accumulation of p27 KIP1 is associated with BMP2-induced growth arrest and neuronal differentiation of human neuroblastoma-derived cell lines. Biochem Biophys Res Commun 307:206–213

Norris MD, Bordow SB, Marshall GM, Haber PS, Cohn SL, Haber M (1996) Expression of the gene for multidrug-resistance-associated protein and outcome in patients with neuroblastoma. N Engl J Med 334:231–238

Nykjaer A, Lee R, Teng KK, Jansen P, Madsen P, Nielsen MS, Jacobsen C, Kliemannel M, Schwarz E, Willnow TE, Hempstead BL, Petersen CM (2004) Sortilin is essential for proNGF-induced neuronal cell death. Nature 427:843–848

Peverali FA et al. (1996) Retinoic acid-induced growth arrest and differentiation of neuroblastoma cells are counteracted by N-myc and enhanced by max overexpressions. Oncogene 12:457–462

Ponzoni M et al. (1995) Differential effects of N-(4-hydroxyphenyl)retinamide and retinoic acid on neuroblastoma cells: apoptosis versus differentiation. Cancer Res 55:853–861

Raaf JH, Cangir A, Luna M (1982) Induction of neuroblastoma maturation by a new chemotherapy protocol. Med Pediatr Oncol 10:275–282

Raffaghello L et al. (2003) Immunoliposomal fenretinide: a novel antitumoral drug for human neuroblastoma. Cancer Lett 197:151–155

Reynolds CP (2004) Detection and treatment of minimal residual disease in high-risk neuroblastoma. Pediatr Transplant 8:56–66

Reynolds CP, Lemons RS (2001) Retinoid therapy of childhood cancer. Hematol Oncol Clin North Am 15:867–910

Reynolds CP et al. (1991) Response of neuroblastoma to retinoic acid in vitro and in vivo. Prog Clin Biol Res 366:203–211

Reynolds CP, Schindler PF, Jones DM, Gentile JL, Proffitt RT, Einhorn PA (1994) Comparison of 13-cis-retinoic acid to trans-retinoic acid using human neuroblastoma cell lines. Prog Clin Biol Res 385:237–244

Reynolds CP, Wang Y, Melton LJ, Einhorn PA, Slamon DJ, Maurer BJ (2000) Retinoic-acid-resistant neuroblastoma cell lines show altered MYC regulation and high sensitivity to fenretinide. Med Pediatr Oncol 35:597–602

Reynolds CP, Maurer BJ, Kolsenick R (2004) Ceramide synthesis and metabolism as a target of cancer chemotherapy. Cancer Lett 206:169–180

Ribatti D et al. (2001) Inhibition of neuroblastoma-induced angiogenesis by fenretinide. Int J Cancer 94:314–321

Sawai S, Shimono A, Wakamatsu Y, Palmes C, Hanaoka K, Kondoh H (1993) Defects of embryonic organogenesis resulting from targeted disruption of the N-myc gene in the mouse. Development 117:1445–1455

Scala S et al. (1996) Brain-derived neurotrophic factor protects neuroblastoma cells from vinblastine toxicity. Cancer Res 56:3737–3742

Schober A, Wolf N, Kahane N, Kalcheim C, Krieglstein K, Unsicker K (1999) Expression of neurotrophin receptors trkB and trkC and their ligands in rat adrenal gland and the intermediolateral column of the spinal cord. Cell Tissue Res 296:271–279

Seeger RC et al. (1985) Association of multiple copies of the N-myc oncogene with rapid progression of neuroblastomas. N Engl J Med 313:1111–1116

Shimada H et al. (1984) Histopathologic prognostic factors in neuroblastic tumors: definition of subtypes of ganglioneuroblastoma and an age-linked classification of neuroblastomas. J Natl Cancer Inst 73:405–416

Sidell N (1982) Retinoic acid-induced growth inhibition and morphologic differentiation of human neuroblastoma cells in vitro. J Natl Cancer Inst 68:589–596

Smith J, Fauquet M (1984) Glucocorticoids stimulate adrenergic differentiation in cultures of migrating and premigratory neural crest. J Neurosci 4:2160–2172

Smith MA et al. (1992a) Phase I and pharmacokinetic evaluation of all-trans-retinoic acid in pediatric patients with cancer (see comments). J Clin Oncol 10:1666–1673

Smith MA, Parkinson DR, Cheson BD, Friedman MA (1992b) Retinoids in cancer therapy. J Clin Oncol 10:839–864

Stanton BR, Perkins AS, Tessarollo L, Sassoon DA, Parada LF (1992) Loss of N-myc function results in embryonic lethality and failure of the epithelial component of the embryo to develop. Genes Dev 6:2235–2247

Sumantran VN, Brederlau A, Funa K (2003) BMP-6 and retinoic acid synergistically differentiate the IMR-32 human neuroblastoma cells. Anticancer Res 23:1297–1303

Teng KK, Hempstead BL (2004) Neurotrophins and their receptors: signaling trios in complex biological systems. Cell Mol Life Sci 61:35–48

Thiele CJ, Israel MA (1988) Regulation of N-myc expression is a critical event controlling the ability of human neuroblasts to differentiate. Exp Cell Biol 56:321–333

Thiele CJ, Reynolds CP, Israel MA (1985) Decreased expression of N-myc precedes retinoic acid-induced morphological differentiation of human neuroblastoma. Nature 313:404–406

Thiele CJ, Deutsch LA, Israel MA (1988) The expression of multiple proto-oncogenes is differentially regulated during retinoic acid induced maturation of human neuroblastoma cell lines. Oncogene 3:281–288

Tweddle DA, Malcolm AJ, Bown N, Pearson AD, Lunec J (2001) Evidence for the development of p53 mutations after cytotoxic therapy in a neuroblastoma cell line. Cancer Res 61:8–13

Villablanca JG et al. (1995) Phase I trial of 13-cis-retinoic acid in children with neuroblastoma following bone marrow transplantation. J Clin Oncol 13:894–901

Villablanca JG, Ames MM, Reid JM, Bagniewski PG, Krailo M, Reynolds CP (2002) Phase I trial of oral N-(4-hydroxyphenyl)retinamide (4-HPR) in children with resistant/recurrent solid tumors: a Childrens Cancer Group Study (CCG 09709). Proc Am Soc Clin Oncol 21:1558

Wakamatsu Y, Watanabe Y, Nakamura H, Kondoh H (1997) Regulation of the neural crest cell fate by N-myc: promotion of ventral migration and neuronal differentiation. Development 124:1953–1962

Warrell RP Jr et al. (1991) Differentiation therapy of acute promyelocytic leukemia with tretinoin (all-trans-retinoic acid). N Engl J Med 324:1385–1393

Wartiovaara K, Barnabe-Heider F, Miller FD, Kaplan DR (2002) N-myc promotes survival and induces S-phase entry of postmitotic sympathetic neurons. J Neurosci 22:815–824

Woo CW, Lucarelli E, Thiele CJ (2004) NGF activation of TrkA decreases N-myc expression via MAPK path leading to a decrease in neuroblastoma cell number. Oncogene 23:1522–1530

Wu J, Saint-Jeannet JP, Klein PS (2003) Wnt-frizzled signaling in neural crest formation. Trends Neurosci 26:40–45

Yamashiro DJ et al. (1997) Expression and function of Trk-C in favourable human neuroblastomas. Eur J Cancer 33:2054–2057

Angiogenesis

Darrell J. Yamashiro, Susan L. Cohn

Contents

16.1 Introduction

It is widely accepted that solid tumors must acquire a new blood supply in order to grow beyond a few millimeters in size (Folkman 2002). This concept has stimulated much interest in identifying factors that promote or impede angiogenesis. Proangiogenic cytokines that appear to play a role in human cancer progression include the vascular endothelial growth factor (VEGF) family, fibroblast growth factor (FGF) family, interleukin-8 (IL-8), and platelet-derived growth factor (PDGF) family. Numerous endogenous inhibitors of angiogenesis have also been identified, including thrombospondin-1, angiostatin, and endostatin. It has also been increasingly recognized that genes implicated in malignant transformation, such as the p53 tumor suppressor or the *MYCN* oncogene, may play an important role in the regulation of angiogenesis (Hatzi et al. 2000; Yu et al. 2002). The multiplicity of these factors and their potential interactions, emphasizes the complexity of the regulation of angiogenesis. Patterns of new vessel growth vary in different tumor types, and vary even in tumors of the same type but of different clinical stage or histologic grade. For example, VEGF blockade appears to be less effective in suppressing growth of experimental neuroblastoma tumors than in parallel models of Wilms' tumor (Kim et al. 2001). In addition, expression of angiogenic factors is increased in neuroblastomas of advanced clinical stage; thus, investigating the specific mechanisms by which neuroblastoma tumors acquire a new blood supply may lead to the identification of potential new targets for treatment of this malignancy.

16.2 Vascularity in Neuroblastoma

Folkman and colleagues were among the first to suggest that the intensity of intratumoral angiogenesis correlates with tumor grade and aggressiveness (Brem et al. 1972). Although the majority of published studies have shown a positive correlation between intratumoral microvessel density and prognosis in solid tumors (Hasan et al. 2002), the prognostic role of angiogenesis in neuroblastoma is unclear. Meitar et al. initially reported in a study of 50 primary tumors that high tumor vascularity strongly correlated with widely disseminated disease, *MYCN* amplification, unfavorable histology, and poor survival (Meitar et al. 1996). Ribatti et al. found similar results in a smaller series of patients, with increased microvessel density associated with advanced-stage tumors (Ribatti et al. 2001). In further support, Erdreich-Epstein and co-workers (2000) have recently demonstrated a significant association between high-risk neuroblastoma and high levels of expression of the integrins $\alpha_v\beta_3$ and $\alpha_v\beta_5$, which are markers of active angiogenesis. In contrast, Canete et al. (2000) in a study of 69 neuroblastoma patients found no correlation of vascular parameters with the prognostic factors of age, stage, histology, TrkA, or *MYCN* amplification or with overall survival. The conflicting results most likely reflect differences in techniques used to measure vessel number, a difficulty encountered in reconciling the results of studies of other solid tumors such as breast cancer (Hasan et al. 2002). Interestingly, all three studies are in concordance, i.e., infants with stage-4S disease have higher levels of vascularity than any of the other stages. The increased vascularity in stage 4S is consistent with the rapid rate of tumor growth in a subset of these patients with widely disseminated disease.

16.3 Expression of Proangiogenic Factors

The ability of neuroblastoma to produce proangiogenic factors was first described by Folkman in 1971, who isolated a "tumor angiogenic factor" from extracts of human neuroblastoma, Wilms' tumor, and hepatoblastoma (Folkman et al. 1971). The tumor extracts caused the formation of new blood vessels in the subcutaneous fascia of rats within 48 h. Since this time, expression of numerous proangiogenic factors, such as VEGF, PDGF, FGF, and angiopoietins, has been found in neuroblastoma.

16.3.1 VEGF and VEGF Receptors

Among the proangiogenic factors VEGF-A has been the best characterized. VEGF-A is a potent mitogen for endothelial cells and can elicit a pronounced angiogenic response in vivo. VEGF-A is also a survival factor for endothelial cells both in vitro and in vivo (Ferrara 2001; Leung et al. 1989). There are numerous isoforms of VEGF-A that are generated by alternative exon splicing that include VEGF-A_{121}, VEGF-A_{165}, VEGF-A_{189}, and VEGF-A_{206} (Clauss 2000; Ferrara 2001). In addition to the different VEGF-A isoforms, there is a family of VEGF-related angiogenic growth factors VEGF-B, VEGF-C, VEGF-D, VEGF-E, and placental growth factor (PlGF; Clauss 2000; Ferrara 2001). The precise function of many of these VEGF-related ligands is currently not known or ambiguous.

VEGF-A is nearly ubiquitously expressed by both neuroblastoma primary tumors and cell lines, with the predominate isoform VEGF-A_{165} (Eggert et al. 2000; Fakhari et al. 2002; Komuro et al. 2001; Meister et al. 1999; Ribatti et al. 1998; Rossler et al. 1999). High expression of VEGF-A has been shown to significantly correlate with advanced stage in several studies (Eggert et al. 2000; Fakhari et al. 2002; Komuro et al. 2001). Elevated serum levels of VEGF-A have also been observed in patients with stage-III tumors (Fakhari et al. 2002). Eggert and co-workers reported that the level of expression of other proangiogenic factors including VEGF-B, VEGF-C, bFGF, angiopoietin-2, transforming growth factor-α (TGF-α), and PDGF-A, was significantly higher in stage-3 and stage-4 neuroblastomas compared to stage-1, stage-2, or stage-4S tumors (Eggert et al. 2000). In this study, high levels of PDGF-A expression was also significantly associated with decreased survival; however, no correlation between VEGF-C or bFGF and stage was seen in a series of tumors analyzed by Komuro and colleagues (2001). In addition, while Fakhari et al. were able to show correlations between high levels of VEGF-A, VEGF-B and VEGF-C mRNA and advanced stage by real-time RT-PCR, only VEGF-A was detectable in tumor material by Western blotting (Fakhari et al. 2002). These observations suggest that VEGF-A is the major ligand of the VEGF family regulating angiogenesis in neuroblastoma. The role of the other VEGF ligands remains to be elucidated.

VEGF family members bind with differential affinity to three signaling VEGF receptors, VEGFR-1 (*Flt-1*), VEGFR-2 (*flk-1/KDR*), and VEGFR-3 (*FLT4*). VEGF binds to both VEGFR-1 and VEGFR-2, while PlGF and VEGF-B bind exclusively to VEGFR-1. VEGF-C and VEGF-D bind to VEGFR-2 and VEGFR-3, and are mitogens for both vascular and lymphatic endothelial cells. VEGFR-2 appears to be the principal receptor on endothelial cells by which VEGF exerts its angiogenic effects (Ferrara 2001). The role of VEGFR-1 is more complex. This receptor may act not only as a ligand-binding molecule but also aid in the recruitment of bone marrow-derived endothelial precursor cells to newly formed tumor vasculature (Lyden et al. 2001), and in promoting metastases by induction of metalloprotease MMP9 (Hiratsuka et al. 2002). VEGF isoforms that have a heparin-binding site can also bind to the semaphorin receptors neuropilin-1 and neuropilin-2 (Neufeld et al. 2002). Their exact role in angiogenesis is not clear, but neuropilins may modulate binding to VEGFR-2 and subsequent bioactivity (Soker et al. 1998). Recently, expression of neuropilin-1 and neuropilin-2 has been detected in vascular endothelial cells of primary neuroblastoma tumors, but their function remains to be determined (Fakhari et al. 2002).

Expression of VEGFR-2 and to a lesser degree VEGFR-1 in primary tumors has been reported in several studies, consistent with the importance of VEGFR-2 in vascular endothelium (Fakhari et al. 2002; Fukuzawa et al. 2002; Langer et al. 2000; Meister et al. 1999); however, the expression of VEGFR-2 in neuroblastoma tumor cells remains unresolved. VEGFR-2 was detected by RT-PCR in either none (Rossler et al. 1999), few (Langer et al. 2000), or all (Meister et al. 1999) of the neuroblastoma cell lines tested. In four cell lines in which VEGFR-2 was expressed, neutralizing antibody to VEGF did not result in inhibition of proliferation of neuroblastoma cells (Meister et al. 1999). In primary tumors, VEGFR-2 has been detected in tumor cells by immunohistochemistry and in situ hybridization (Fukuzawa et al. 2002); however, VEGFR-2 could not be detected in Western blot analysis of tumor lysates suggesting either a limited expression of VEGFR-2 (e.g., in the vasculature) or a very low/minimal expression in the tumor cells.

16.3.2 Matrix Metalloproteinases

The matrix metalloproteinases (MMPs) are a family of endopeptidases that play a key role in maintaining the balance between deposition and degradation of extracellular matrix. Activity of MMP-2 and MMP-9 is associated with tumor progression and metastasis in many cancers, presumably facilitating the invasion of tumor cells and sprouting of new vasculature (Overall and Lopez-Otin 2002). Consistent with these functions, inhibitors of MMPs have been shown to suppress both tumor invasion and angiogenesis. In neuroblastoma, an association between increased levels of MMP-2 (gelatinase A) and MMP-9 (gelatinase B) in patients with advanced stage has been reported (Ribatti et al. 2001; Sugiura et al. 1998). In addition, decreased expression of the tissue inhibitor metalloproteinase TIMP-2, a specific inhibitor of MMP-2 and MMP-9, has been significantly related to advanced disease (Ara et al. 1998). Lastly, Sakakibara et al. have demonstrated that higher ratios of gelatinase activation resulting from high expression of membrane-type matrix metalloproteinase-1 (MT-MMP-1) is associated with stage-IV disease and unfavorable outcome (Sakakibara et al. 1999).

16.4 Expression of Angiogenesis Inhibitors

Tumor angiogenesis is regulated by the balance of angiogenesis stimulators and inhibitors produced by tumor cells, the surrounding stoma, and host cells (Bergers and Benjamin 2003). Neuroblastomas are biologically heterogeneous tumors that consist of two main cell populations: neuroblastic/ganglionic cells and Schwann cells. Regulation of angiogenesis by Schwann cells is suggested by the finding that Schwannian stroma rich/stroma dominant tumors are associated with decreased tumor vascularity (Meitar et al. 1996). Further evidence suggests that Schwann cells can influence angiogenesis by producing inhibitors that can induce endothelial cell apoptosis and inhibit angiogenesis in vivo (Huang et al. 2000).

16.4.1 Pigment Epithelium-Derived Factor

One of the factors isolated from Schwann cells is the endogenous angiogenesis inhibitor, pigment epithelium-derived factor (PEDF) (Crawford et al. 2001). PEDF can inhibit angiogenesis both in vitro and in vivo, promote growth and survival of Schwann cells, and induce tumor cell differentiation; thus, PEDF may regulate neuroblastoma growth by inhibiting new blood vessel growth and by supporting the survival of differentiated cell types.

16.4.2 Secreted Protein Acidic and Rich in Cysteine

Recently, another angiogenic inhibitor was isolated from Schwann cell-conditioned media, identified as secreted protein acidic and rich in cysteine (SPARC) (Chlenski et al. 2002). SPARC, also known as osteonectin, BM-40, and 43 K protein, is a highly conserved calcium-binding glycoprotein that plays a modulatory role in cell-matrix interactions and appears to contribute to vascular morphogenesis (Brekken and Sage 2001). SPARC is generally considered an antiangiogenic protein because it blocks VEGF- and FGF-2-induced proliferation of endothelial cells and can inhibit PDGF activity on stromal cells (Brekken and Sage 2001).

SPARC expression is inversely correlated with the degree of malignant progression in neuroblastoma tumors (Chlenski et al. 2002). In favorable histology Schwannian stroma-rich/stroma-dominant tumors, SPARC was detected in Schwann cells as well as differentiating neuroblast/ganglion cells. In contrast, minimal to no staining for SPARC was observed in Schwannian stroma-poor tumors. SPARC was critical for the anti-angiogenic phenotype of cultured Schwann cells, as the addition of anti-SPARC neutralizing antibodies largely reversed the anti-angiogenic activity of Schwann cell-conditioned media. Furthermore, at concentrations found in Schwann cell-conditioned media, purified SPARC inhibited angiogenesis and impaired neuroblastoma tumor growth in vivo.

16.4.3 Thrombospondin-1

Thrombospondin-1 (TSP-1), a well-characterized endogenous inhibitor of angiogenesis, was initially isolated as a constituent of extracellular matrix, and shown to interact with wild-type p53 to regulate angiogenesis (Dameron et al. 1994). More recently, TSP-1 has been shown to modulate mobilization of VEGF directly (Rodriguez-Manzaneque et al. 2001). A number of workers have reported that TSP-1 plays an important role in the differentiation of neuroblasts induced by retinoic acid treatment (Castle et al. 1992; Pijuan-Thompson et al. 1999). Castle and co-workers reported a rapid induction of TSP-1 when cultured human neuroblastoma cells were treated with retinoic acid (Castle et al. 1992). Furthermore, differentiation was partially prevented by anti-TSP-1 antibody. Because TSP-1 is a negative regulator of VEGF, these findings suggest that differentiation of neuroblasts may be linked to a decrease in proangiogenic signaling. The recent development of TSP-1 mimetic peptides with anti-angiogenic activity is therefore intriguing (Reiher et al. 2002) as such agents may promote neuroblastoma differentiation and inhibit VEGF-stimulated angiogenesis.

16.5 Regulation of Angiogenesis by *MYCN*

MYCN amplification is a poor prognostic factor in children with neuroblastoma, and is associated with advanced tumor stage and metastasis. *MYCN* appears to play a significant role in neuroblastoma angiogenesis. Amplification of *MYCN* has been shown to correlate with mean vascular density (Meitar et al. 1996), and the expression of PDGF (but not with VEGF-A) (Eggert et al. 2000). Angiogenic activity of biopsy samples was significantly higher in those with *MYCN*-amplified tumors when tested in a chick embryo chorioallantoic membrane assay (Ribatti et al. 2002). It remains unclear if *MYCN* directly upregulates cytokines that promote neovascular development.

MYCN may also decrease the expression of endogenous inhibitors of angiogenesis. In cultured neuroblastoma cells *MYCN* causes decreased expression of interleukin-6 (IL-6), leukemia inhibitory factor, and activin A (Breit et al. 2000; Hatzi et al. 2000, 2002a,b). Over-expression of IL-6 in neuroblastoma xenografts results in decreased tumor angiogenesis and growth inhibition (Hatzi et al. 2002b); thus, current evidence suggests that *MYCN* promotes angiogenesis in neuroblastoma at least in part by decreasing expression of genes that normally function to restrain new blood vessel growth.

16.6 Preclinical Testing of Antiangiogenic Agents

16.6.1 VEGF Blockade

Inhibition of VEGF has recently been shown to be effective in clinical trials of some human cancers (Glade-Bender et al. 2003). VEGF blockade has also shown efficacy in preclinical models of human neuroblastoma, using agents that target the ligand or its VEGFR2 receptor (Davidoff et al. 2001b; Klement et al. 2000; Rowe et al. 2000). More recent reports demonstrate that neuroblastoma tumors may co-opt host vasculature early in development (Kim et al. 2002a). Partial blockade of VEGF may prolong co-option, which presumably contributes to tumor perfusion and supports continued, although reduced, tumor growth. Use of very high-affinity VEGF-binding molecules, such as the recently described novel fusion construct VEGF-Trap, can cause regression of such co-opted vessels (Holash et al. 2002; Kim et al. 2002a); thus, selection of optimal VEGF blocking strategies for testing in patients with neuroblastoma may require selection of agents based on specific biochemical and pharmacologic properties.

16.6.2 TNP-470

One of the first anti-angiogenic molecules proposed was TNP-470 (AGM-1470), an analog of fumagillin, a naturally secreted antibiotic of the fungus *Aspergillus fumigatus fresenius* (Ingber et al. 1990), identified by its ability to inhibit endothelial proliferation in vitro. Subsequently, its TNP-470 analog was shown to inhibit tumor growth in multiple xenograft models (Ingber et al. 1990; Kurebayashi et al. 1994; Kusaka et al. 1991; Yamaoka et al. 1993a,b). Based on these experiments, TNP-470 aroused much interest as a potential anti-angiogenic agent; however, testing in preclinical models of neuroblastoma has demonstrated relatively modest anti-tumor effects (Katzenstein et al. 1999; Nagabuchi et al. 1997; Shusterman et al. 2001). Some investigators indicate that TNP-470 is most effective when small neuroblastoma tumors are treated (Katzenstein et al. 1999; Shusterman et al. 2001), suggesting that this agent may be more effective in the setting of minimal residual disease.

16.6.3 Endostatin

Endostatin, a peptide fragment of collagen XVIII, was initially purified from a hemangioendothelioma based on its ability to inhibit endothelial proliferation in vitro and tumor growth in vivo (O'Reilly et al. 1997). Endostatin appears to act by disrupting endothelial interactions with anchoring proteins in extracellular matrix (Dixelius et al. 2002; Kim et al. 2000; Rehn et al. 2001). Another report suggests that endostatin may also directly block VEGFR2 signaling (Kim et al. 2002b). Despite these findings, activity of endostatin in murine models of neuroblastoma has not been consistently demonstrated, with groups detecting either modest or no effect on tumor growth

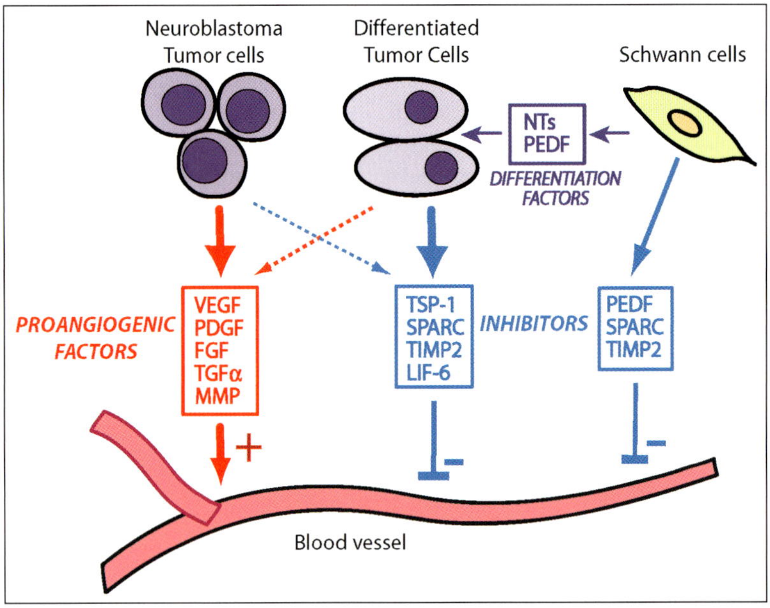

Figure 16.1

Model of angiogenesis in neuroblastoma. Tumor cells produce both proangiogenic factors and inhibitors of angiogenesis. The relative expression of these factors may depend on the differentiation status of the tumor cells. More differentiated tumors may express more angiogenesis inhibitors. Schwann cells produce not only inhibitors of angiogenesis, but also factors, e.g., neurotrophins (*NTs*) and pigment epithelium-derived factor (*PEDF*), that promote differentiation of neuroblastoma tumor cells. *VEGF* vascular endothelial growth factor, *PDGF* platelet-derived growth factor, *SPARC* secreted protein acidic and rich in cysteine, *FGF* fibroblast growth factor, *TGF* transforming growth factor, *MMP* metalloprotease, *TSP* thrombospondin, *TIMP* tissue inhibitor metalloproteinase

(Davidoff et al. 2001a; Jouanneau et al. 2001; Kuroiwa et al. 2001). Davidoff and colleagues report enhancement of a modest anti-tumor effect of endostatin in experimental neuroblastoma by combination of this agent with an immunomodulatory strategy (Davidoff et al. 2001a).

16.7 Conclusions

Investigations of angiogenesis in neuroblastoma to date reflect the complexity that results from the combined influences of genetic and epigenetic factors on tumor vessel formation. Tumors that are clinically aggressive may express higher levels of proangiogenic cytokines, while concurrently expressing decreased levels of factors that function to restrain new blood vessel growth (Fig. 16.1). Conversely, the more benign nature of ganglioneuroblastomas and other relatively indolent, differentiated tumors may reflect the influence of secreted angiogenesis inhibitors. Such factors may be elaborated by Schwann cells in the tumor stroma, or possibly by tumor cells that have undergone further differentiation.

Preclinical studies suggest that neuroblastoma may be susceptible to certain anti-angiogenic strategies. For example, blockade of VEGF in neuroblastoma has shown consistent effectiveness between experimental models and investigators. In addition, this approach has recently been shown to have efficacy in clinical trials of adult human cancers (Glade-Bender et al. 2003); however, even the most promising reports suggest that neuroblastoma may be able to partially evade anti-VEGF agents by co-opting host vessels (Kim et al. 2002a). Understanding such events will require further dissection of the unique interactions between neuroblastoma cells and developing vasculature. Such studies are essential if patients with advanced neuroblastoma are to benefit from this area of investigation.

Acknowledgements. The authors thank J. Kandel and J. Glade-Bender for reviewing the chapter. This work was supported in part by NCI grant number CA088951 (D.J.Y.), the Neuroblastoma Children's Cancer Society (S.L.C.), Friends for Steven Pediatric Cancer Research Fund (S.L.C.), and the Elise Anderson Neuroblastoma Research Fund (S.L.C.)

References

Ara T, Fukuzawa M, Kusafuka T, Komoto Y, Oue T, Inoue M, Okada A (1998) Immunohistochemical expression of MMP-2, MMP-9, and TIMP-2 in neuroblastoma: association with tumor progression and clinical outcome. J Pediatr Surg 33:1272–1278

Bergers G, Benjamin LE (2003) Angiogenesis: tumorigenesis and the angiogenic switch. Nat Rev Cancer 3:401–410

Breit S, Ashman K, Wilting J, Rossler J, Hatzi E, Fotsis T, Schweigerer L (2000) The N-myc oncogene in human neuroblastoma cells: down-regulation of an angiogenesis inhibitor identified as activin A. Cancer Res 60:4596–4601

Brekken RA, Sage EH (2001) SPARC, a matricellular protein: at the crossroads of cell-matrix communication. Matrix Biol 19:816–827

Brem S, Cotran R, Folkman J (1972) Tumor angiogenesis: a quantitative method for histologic grading. J Natl Cancer Inst 48:347–356

Canete A, Navarro S, Bermudez J, Pellin A, Castel V, Llombart-Bosch A (2000) Angiogenesis in neuroblastoma: relationship to survival and other prognostic factors in a cohort of neuroblastoma patients. J Clin Oncol 18:27–34

Castle VP, Ou X, O'Shea S, Dixit VM (1992) Induction of thrombospondin 1 by retinoic acid is important during differentiation of neuroblastoma cells. J Clin Invest 90:1857–1863

Chlenski A, Liu S, Crawford SE, Volpert OV, DeVries GH, Evangelista A, Yang Q, Salwen HR, Farrer R, Bray J, Cohn SL (2002) SPARC is a key Schwannian-derived inhibitor controlling neuroblastoma tumor angiogenesis. Cancer Res 62:7357–7363

Clauss M (2000) Molecular biology of the VEGF and the VEGF receptor family. Semin Thromb Hemost 26:561–569

Crawford SE, Stellmach V, Ranalli M, Huang X, Huang L, Volpert O, De Vries GH, Abramson LP, Bouck N (2001) Pigment epithelium-derived factor (PEDF) in neuroblastoma: a multifunctional mediator of Schwann cell antitumor activity. J Cell Sci 114:4421–4428

Dameron KM, Volpert OV, Tainsky MA, Bouck N (1994) Control of angiogenesis in fibroblasts by p53 regulation of thrombospondin-1. Science 265:1582–1584

Davidoff AM, Leary MA, Ng CY, Spurbeck WW, Frare P, Vanhove M, Nienhuis AW, Vanin EF (2001a) Autocrine expression of both endostatin and green fluorescent protein provides a synergistic antitumor effect in a murine neuroblastoma model. Cancer Gene Ther 8:537–545

Davidoff AM, Leary MA, Ng CY, Vanin EF (2001b) Gene therapy-mediated expression by tumor cells of the angiogenesis inhibitor flk-1 results in inhibition of neuroblastoma growth in vivo. J Pediatr Surg 36:30–36

Dixelius J, Cross M, Matsumoto T, Sasaki T, Timpl R, Claesson-Welsh L (2002) Endostatin regulates endothelial cell adhesion and cytoskeletal organization. Cancer Res 62:1944–1947

Eggert A, Ikegaki N, Kwiatkowski J, Zhao H, Brodeur GM, Himelstein BP (2000) High-level expression of angiogenic factors is associated with advanced tumor stage in human neuroblastomas. Clin Cancer Res 6:1900–1908

Erdreich-Epstein A, Shimada H, Groshen S, Liu M, Metelitsa LS, Kim KS, Stins MF, Seeger RC, Durden DL (2000) Integrins alpha(v)beta3 and alpha(v)beta5 are expressed by endothelium of high-risk neuroblastoma and their inhibition is associated with increased endogenous ceramide. Cancer Res 60:712–721

Fakhari M, Pullirsch D, Abraham D, Paya K, Hofbauer R, Holzfeind P, Hofmann M, Aharinejad S (2002) Selective upregulation of vascular endothelial growth factor receptors neuropilin-1 and -2 in human neuroblastoma. Cancer 94:258–263

Fakhari M, Pullirsch D, Paya K, Abraham D, Hofbauer R, Aharinejad S (2002) Upregulation of vascular endothelial growth factor receptors is associated with advanced neuroblastoma. J Pediatr Surg 37:582–587

Ferrara N (2001) Role of vascular endothelial growth factor in regulation of physiological angiogenesis. Am J Physiol Cell Physiol 280:C1358–C1366

Folkman J (2002) Role of angiogenesis in tumor growth and metastasis. Semin Oncol 29:15–18

Folkman J, Merler E, Abernathy C, Williams G (1971) Isolation of a tumor factor responsible or angiogenesis. J Exp Med 133:275–288

Fukuzawa M, Sugiura H, Koshinaga T, Ikeda T, Hagiwara N, Sawada T (2002) Expression of vascular endothelial growth factor and its receptor Flk-1 in human neuroblastoma using in situ hybridization. J Pediatr Surg 37:1747–1750

Glade-Bender J, Kandel JJ, Yamashiro DJ (2003) VEGF blocking therapy in the treatment of cancer. Exp Opin Biol Ther 3:263–276

Hasan J, Byers R, Jayson GC (2002) Intra-tumoural microvessel density in human solid tumours. Br J Cancer 86:1566–1577

Hatzi E, Breit S, Zoephel A, Ashman K, Tontsch U, Ahorn H, Murphy C, Schweigerer L, Fotsis T (2000) MYCN oncogene and angiogenesis: down-regulation of endothelial growth inhibitors in human neuroblastoma cells. Purification, structural, and functional characterization. Adv Exp Med Biol 476:239–248

Hatzi E, Murphy C, Zoephel A, Ahorn H, Tontsch U, Bamberger AM, Yamauchi-Takihara K, Schweigerer L, Fotsis T (2002a) N-myc oncogene overexpression down-regulates leukemia inhibitory factor in neuroblastoma. Eur J Biochem 269:3732–3741

Hatzi E, Murphy C, Zoephel A, Rasmussen H, Morbidelli L, Ahorn H, Kunisada K, Tontsch U, Klenk M, Yamauchi-Takihara K, Ziche M, Rofstad EK, Schweigerer L, Fotsis T (2002b) N-myc oncogene overexpression down-regulates IL-6; evidence that IL-6 inhibits angiogenesis and suppresses neuroblastoma tumor growth. Oncogene 21:3552–3561

Hiratsuka S, Nakamura K, Iwai S, Murakami M, Itoh T, Kijima H, Shipley JM, Senior RM, Shibuya M (2002) MMP9 induction by vascular endothelial growth factor receptor-1 is involved in lung-specific metastasis. Cancer Cell 2:289–300

Holash J, Davis S, Papadopoulos N, Croll SD, Ho L, Russell M, Boland P, Leidich R, Hylton D, Burova E, Ioffe E, Huang T, Radziejewski C, Bailey K, Fandl JP, Daly T, Wiegand SJ, Yancopoulos GD, Rudge JS (2002) VEGF-Trap: A VEGF blocker with potent antitumor effects. Proc Natl Acad Sci USA 99:11393–11398

Huang D, Rutkowski JL, Brodeur GM, Chou PM, Kwiatkowski JL, Babbo A, Cohn SL (2000) Schwann cell-conditioned medium inhibits angiogenesis. Cancer Res 60:5966–5971

Ingber D, Fujita T, Kishimoto S, Sudo K, Kanamaru T, Brem H, Folkman J (1990) Synthetic analogues of fumagillin that inhibit angiogenesis and suppress tumour growth. Nature 348:555–557

Jouanneau E, Alberti L, Nejjari M, Treilleux I, Vilgrain I, Duc A, Combaret V, Favrot M, Leboulch P, Bachelot T (2001) Lack of antitumor activity of recombinant endostatin in a human neuroblastoma xenograft model. J Neurooncol 51:11–18

Katzenstein HM, Rademaker AW, Senger C, Salwen HR, Nguyen NN, Thorner PS, Litsas L, Cohn SL (1999) Effectiveness of the angiogenesis inhibitor TNP-470 in reducing the growth of human neuroblastoma in nude mice inversely correlates with tumor burden. Clin Cancer Res 5:4273–4278

Kim YM, Jang JW, Lee OH, Yeon J, Choi EY, Kim KW, Lee ST, Kwon YG (2000) Endostatin inhibits endothelial and tumor cellular invasion by blocking the activation and catalytic activity of matrix metalloproteinase. Cancer Res 60:5410–5413

Kim E, Moore J, Huang J, Soffer S, Manley CA, O'Toole K, Middlesworth W, Stolar CJ, Kandel JJ, Yamashiro DJ (2001) All angiogenesis is not the same: distinct patterns of response to antiangiogenic therapy in experimental neuroblastoma and Wilms tumor. J Pediatr Surg 36:287–290

Kim ES, Serur A, Huang J, Manley CA, McCrudden KW, Frischer JS, Soffer SZ, Ring L, New T, Zabski S, Rudge JS, Holash J, Yancopoulos GD, Kandel JJ, Yamashiro DJ (2002a) Potent VEGF blockade causes regression of coopted vessels in a model of neuroblastoma. Proc Natl Acad Sci USA 99:11399–11404

Kim YM, Hwang S, Pyun BJ, Kim TY, Lee ST, Gho YS, Kwon YG (2002b) Endostatin blocks vascular endothelial growth factor-mediated signaling via direct interaction with KDR/Flk-1. J Biol Chem 277:27872–27879

Klement G, Baruchel S, Rak J, Man S, Clark K, Hicklin DJ, Bohlen P, Kerbel RS (2000) Continuous low-dose therapy with vinblastine and VEGF receptor-2 antibody induces sustained tumor regression without overt toxicity. J Clin Invest 105:R15–R24

Komuro H, Kaneko S, Kaneko M, Nakanishi Y (2001) Expression of angiogenic factors and tumor progression in human neuroblastoma. J Cancer Res Clin Oncol 127:739–743

Kurebayashi J, Kurosumi M, Dickson RB, Sonoo H (1994) Angiogenesis inhibitor O-(Chloroacetyl-carbamoyl) fumagillol (TNP-470) inhibits tumor angiogenesis, growth and spontaneous metastasis of MKL-4 human breast cancer cells in female athymic nude mice. Breast Cancer 1:109–115

Kuroiwa M, Ikeda H, Hongo T, Tsuchida Y, Hirato J, Kaneko Y, Suzuki N, Obana K, Makino SI (2001) Effects of recombinant human endostatin on a human neuroblastoma xenograft. Int J Mol Med 8:391–396

Kusaka M, Sudo K, Fujita T, Marui S, Itoh F, Ingber D, Folkman J (1991) Potent anti-angiogenic action of AGM-1470: comparison to the fumagillin parent. Biochem Biophys Res Commun 174:1070–1076

Langer I, Vertongen P, Perret J, Fontaine J, Atassi G, Robberecht P (2000) Expression of vascular endothelial growth factor (VEGF) and VEGF receptors in human neuroblastomas. Med Pediatr Oncol 34:386–393

Leung DW, Cachianes G, Kuang WJ, Goeddel DV, Ferrara N (1989) Vascular endothelial growth factor is a secreted angiogenic mitogen. Science 246:1306–1309

Lyden D, Hattori K, Dias S, Costa C, Blaikie P, Butros L, Chadburn A, Heissig B, Marks W, Witte L, Wu Y, Hicklin D, Zhu Z, Hackett NR, Crystal RG, Moore MA, Hajjar KA, Manova K, Benezra R, Rafii S (2001) Impaired recruitment of bone-marrow-derived endothelial and hematopoietic precursor cells blocks tumor angiogenesis and growth. Nat Med 7:1194–1201

Meister B, Grunebach F, Bautz F, Brugger W, Fink FM, Kanz L, Mohle R (1999) Expression of vascular endothelial growth factor (VEGF) and its receptors in human neuroblastoma. Eur J Cancer 35:445–449

Meitar D, Crawford SE, Rademaker AW, Cohn SL (1996) Tumor angiogenesis correlates with metastatic disease, N-myc amplification, and poor outcome in human neuroblastoma. J Clin Oncol 14:405–414

Nagabuchi E, VanderKolk WE, Une Y, Ziegler MM (1997) TNP-470 antiangiogenic therapy for advanced murine neuroblastoma. J Pediatr Surg 32:287–293

Neufeld G, Cohen T, Shraga N, Lange T, Kessler O, Herzog Y (2002) The neuropilins: multifunctional semaphorin and VEGF receptors that modulate axon guidance and angiogenesis. Trends Cardiovasc Med 12:13–19

O'Reilly MS, Boehm T, Shing Y, Fukai N, Vasios G, Lane WS, Flynn E, Birkhead JR, Olsen BR, Folkman J (1997) Endostatin: an endogenous inhibitor of angiogenesis and tumor growth. Cell 88:277–285

Overall CM, Lopez-Otin C (2002) Strategies for MMP inhibition in cancer: innovations for the post-trial era. Nat Rev Cancer 2:657–672

Pijuan-Thompson V, Grammer JR, Stewart J, Silverstein RL, Pearce SF, Tuszynski GP, Murphy-Ullrich JE, Gladson CL (1999) Retinoic acid alters the mechanism of attachment of malignant astrocytoma and neuroblastoma cells to thrombospondin-1. Exp Cell Res 249:86–101

Rehn M, Veikkola T, Kukk-Valdre E, Nakamura H, Ilmonen M, Lombardo C, Pihlajaniemi T, Alitalo K, Vuori K (2001) Interaction of endostatin with integrins implicated in angiogenesis. Proc Natl Acad Sci USA 98:1024–1029

Reiher FK, Volpert OV, Jimenez B, Crawford SE, Dinney CP, Henkin J, Haviv F, Bouck NP, Campbell SC (2002) Inhibition of tumor growth by systemic treatment with thrombospondin-1 peptide mimetics. Int J Cancer 98:682–689

Ribatti D, Alessandri G, Vacca A, Iurlaro M, Ponzoni M (1998) Human neuroblastoma cells produce extracellular matrix-degrading enzymes, induce endothelial cell proliferation and are angiogenic in vivo. Int J Cancer 77:449–454

Ribatti D, Surico G, Vacca A, De Leonardis F, Lastilla G, Montaldo PG, Rigillo N, Ponzoni M (2001) Angiogenesis extent and expression of matrix metalloproteinase-2 and -9 correlate with progression in human neuroblastoma. Life Sci 68:1161–1168

Ribatti D, Raffaghello L, Pastorino F, Nico B, Brignole C, Vacca A, Ponzoni M (2002) In vivo angiogenic activity of neuroblastoma correlates with MYCN oncogene overexpression. Int J Cancer 102:351–354

Rodriguez-Manzaneque JC, Lane TF, Ortega MA, Hynes RO, Lawler J, Iruela-Arispe ML (2001) Thrombospondin-1 suppresses spontaneous tumor growth and inhibits activation of matrix metalloproteinase-9 and mobilization of vascular endothelial growth factor. Proc Natl Acad Sci USA 98: 12485–12490

Rossler J, Breit S, Havers W, Schweigerer L (1999) Vascular endothelial growth factor expression in human neuroblastoma: up-regulation by hypoxia. Int J Cancer 81:113–117

Rowe DH, Huang J, Li J, Manley C, O'Toole KM, Stolar CJ, Yamashiro DJ, Kandel JJ (2000) Suppression of primary tumor growth in a mouse model of human neuroblastoma. J Pediatr Surg 35:977–981

Sakakibara M, Koizumi S, Saikawa Y, Wada H, Ichihara T, Sato H, Horita S, Mugishima H, Kaneko Y, Koike K (1999) Membrane-type matrix metalloproteinase-1 expression and activation of gelatinase A as prognostic markers in advanced pediatric neuroblastoma. Cancer 85:231–239

Shusterman S, Grupp SA, Barr R, Carpentieri D, Zhao H, Maris JM (2001) The angiogenesis inhibitor TNP-470 effectively inhibits human neuroblastoma xenograft growth, especially in the setting of subclinical disease. Clin Cancer Res 7:977–984

Soker S, Takashima S, Miao HQ, Neufeld G, Klagsbrun M (1998) Neuropilin-1 is expressed by endothelial and tumor cells as an isoform-specific receptor for vascular endothelial growth factor. Cell 92:735–745

Sugiura Y, Shimada H, Seeger RC, Laug WE, DeClerck YA (1998) Matrix metalloproteinases-2 and -9 are expressed in human neuroblastoma: contribution of stromal cells to their production and correlation with metastasis. Cancer Res 58:2209–2216

Yamaoka M, Yamamoto T, Ikeyama S, Sudo K, Fujita T (1993a) Angiogenesis inhibitor TNP-470 (AGM-1470) potently inhibits the tumor growth of hormone-independent human breast and prostate carcinoma cell lines. Cancer Res 53: 5233–5236

Yamaoka M, Yamamoto T, Masaki T, Ikeyama S, Sudo K, Fujita T (1993b) Inhibition of tumor growth and metastasis of rodent tumors by the angiogenesis inhibitor O-(chloroacetyl-carbamoyl)fumagillol (TNP-470; AGM-1470). Cancer Res 53:4262–4267

Yu JL, Rak JW, Coomber BL, Hicklin DJ, Kerbel RS (2002) Effect of p53 status on tumor response to antiangiogenic therapy. Science 295:1526–1528

Experimental Therapeutics and Preclinical Models

Jennifer K. Peterson, Peter J. Houghton

Contents

17.1 Introduction

Although the treatment outcome for children with advanced-stage neuroblastoma has improved, 5-year event-free survival in most studies is less than 30% (Castel et al. 2001). In a few studies (e.g., Kaneko et al. 2002) survival reaching 34% for patients with *MYCN* amplification (more than ten copies) receiving intensified regimens of cytotoxic agents has been reported. While the survival rate is significantly increased over that of less intensive regimens, two-thirds of high-risk patients with *MYCN* amplification succumb to their disease. Furthermore, the survival of patients with advanced disease without MYCN amplification (less than ten copies) is not much greater (Kaneko et al. 2002); thus, there is still a need to develop more effective, less toxic therapies that will boost survival probability for these children (Brodeur 2002; Tsuchida et al. 2003).

This chapter focuses on the potential of preclinical animal model systems in development of new therapies. Each model has both limitations and uses; the art is to recognize the model attributes and not to extrapolate results beyond the true useful range for that model, i.e., each type of model has a functional use and it is likely that no one class of model will be useful for all applications. For example, syngeneic animal tumor models may have particular value in development of active immunity approaches, whereas heterotransplant models, such as human tumors in immune-deficient mice, have a more restricted application.

Cytotoxic therapies still play the major role in neuroblastoma treatment inducing high complete response rates even in a subset of patients with stage-4

MYCN amplified disease (Castel and Canete 2004; Donfrancesco et al. 2004). Bone marrow or peripheral blood stem cell transplants appear to have some value increasing relapse-free survival, at least in some studies (Goldsby and Matthay 2004; Imaizumi et al. 2001; Valteau-Couanet et al. 2000; Matthay et al. 1999). Differentiation agents and immunotherapies may also increase survival in patients having a complete or good partial response during induction therapy. It is against this background that we consider the use of preclinical models with particular emphasis on contemporary approaches to therapy with novel cytotoxic agents, "molecularly targeted" agents, antiangiogenic agents, and immunotherapy approaches to treating neuroblastoma.

17.2 Heterotransplant Models

17.2.1 Cytotoxic Agents

Human tumors heterografted into immune-deficient mice have provided the major models for drug identification and development over the past two decades. While such models are often criticized as being inadequate, or for failing to predict responsiveness of human cancers, specifically adult malignancies of epithelial origin (Johnson et al. 2001), the experience with models of childhood cancer has been more positive (Peterson and Houghton 2004). In part this may be because tumors such as neuroblastoma are more chemoresponsive; hence, it may be easier to assess response in the clinical situation. For example, the identification of topotecan and irinotecan, DNA topoisomerase-I poisons, as being highly active in preclinical models of rhabdomyosarcoma and neuroblastoma has translated accurately in clinical phase-II trials (Furman et al. 1999; Houghton et al. 1992, 1996, 2002; Santana et al. 2003; Thompson et al. 1997). Similarly, drugs known to be active against clinical neuroblastoma are identified in these models (Houghton et al. 2002; Tsuchida et al. 1984). Yet despite numerous neuroblastoma xenografts propagated either as subcutaneous implants or as disseminated disease following parenteral inoculation of cells, relatively few therapeutic studies have been reported. One exception is the work of Tsuchida and colleagues (1984), who have characterized the chemosensitivity of subcutaneously propagated neuroblastoma xenografts in athymic nude mice. Consistent with clinical experience, cisplatin and cyclophosphamide were identified as most active in this panel of tumors. One advantage of the xenograft system, compared with syngeneic models, is that tumors can be established from patients either at diagnosis or relapse. Identification of novel agents that retain activity against chemorefractory disease is of particular interest. The biological characteristics and treatment status at the time of tumor establishment for a panel of neuroblastoma xenografts is shown in Table 17.1. The chemosensitivity profile of these neuroblastoma xenografts is shown in Table 17.2. Notably, the camptothecin analog topotecan demonstrated good activity against several of these tumors derived from relapsed samples within the panel, although tumors established at diagnosis were more sensitive to topotecan. Recent clinical results in Japan with irinotecan, another camptothecin analog, and in phase-I and phase-II trials at St. Jude (Furman et al. 1999; Santana et al. 2003), indicate that irinotecan and topotecan have significant activity against neuroblastoma. The DNA methylating agent temozolomide also showed promising activity in both diagnosis and relapse models. Sensitivity to temozolomide has been associated with cells that have functional DNA mismatch repair (MMR), and low levels of the DNA repair protein O^6 methylguanine DNA methyltransferase (MGMT). Determination of whether the MMR/MGMT status of xenografts accurately represents the patient tissue may be important in translating these preclinical results (Middlemas et al. 2000; Wagner et al. 2002).

These data suggest that neuroblastoma xenografts respond to known and experimental drugs in a manner similar to that in patients; at least to cytotoxic agents. The potential pitfalls of translating these results have been reviewed recently (Kirstein et al. 2001; Peterson and Houghton 2004). Clearly there are examples of agents that demonstrate very significant activity in such models but fail to fulfill such promise in clinical trials. Retrospective analysis shows that in many instances this disconnect is a consequence of differential host sensitivity: if the mouse is hyper-tol-

Table 17.1. Characteristics of neuroblastoma xenografts

Tumor designation	Clinical stage	*MYCN*	Status/treatment	Doubling time (days)
NB-1382	Local–regional	Amplified	Relapse[a]	11
NB-1643	Stage 4	Amplified	Diagnosis	18
NB-1691	Stage 4	Amplified	Relapse[b]	7
NB-1771	Stage 4	Amplified	Diagnosis	15
NB-EB	Stage 4	Not amplified	Relapse[c]	5
NB-SD	Stage 4	Amplified	Relapse[c]	7

[a] Vincristine, etoposide, cytoxan, cisplatin, carboplatin
[b] Cytarabine, daunorubicin, 6-TG, etoposide, 5-azacytidine
[c] Cytoxan, doxorubicin, cisplatin, etoposide

Table 17.2. Chemosensitivity of neuroblastoma xenografts

Agent	Tumor line NB-1382	NB-1643	NB-1691	NB-1771	NB-EB	NB-SD
Vincristine	++++	++	–	+	–	–
Topotecan	++++++	+++++	+++	++++++	+++++	+++
Temozolomide	++++++	++++++	+	++++++	++++	+++
CPT-11	++++	+++++	++	++++	++++++	++++++
MG1-114	++++++	+++++	++++	++++?	++++	+
VP-16	+++	+++(+)	++(+)	+	++	+/–
CDDP	+	+	ND	ND	–	+/–
Carboplatin	+	ND	+(+)	ND	ND	+(+)
Cytoxan	++	++++	+	+	–	+/–
Doxorubicin	++	+	–		–	++
BMS247550	++++++	++++	++			
ZD1839	++	–	–		–	
SU6668	++		++	+		

Tumor response:
– No growth inhibition
± Transient response, inhibition $<Td_2$ (=mean time for tumor volume to double)
+ Growth inhibition $\geq Td_2$
++ Growth inhibition $\geq 2\times Td_2$
+++ Growth inhibition $\geq 3\times Td_2$
++++ Growth inhibition $\geq 3\ Td_2$+volume regression ≥50%
+++++ Complete regression with subsequent growth
++++++ Complete regression with no regrowth of any tumors during the period of observation (≥84 days)

erant to a drug, relative to human, then the mouse models will overpredict activity (Leggas et al. 2002). If the converse holds, then the mouse models may fail to identify potentially useful agents for clinical disease; thus, it is critical to determine whether drug doses inducing tumor regressions in the models achieve systemic exposures that are relevant to clinical exposures at tolerated doses (Boland et al. 1999; Zamboni et al. 1998). In most instances drug pharmacokinetic data are available from phase-I trials in adult patients prior to initiating pediatric clinical trials; hence, these comparisons can be used to prioritize or de-emphasize development of a specific agent in pediatric trials.

17.2.2 Signal Transduction Inhibitors

Perhaps a greater challenge will be identifying agents that are targeted to components of signaling pathways that regulate proliferation and survival. To be of value such models must accurately mimic the cellular metabolic characteristics of the clinical disease, i.e., unless the pathways accurately recapitulate the function in clinical cancer, the models may have limited value in identifying active agents, or in accurately defining the activity of drug combinations. In an attempt to characterize current preclinical models the Cancer Treatment Evaluation Program at the National Cancer Institute has initiated a Project (POPPTAP – Pediatric Oncology Preclinical Tissue Array Project) to molecularly characterize preclinical models by expression profiling and proteomics profiling. The goal of this project is to determine whether expression profiles of xenografts is similar to that of the respective tumor type in children (i.e., do neuroblastoma xenograft samples cluster with clinical neuroblastoma?). The proteomics component will establish tissue arrays that will allow definition of pathways that are activated, and it is anticipated that such data may allow new target identification. This raises a question as to whether orthotopic models will have to be used to accurately recapitulate gene expression profiles found in clinical tumors. (Khanna et al. 2002) have suggested that human neuroblastoma orthotopically grown in the adrenal gland of Beige-SCID mice demonstrates more relevant tumor biology including an angiogenic phenotype and enhanced distant metastases compared with heterotopic (subcutaneous) tumors and tumors at different sites were associated with differences in expression of angiogenesis-associated genes. A similar analysis has not been undertaken with other models of disseminated neuroblastoma, where cells are injected intravenously or into the heart. Although there are many reports of such specialized models (Gilbert et al. 1988; Martinez et al. 1996; Turner et al. 1990), they tend to be labor intensive and few therapeutic studies have been reported (Thompson et al. 2001). A similar concern over the site of tumor growth exists when one considers evaluation of novel signaling inhibitors. For example, the indolocarbazole CEP-751 inhibits Trk receptors expressed on neuroblastoma and medulloblastoma cells. Interestingly, whereas treatment significantly inhibited growth of IMR-5, NBL-S, and CHP-134 when therapy was started against palpable tumor, it was less effective in a setting of preclinical disease where treatment started 4–6 days after inoculation of cells (Evans et al. 1999). Whether such differences reflect expression levels of the receptor is unknown. In other studies it was shown that CEP-751 had greater inhibitory activity against clones of SY5Y neuroblastoma engineered to express TrkB (Evans et al. 2001), suggesting some specificity of the antitumor activity, although clearly there are other targets for CEP-751 other than Trk receptors. That certain kinase inhibitors may have promiscuous activities, however, is demonstrated by the synergistic activity of the ErbB1 inhibitor gefitinib (Iressa, ZD1839) when combined with the topoisomerase-I poison irinotecan (Stewart et al. 2004) against both neuroblastoma and other xenografts that do not express detectable levels of ErbB-family receptors. In this case the enhanced activity of irinotecan appears to be due to potent inhibition of an ABC transporter (ABCG2/BCRP) that confers cellular resistance to SN-38, the active metabolite of irinotecan (Wierdl et al. 2003). Similarly, imatinib mesylate, an inhibitor of c-KIT, PDGFR, and BCR-ABL, potently inhibits the ABCG2 transporter, reversing resistance to topotecan in vitro (Houghton et al. 2004). It will be important to compare gene expression profiles for micrometastases growing in different organs to determine whether tumor site may ultimately determine the effectiveness of particular signaling inhibitors, adding yet another level of complexity to developing novel therapies for these tumors.

17.2.3 Angiogenesis Inhibitors

Tumor vascularity is highly correlated with outcome. The role for anti-angiogenic, and in vivo angiogenic, activity of neuroblastoma correlates with *MYCN* oncogene overexpression (Ribatti et al. 2002). Consequently, anti-angiogenic agents have been extensively investigated in neuroblastoma xenograft models. Results have been variable. In the study by Katzenstein et al. (1999) initiating therapy with TNP-470 before tumors were clinically evident resulted in 53% of mice being tumor free at 12 weeks. When tumors were staged (<400 mm^3) drug treatment significantly retarded growth of NBL-W-N neuroblastomas, whereas treatment had no effect when tumors were larger (>400 mm^3) at the start of treatment. Similar results were obtained with CHP-134 xenografts (Shusterman et al. 2000, 2001). Other studies (Kim et al. 2002) demonstrated that blockade of VEGF using anti-human VEGF(165) RNA-based fluoropyrimidine aptamer, a monoclonal anti-human VEGF antibody and a VEGFR-1 and VEGFR-2 decoy receptor (VEGF-Trap), inhibited growth NGP-GFP neuroblastomas. Of these the VEGF-Trap approach gave the greatest tumor inhibition; however, in the presence of prolonged inhibition of VEGF function tumors persisted in cooption of blood vessels. This may explain why experimental neuroblastoma may be less sensitive to inhibiting VEGF than another model of Wilms' tumor. Recombinant human and murine endostatin has been evaluated against TNB9 and SKNAS neuroblastoma models, respectively (Jouanneau et al. 2001; Kuroiwa et al. 2001). Both studies initiated therapy when tumors were relatively small, but neither study showed a significant inhibition of tumor growth. Similarly, the VEGFR-2 receptor inhibitor SU6668 demonstrated little activity against several neuroblastoma xenografts (Table 17.2). In contrast, another VEGFR-2 inhibitor SU5416 did inhibit growth of SH-SY5Y tumors by 65% (Backman et al. 2002). A novel approach to controlling angiogenesis through inhibition of hypoxia-inducible factor 1α (HIF-1α) has been tested in various xenograft models including neuroblastoma (Yeo et al. 2003). YC-1, an inhibitor of HIF-1α significantly retarded growth of SK-N-MC PNET xenografts and decreased vascularization. These diverse results reported with different anti-angiogenic agents raises the question of how best to evaluate anti-angiogenic agents in mice; indeed, what constitutes the best model systems? Should orthotopic models be prioritized for these studies, or should established tumors be de-bulked by chemotherapy prior to starting the antiangiogenic treatment? These "secondary" screening models would more readily mimic a clinical situation; however, one still has a hybrid model in which it is murine endothelial elements that are targeted in a human tumor. A more extensive evaluation of anti-angiogenic therapies in a panel of subcutaneous or orthotopic neuroblastoma models is required to address these issues.

17.2.4 Viral-Based Therapies

Adenoviral vectors have been used to deliver angiostatin, an internal fragment of plasminogen containing the first four kringle structures fused to human serum albumin (K3-HAS) (Joseph et al. 2003). Mice bearing IGR-N835 neuroblastomas were administered 5×10^9 PFU (plaque forming units) by intravenous injection when tumors were either early stage, established, or at a state of minimal residual disease. No delay in tumor growth in animals treated with AdK3-HAS was observed compared with control empty virus. K3-HAS was found to be expressed at high levels; hence, it would appear that this approach may not be successful. Instead, IGR-N835 tumors were found to secrete high concentrations of VEGF suggesting that targeting this ligand or its receptor system may be more useful.

A novel approach to treatment of neuroblastoma has been to administer the avian paramyxovirus Newcastle disease virus either by direct intratumoral injection or by intraperitoneal injection (Phuangsab et al. 2001). After a single intraperitoneal injection of 5×10^9 PFU complete regression of IMR-32 neuroblastomas was observed in 9 of 12 mice without recurrence for 3–9 months. In half of those mice where tumor recurred complete response was achieved with three additional courses of treatment. Viral-dependent enzyme prodrug therapy (VDEPT) has also been used to selectively purge neuroblastoma-contaminated human or murine bone marrow. Adenovirus encoding a carboxylesterase that efficiently activates the DNA topoisomerase-I poison irinotecan (CPT-11) was used to selectively activate drug in NB-1691 neuroblastoma cells. Purged marrows were bioassayed by injecting cells into SCID mice. Interestingly, marrows having up to 10% tumor cells were successfully purged, as determined by loss of detection of neuroblastoma markers tyrosine hydroxylase and *MYCN*, and failure to establish disease in mice (Wagner et al. 2002).

17.2.5 Immunotherapy and Radioimmunotherapy

Heterotransplant models have also been used to probe the role of antibodies and antibody-conjugates in the treatment of neuroblastoma for both subcutaneous (Cheung et al. 1986; Cheung and Modak 2002), leptomeningeal (Bergman et al. 1999) as well as metastatic models (Raffaghello et al. 2003). Several promising strategies are being tested in the clinic.

17.3 Transgenic Models

The transgenic neuroblastoma model (Weiss et al. 1997), in which the human *MYCN* gene is expressed in neuroectodermal cells under control of the tyrosine hydroxylase promoter, represents a novel syngeneic model of human disease. Because overexpression of the human *MYCN* oncogene in murine neuroblastoma models is one of the relatively few genetic mutations associated with NB tumorigenesis, it is a potential target for manipulation by investigational therapies. The consequences of amplified human *MYCN* expression in the preclinical setting are of particular importance because a recapitulation of histological and pathological aspects of clinical disease has been shown (Hackett et al. 2003; Weiss et al. 1997). Even though these studies suggest that numerous *other* genetic characteristics of clinical neuroblastoma are also present in mice expressing a human *MYCN* oncogene, this particular characteristic (human *MYCN* overexpression) is the only one associated consistently with enhanced tumorigenesis both in the preclinical and clinical settings (Hackett et al. 2003; Weiss et al. 2000). The mechanism by which human *MYCN* overexpression contributes to the pathogenesis of neuroblastoma is not completely understood but likely involves an alteration in potential for malignancy via gene expression regulation [e.g., *MYCN* regulates the expression of the genes that encode the multidrug resistance associated protein 1 (MRP1) and ornithine decarboxylase (ODC) and possibly expression of the type-1 insulin-like growth factor receptor]. Whatever the mechanism, it seems logical that inhibiting expression of the oncogene would ultimately limit the cell proliferation abilities of the tumor. In fact, Burkhart et al. (2003) found that inhibition of the human *MYCN* oncogene in vivo through antisense oligonucleotide administration was associated with decreases in tumor incidence as well as tumor mass. The results appeared to be directly due to human *MYCN* inhibition since expression/activity of the closely related *MYC* gene family was unaffected. Furthermore, because expression of the gene is virtually absent from adult tissues (restricted to stages of embryogenesis), antisense inhibition of the human *MYCN* oncogene would likely be void of serious adverse events. This study not only stresses the significance of the role of human *MYCN* in neuroblastoma, but also highlights its importance as a potential target for future antisense therapies (Burkhart et al. 2003). It is noteworthy that novel therapies, such as targeted oligonucleotide administration, are not without limitation. Applicability in vivo is impaired by significant instability; oligonucleotides in general are highly sensitive to cellular nuclease degradation. Brignole et al. (2003) suggest that lipid encapsulation of the oligonucleotides prior to administration improves stability and enhances antitumor response. Such a formulation showed good cell binding and relatively desirable tumor cell specificity; however, although antisense, or inhibitory, RNA approaches appear useful in vitro, they face significant hurdles before achieving acceptance as therapeutic modalities for treatment of systemic disease. Instead, at this time they serve as reagents for proof of principle studies in the transgenic mouse models.

17.4 Syngeneic Models

Syngeneic models of neuroblastoma, most frequently derived from the C1300 tumor, have been used to probe the role of immunotherapy. This tumor arose spontaneously in the spinal cord region of a strain-A mouse (Ishizu et al. 1994; Ziegler et al. 1997) and as a subcutaneous implant shows local invasion but rarely metastasizes. A variant of C-1300, TBJ, grows more rapidly and metastasizes extensively, and C-1300 cells inoculated into a subcutaneously translocated spleen gives rise to hepatic metastases. Against C-1300 tumors both rIFN-γ and rIL-2 prolong tumor latency, and enhance tumor lysis in vitro by natural killer cells. The variant neuro-2a tumor has also been used to evaluate the role of expressing both B-7-1 costimulator and IFN-γ. This resulted in upregulation of expression of class-1 MHC and a CD8-positive T-cell response that effectively induced tumor rejection (Katsanis et al. 1996). A variant of C-1300, NX31T28, engineered to express GD2 ganglioside has been used to evaluate biodistribution and activity of a novel fusion protein consisting of mouse chimeric anti-GD2 antibody ch14.18 fused to IL-2 (Lode et al. 1999). This fusion protein, but not the antibody alone or IL-2 plus antibody, was effective in suppressing development of bone marrow and liver disease. The same group showed that CD8+ T cells genetically engineered to produce a single chain IL-12 fusion protein significantly protect syngeneic A/J mice from disseminated neuroblastoma growth (to bone marrow and liver) (Lode et al. 1998a). Local release of cytokines in the tumor microenvironment is the mechanism thought to be responsible for inhibition of malignant growth and thus successful therapy. The NX31T28 model engineered to express IL-12 has also been used to induce CD8 positive-dependent protective immunity, prevented growth of wild-type cells, and eradicated established disease. The same model as been used to evaluate anti-GD2 antibody conjugated to the cytotoxic antibiotic calicheamycin $\theta^1{}_1$ (Lode et al. 1998b). Other approaches evaluated in syngeneic models include immunotherapy with a modified DNA vaccine where mice were immunized with a tyrosine hydroxylase-based DNA vaccine enhanced with the posttranscriptional regulatory acting RNA element derived from the woodchuck hepatitis virus in combination with an antibody-cytokine fusion protein ch14.18-IL-2. This DNA vaccine was delivered using attenuated *Salmonella typhimurium* and administered by oral gavage (Pertl et al. 2003). This facultative intracellular parasite that colonizes the liver has been shown to accumulate within extrahepatic malignancies (Soto et al. 2004). Other researchers have investigated the use of IL-12 or IL-2 plus IL-18 transduced dendritic cells as vaccines for neuroblastoma treatment (Redlinger et al. 2003a,b), the effect of cytokine expression on neuroblastoma growth (Siapati et al. 2003), and alteration in tumors recurrent after suboptimal dosing of a humanized IL-2 immunocytokine targeted to the GD2-ganglioside. The antitumor effect of retinoic acid on the susceptibility of neuroblastoma to CTL-mediated killing has recently been reported to act through stabilization of MHC class-1 complexes, and independently of IFN-γ or TNF-α (Vertuani et al. 2003).

17.5 Conclusion

There is now an increasing selection of animal models in which to evaluate experimental therapy of neuroblastoma. No one model fits all. Instead, a specific model may have a restricted but valuable role. As yet, there is limited data on the role of the transgenic *MYCN* model in developmental therapeutics, but undoubtedly this will emerge; however, retrospective analysis of why the significant efficacy of cytotoxic or other agents in mice fail to translate into clinical responses suggests that direct translation from any murine model to humans needs considerable caution irrespective of the tumor model being used. Despite the limitations, clearly these models are useful in identifying novel approaches to neuroblastoma treatment.

Acknowledgements. Work from this laboratory was supported by CA23099 and CA21765 (Cancer Center Support) grants from NIH.

References

Backman U, Svensson A, Christofferson R (2002) Importance of vascular endothelial growth factor A in the progression of experimental neuroblastoma. Angiogenesis 5:267–274

Bergman I, Barmada MA, Heller G, Griffin JA, Cheung NK (1999) Treatment of neoplastic meningeal xenografts by intraventricular administration of an antiganglioside monoclonal antibody 3F8. Int J Cancer 82:538–548

Boland I, Vassal G, Morizet J, Terrier-Lacombe MJ, Valteau-Couanet D, Kalifa C, Hartmann O, Gouyette A (1999) Busulphan is active against neuroblastoma and medulloblastoma xenografts in athymic mice at clinically achievable plasma drug concentrations. Br J Cancer 79:787–792

Brignole C, Pagnan G, Marimpietri D, Cosimo E, Allen TM, Ponzoni M, Pastorino F (2003) Targeted delivery system for antisense oligonucleotides: a novel experimental strategy for neuroblastoma treatment. Cancer Lett 197:231–235

Brodeur GM (2002) Commentary on Kaneko et al.: Intensified chemotherapy increases the survival rates in patients with stage 4 neuroblastoma with MYCN amplification. Int J Pediatr Hematol Oncol 24:608–609

Burkhart CA, Cheng AJ, Madafiglio J, Kavallaris M, Mili M, Marshall GM, Weiss WA, Khachigian LM, Norris MD, Haber M (2003) Effects of MYCN antisense oligonucleotide administration on tumorigenesis in a murine model of neuroblastoma. Int J Natl Cancer Inst 95:1394–1403

Castel V, Canete A (2004) A comparison of current neuroblastoma chemotherapeutics. Exp Opin Pharmacother 5:71–80

Castel V, Canete A, Navarro S, Garcia-Miguel P, Melero C, Acha T, Navajas A, Badal MD (2001) Outcome of high-risk neuroblastoma using a dose intensity approach: improvement in initial but not in long-term results. Med Pediatr Oncol 37:537–542

Cheung NK, Modak S (2002) Oral (1→3),(1→4)-β-D-glucan synergizes with anti-ganglioside GD2 monoclonal antibody 3F8 in the therapy of neuroblastoma. Clin Cancer Res 8:1217–1223

Cheung NK, Landmeier B, Neely J, Nelson AD, Abramowsky C, Ellery S, Adams RB, Miraldi F (1986) Complete tumor ablation with iodine 131-radiolabeled disialoganglioside GD2 specific monoclonal antibody against human neuroblastoma xenografted in nude mice. J Natl Cancer Inst 77:739–745

Donfrancesco A, Jenkner A, Castellano A, Ilari I, Milano GM, Sio L, de Cozza R, Fidani P, Deb G, de Laurentis C et al. (2004) Ifosfamide/carboplatin/etoposide (ICE) as front-line, topotecan/cyclophosphamide as second-line and oral temozolomide as third-line treatment for advanced neuroblastoma over one year of age. Acta Paediatr (Suppl) 93:6–11

Evans AE, Kisselbach KD, Yamashiro DJ, Ikegaki N, Camoratto AM, Dionne CA, Brodeur GM (1999) Antitumor activity of CEP-751 (KT-6587) on human neuroblastoma and medulloblastoma xenografts. Clin Cancer Res 36:3594–3602

Evans AE, Kisselbach KD, Liu X, Eggert A, Ikegaki N, Camoratto AM, Dionne C, Brodeur GM (2001) Effect of CEP-751 (KT-6587) on neuroblastoma xenografts expressing TrkB. Med Pediatr Oncol 5:181–184

Furman WL, Stewart CF, Poquette CA, Pratt CB, Santana VM, Zamboni WC, Bowman LC, Ma MK, Hoffer FA, Meyer WH et al. (1999) Direct translation of a protracted irinotecan schedule from a xenograft model to a phase I trial in children. J Clin Oncol 171815–1824

Gilbert F, Tsao KL, LaLatta F, Xu L, Potluri VR, LaBadie G (1988) Human neuroblastoma metastases in a nude mouse model: tumor progression and onc gene amplification. Prog Clin Biol Res 271:17–29

Goldsby RE, Matthay KK (2004) Neuroblastoma: evolving therapies for a disease with many faces. Paediatr Drugs 6:107–122

Hackett CS, Hodgson JG, Law ME, Fridlyand J, Osoegawa K, de Jong PJ, Nowak NJ, Pinkel D, Albertson DG, Jain A et al. (2003) Genome-wide array CGH analysis of murine neuroblastoma reveals distinct genomic aberrations which parallel those in human tumors. Cancer Res 63:5266–5273

Houghton PJ, Stewart CF, Zamboni WC, Thompson J, Luo X, Danks MK, and Houghton JA (1996) Schedule-dependent efficacy of camptothecins in models of human cancer. Ann NY Acad Sci 803:188–201

Houghton PJ, Cheshire PJ, Myers L, Stewart CF, Synold TW, Houghton JA (1992) Evaluation of 9-dimethylaminomethyl-10-hydroxycamptothecin against xenografts derived from adult and childhood solid tumors. Cancer Chemother Pharmacol 31:229–239

Houghton PJ, Adamson PC, Blaney S, Fine HA, Gorlick R, Haber M, Helman L, Hirschfeld S, Hollingshead MG, Israel MA et al. (2002) Testing of new agents in childhood cancer preclinical models: meeting summary. Clin Cancer Res 8:3646–3657

Houghton PJ, Germain GS, Harwood FC, Schuetz JD, Stewart CF, Buchdunger E, Traxler P (2004) Imatinib mesylate is a potent inhibitor of the ABCG2 (BCRP) transporter and reverses resistance to topotecan and SN-38 in vitro. Cancer Res 64:2333–2337

Imaizumi M, Watanabe A, Kikuta A, Takano T, Ito E, Shimizu T, Tsuchiya S, Iinuma K, Konno T, Ohi R, Hayashi Y (2001) Improved survival of children with advanced neuroblastoma treated by intensified therapy including myeloablative chemotherapy with stem cell transplantation: a retrospective analysis from the Tohoku Neuroblastoma Study Group. Tohoku J Exp Med 195:3–83

Ishizu H, Bove KE, Ziegler MM, Arya G (1994) Immune-mediated regression of "metastatic" neuroblastoma in the liver. J Pediatr Surg 29:55–160

Johnson JI, Decker S, Zaharevitz D, Rubinstein LV, Venditti JM, Schepartz S, Kalyandrug S, Christian M, Arbuck S, Hollingshead M, Sausville EA (2001) Relationships between drug activity in NCI preclinical in vitro and in vivo models and early clinical trials. Br J Cancer 84:424–431

Joseph JM, Bouquet C, Opolon P, Morizet J, Aubert G, Rossler J, Gross N, Griscelli F, Perricaudet M, Vassal G (2003) High level of stabilized angiostatin mediated by adenovirus delivery does not impair the growth of human neuroblastoma xenografts. Cancer Gene Ther 10:859–866

Jouanneau E, Alberti L, Nejjari M, Treilleux I, Vilgrain I, Duc A, Combaret V, Favrot M, Leboulch P, Bachelot T (2001) Lack of antitumor activity of recombinant endostatin in a human neuroblastoma xenograft model. J Neurooncol 51:11–18

Kaneko M, Tsuchida Y, Mugishima H, Ohnuma N, Yamamoto K, Kawa K, Iwafuchi M, Sawada T, Suita S (2002) Intensified chemotherapy increases the survival rates in patients with stage 4 neuroblastoma with MYCN amplification. J Pediatr Hematol Oncol 24:613–621

Katsanis E, Bausero MA, Panoskaltsis-Mortari A, Dancisak BB, Xu Z, Orchard PJ, Davis CG, Blazar BR (1996) Irradiation of singly and doubly transduced murine neuroblastoma cells expressing B7-1 and producing interferon-gamma reduces their capacity to induce systemic immunity. Cancer Gene Ther 3:75–82

Katzenstein HM, Rademaker AW, Senger C, Salwen HR, Nguyen NN, Thorner PS, Litsas L, Cohn SL (1999) Effectiveness of the angiogenesis inhibitor TNP-470 in reducing the growth of human neuroblastoma in nude mice inversely correlates with tumor burden. Clin Cancer Res 5:4273–4278

Khanna C, Jaboin JJ, Drakos E, Tsokos M, Thiele CJ (2002) Biologically relevant orthotopic neuroblastoma xenograft models: primary adrenal tumor growth and spontaneous distant metastasis. In Vivo 16:77–85

Kim ES, Serur A, Huang J, Manley CA, McCrudden KW, Frischer JS, Soffer SZ, Ring L, New T, Zabski S et al. (2002) Potent VEGF blockade causes regression of coopted vessels in a model of neuroblastoma. Proc Natl Acad Sci USA 99: 11399–11404

Kirstein MN, Houghton PJ, Cheshire PJ, Richmond LB, Smith AK, Hanna SK, Stewart CF (2001) Relation between 9-aminocamptothecin systemic exposure and tumor response in human solid tumor xenografts. Clin Cancer Res 7:358–366

Kuroiwa M, Ikeda H, Hongo T, Tsuchida Y, Hirato J, Kaneko Y, Suzuki N, Obana K, Makino SI (2001) Effects of recombinant human endostatin on a human neuroblastoma xenograft. Int J Mol Med 8:391–396

Leggas M, Stewart CF, Woo MH, Fouladi M, Cheshire PJ, Peterson JK, Friedman HS, Billups C, Houghton PJ (2002) Relation between Irofulven (MGI-114) systemic exposure and tumor response in human solid tumor xenografts. Clin Cancer Res 8:3000–3007

Lode HN, Dreier T, Xiang R, Varki NM, Kang AS, Reisfeld RA (1998a) Gene therapy with a single chain interleukin 12 fusion protein induces T cell-dependent protective immunity in a syngeneic model of murine neuroblastoma. Proc Natl Acad Sci USA 95:2475–2480

Lode HN, Reisfeld RA, Handgretinger R, Nicolaou KC, Gaedicke G, Wrasidlo W (1998b) Targeted therapy with a novel enediyene antibiotic calicheamicin theta(I)1 effectively suppresses growth and dissemination of liver metastases in a syngeneic model of murine neuroblastoma. Cancer Res 58:2925–2928

Lode HN, Xiang R, Duncan SR, Theofilopoulos AN, Gillies SD, Reisfeld RA (1999) Tumor-targeted IL-2 amplifies T cell-mediated immune response induced by gene therapy with single-chain IL-12. Proc Natl Acad Sci USA 96:8591–8596

Martinez DA, Kahwash S, O"Dorisio MS, Lloyd TV, McGhee RB Jr, Qualman SJ (1996) Disseminated neuroblastoma in the nude rat. A xenograft model of human malignancy. Cancer 77:409–419

Matthay KK, Villablanca JG, Seeger RC, Stram DO, Harris RE, Ramsay NK, Swift P, Shimada H, Black CT, Brodeur GM, Gerbing RB, Reynolds CP (1999) Treatment of high-risk neuroblastoma with intensive chemotherapy, radiotherapy, autologous bone marrow transplantation, and 13-cis-retinoic acid. Children's Cancer Group. N Engl J Med 341: 1165–1173

Middlemas DS, Stewart CF, Kirstein MN, Poquette C, Friedman HS, Houghton PJ, Brent TP (2000) Biochemical correlates of temozolomide sensitivity in pediatric solid tumor xenograft models. Clin Cancer Res 6:998–1007

Pertl U, Wodrich H, Ruehlmann JM, Gillies SD, Lode HN, Reisfeld RA (2003) Immunotherapy with a posttranscriptionally modified DNA vaccine induces complete protection against metastatic neuroblastoma. Blood 101:649–654

Peterson JK, Houghton PJ (2004) Integrating pharmacology and in vivo cancer models in preclinical and clinical drug development. Eur J Cancer 40:837–844

Phuangsab A, Lorence RM, Reichard KW, Peeples ME, Walter RJ (2001) Newcastle disease virus therapy of human tumor xenografts: antitumor effects of local or systemic administration. Cancer Lett 172:27–36

Raffaghello L, Marimpietri D, Pagnan G, Pastorino F, Cosimo E, Brignole C, Ponzoni M, Montaldo PG (2003) Anti-GD2 monoclonal antibody immunotherapy: a promising strategy in the prevention of neuroblastoma relapse. Cancer Lett 197:205–209

Redlinger RE Jr, Mailliard RB, Lotze MT, Barksdale EM Jr (2003a) Synergistic interleukin-18 and low-dose interleukin-2 promote regression of established murine neuroblastoma in vivo. J Pediatr Surg 38:301–307

Redlinger RE Jr, Shimizu T, Remy T, Alber S, Watkins SC, Barksdale EM Jr (2003b) Cellular mechanisms of interleukin-12-mediated neuroblastoma regression. J Pediatr Surg 38:199–204

Ribatti D, Raffaghello L, Pastorino F, Nico B, Brignole C, Vacca A, Ponzoni M (2002) In vivo angiogenic activity of neuroblastoma correlates with MYCN oncogene overexpression. Int J Cancer 102:351–354

Santana VM, Zamboni WC, Kirstein MN, Tan M, Liu T, Gajjar A, Houghton PJ, Stewart CF (2003) A pilot study of protracted topotecan dosing using a pharmacokinetically guided dosing approach in children with solid tumors. Clin Cancer Res 9:633–640

Shusterman S, Grupp SA, Maris JM (2000) Inhibition of tumor growth in a human neuroblastoma xenograft model with TNP-470. Med Pediatr Oncol 35:673–676

Shusterman S, Grupp SA, Barr R, Carpentieri D, Zhao H, Maris JM (2001) The angiogenesis inhibitor tnp-470 effectively inhibits human neuroblastoma xenograft growth, especially in the setting of subclinical disease. Clin Cancer Res 7:977–984

Siapati KE, Barker S, Kinnon C, Michalski A, Anderson R, Brickell P, Thrasher AJ, Hart SL (2003) Improved antitumour immunity in murine neuroblastoma using a combination of IL-2 and IL-12. Br J Cancer 88:1641–1648

Soto LJ III, Sorenson BS, Nelson BW, Solis SJ, Leonard AS, Saltzman DA (eds) (2004) Preferential proliferation of attenuated *Salmonella typhimurium* within neuroblastoma. J Pediatr Surg 39:937–940

Stewart CF, Leggas M, Schuetz JD, Panetta JC, Cheshire PJ, Peterson J, Daw N, Jenkins JJ III, Gilbertson R, Germain GS, Harwood FC, Houghton PJ (2004) Gefitinib enhances the antitumor activity and oral bioavailability of irinotecan in mice. Cancer Res 64:7491–7499

Thompson J, Zamboni WC, Cheshire PJ, Lutz L, Luo X, Li Y, Houghton JA, Stewart CF, Houghton PJ (1997) Efficacy of systemic administration of irinotecan against neuroblastoma xenografts. Clin Cancer Res 3:423–431

Thompson J, Guichard SM, Cheshire PJ, Richmond LB, Poquette CA, Ragsdale ST, Webber B, Lorsbach R, Danks MK, Houghton PJ (2001) Development, characterization and therapy of a disseminated model of childhood neuroblastoma in SCID mice. Cancer Chemother Pharmacol 47:211–221

Tsuchida Y, Yokomori K, Iwanaka T, Saito S (1984) Nude mouse xenograft study for treatment of neuroblastoma: effects of chemotherapeutic agents and surgery on tumor growth and cell kinetics. J Pediatr Surg 19:72–76

Tsuchida Y, Shitara T, Kuroiwa M, Ikeda H (2003) Current treatment and future directions in neuroblastoma. Indian J Pediatr 70:809–812

Turner WJ, Chatten J, Lampson LA (1990) Human neuroblastoma cell growth in xenogeneic hosts: comparison of T cell-deficient and NK-deficient hosts, and subcutaneous or intravenous injection routes. J Neurooncol 8:121–132

Valteau-Couanet D, Benhamou E, Vassal G, Stambouli F, Lapierre V, Couanet D, Lumbroso J, Hartmann O (2000) Consolidation with a busulfan-containing regimen followed by stem cell transplantation in infants with poor prognosis stage 4 neuroblastoma. Bone Marrow Transplant 25:937–942

Vertuani S, de Geer A, Levitsky V, Kogner P, Kiessling R, Levitskaya J (2003) Retinoids act as multistep modulators of the major histocompatibility class I presentation pathway and sensitize neuroblastomas to cytotoxic lymphocytes. Cancer Res 63:8006–8013

Wagner LM, Guichard SM, Burger RA, Morton CL, Straign CM, Ashmun RA, Harris LC, Houghton PJ, Potter PM, Danks MK (2002) Efficacy and toxicity of a virus-directed enzyme prodrug therapy purging method: preclinical assessment and application to bone marrow samples from neuroblastoma patients. Cancer Res 62:5001–5007

Weiss WA, Aldape K, Mohapatra G, Feuerstein BG, Bishop JM (1997) Targeted expression of MYCN causes neuroblastoma in transgenic mice. EMBO J 16:2985–2995

Weiss WA, Godfrey T, Francisco C, Bishop JM (2000) Genome-wide screen for allelic imbalance in a mouse model for neuroblastoma. Cancer Res 60:2483–2487

Wierdl M, Wall A, Morton CL, Sampath J, Danks MK, Schuetz JD, Potter PM (2003) Carboxylesterase-mediated sensitization of human tumor cells to CPT-11 cannot override ABCG2-mediated drug resistance. Mol Pharmacol 64:279–288

Yeo EJ, Chun YS, Cho YS, Kim J, Lee JC, Kim MS, Park JW (2003). YC-1: a potential anticancer drug targeting hypoxia-inducible factor 1. J Natl Cancer Inst 95:516–525

Zamboni WC, Stewart CF, Thompson J, Santana VM, Cheshire PJ, Richmond LB, Luo X, Poquette C, Houghton JA, Houghton PJ (1998) Relationship between topotecan systemic exposure and tumor response in human neuroblastoma xenografts. J Natl Cancer Inst 90:505–511

Ziegler MM, Ishizu H, Nagabuchi E, Takada N, Arya G (1997) A comparative review of the immunobiology of murine neuroblastoma and human neuroblastoma. Cancer 79:1757–1766

Late Effects of Treatment

Caroline Laverdière, James Gurney,
Charles A. Sklar

Contents

18.1 Introduction

Neuroblastoma is a cancer with heterogeneous clinical manifestations and behaviors. Localized tumors can usually be cured by surgical resection alone (Kushner et al. 1996b; Perez et al. 2000; Brodeur and Maris 2002). At the other end of the spectrum, aggressive metastatic tumors frequently progress despite intensive chemoradiotherapy (Brodeur and Maris 2002). The overall prognosis of high-risk neuroblastoma patients remains poor, with an overall survival rate of less than 30% at 5 years (Brodeur and Maris 2002); however, with the use of high-dose chemotherapy regimens, plus new drugs, such as cis-retinoic acid, and new modalities of treatment, such as targeted immunotherapy, a subset of patients with high-risk disease achieve and maintain a complete remission (Kushner et al. 1994; Cheung et al. 1998; Matthay et al. 1999; Cheung et al. 2001). Survivors of high-risk neuroblastoma, therefore, face the long-term consequences of intensive multimodality therapy given, often, at a young age.

Only a limited number of studies have assessed the long-term clinical late effects that are specific to survivors of neuroblastoma. The data are particularly scanty on those who have been treated for high-risk disease (Willi et al. 1992; Olshan et al. 1993; Kaste et al. 1998; Kushner et al. 1998; Hovi et al. 1999; Nève et al. 1999; Barr et al. 2000; Koyle et al. 2001; Hölttä et al. 2002; Van Santen et al. 2002; Weiss et al. 2003).

In this chapter we review the major and most frequent late complications observed in low/intermediate-risk and high-risk neuroblastoma survivors. Since the radiation fields and the chemotherapeutic agents adopted in neuroblastoma treatment protocols are commonly used to treat other pediatric cancers, published data on late effects in these cancer survivors are highly relevant for children with neuroblastoma. Additionally, we discuss the late effects observed in a cohort of 65 neuroblastoma survivors, predominantly survivors treated for high-risk disease, who are followed in the Long-Term Follow-Up Clinic at Memorial Sloan Kettering Cancer Center (MSKCC).

18.2 Long-Term Complications for Low- and Intermediate-Risk Neuroblastoma Survivors

Recent studies in neuroblastoma have allowed for the development of a risk-stratification system for treatment, based on clinical and biological factors (Brodeur 2003). Low-risk patients have localized tumors with favorable biological features and can be cured by surgical removal of the primary tumor (Matthay et al. 1989; Kushner et al. 1996b; Perez et al. 2000). The intermediate-risk group includes mainly patients with locally invasive tumors with favorable biological features. The current management of these patients is conservative and for most patients overaggressive initial surgery is not preferred (Cruccetti et al. 2000). Instead, moderate-dose chemotherapy is used to render the primary tumor resectable at second-look surgery (Matthay et al. 1998). External radiation therapy is more controversial (Kushner et al. 1996a; Matthay et al. 1998).

In previous decades, these two groups of patients were more heavily treated with combinations of radical surgery, radiation therapy, and chemotherapy (Brodeur and Maris 2002). A few studies discuss the late effects in these survivors who were treated between 1950 and 1990 (Meadows et al. 1975; Mayfield et al. 1981; Pastore et al. 1982; Kajanti 1983; Pastore et al. 1987; Paulino et al. 2002). The most common long-term complications reported were musculoskeletal and neurological problems.

18.2.1 Musculoskeletal

Musculoskeletal effects include scoliosis, kyphosis, hypoplasia, and fibrosis of bone and soft tissues, as well as slipped capital femoral epiphysis (Mayfield et al. 1981; Pastore et al. 1982; Kajanti 1983). Most of the patients who develop scoliosis have been treated with moderate to high doses of orthovoltage radiation therapy (1500–5000 cGy) and received asymmetric irradiation of the spine. Some patients were also irradiated under 6 months of age, while others underwent laminectomy for epidural disease (Mayfield et al. 1981; Pastore et al. 1982; Kajanti 1983).

18.2.2 Neurological

Neurological problems include paresthesias, mild to severe paresis, paraplegia, and neurogenic bladder (Pastore et al. 1982; Pastore et al. 1987). These complications are related to the disease itself (intraspinal tumors) and/or to surgery. Surgical complications in neuroblastoma are reported in 5–25% of these cases, especially when aggressive resections of thoracic or abdominal tumors were attempted (Azizkhan et al. 1985; Nitschke et al. 1988; Cruccetti et al. 2000). The incidence of intraspinal tumors is higher in children with local-regional disease than in patients with widely disseminated neuroblastoma (Katzenstein et al. 2001, De Bernardi et al. 2001, Plantaz et al. 1996). Neurological recovery correlates inversely with the severity of the presenting neurological deficits (Hoover et al. 1999; De Bernardi et al. 2001; Katzenstein et al. 2001). Recent studies suggest that chemotherapy is as effective as laminectomy and radiation therapy for the treatment of spinal cord compression and is associated with less long-term skeletal sequelae than the two other modalities (Plantaz et al. 1996; Hoover et al. 1999; Katzenstein et al. 2001).

18.3 Long-Term Complications for Survivors of High-Risk Neuroblastoma

High-risk neuroblastoma survivors commonly develop long-term complications due primarily to the intensive multimodality therapy they receive. We recently reviewed the data of a cohort of neuroblastoma survivors followed at our Long Term Follow-Up Clinic at MSKCC. Since 1991, 65 neuroblastoma survivors have been seen. The clinical and treatment data on these patients are summarized in Table 18.1. The majority of these individuals were treated for high-risk disease. Long-term complications were noted in 58 of the 65 (89%) patients, and 40 (62%) experienced more than one complication. Sixteen of these 65 patients (25%) had more than three complications. The more frequent late effects observed are listed in Table 18.2. The late effects that can arise following successful therapy for high-risk neuroblastoma, as well as the specific risk factors associated with these adverse outcomes, are discussed by organ systems in the next section.

18.3.1 Audiological

The ototoxicity of platinum compounds is well described and is more common with cisplatin (CDDP) than with carboplatin (Piel et al. 1974; Schell et al. 1989; Skinner et al. 1990). Platinum compounds are key components of the chemotherapeutic regimens for high-risk neuroblastoma, and many protocols included dose-intensive cisplatin or carboplatin (Kushner et al. 1994; Matthay et al. 1999; Cheung et al. 2001). The overall incidence of cisplatin-induced hearing loss in the pediatric cancer population, including neuroblastoma patients, ranges from 20 to 80% (Schell et al. 1989; Skinner et al. 1990; Weatherly et al. 1991; Parsons et al. 1998; Simon et al. 2002). The hearing loss is more pronounced in the high-frequency

Table 18.1. Clinical and treatment characteristics of neuroblastoma survivors followed in the Long-Term Follow-Up Clinic at MSKCC (n=65). *ABMT* Autologous bone marrow transplantation, *TBI* total-body irradiation

Characteristic	No. of patients	Percentage
Gender		
Male	33	51
Female	32	49
Stage of neuroblastoma		
Stage 2	1	1.5
Stage 3	10	15
Stage 4	53	82
Stage 4S	1	1.5
Median age at diagnosis	3.8 years (range 0.07–23.5 years)	
Median follow-up	7.3 years (range 1.9–25.5 years)	
Treatment		
Surgery	65	100
Chemotherapy	64	98
Radiation therapy	56	86
ABMT	35	54
TBI	5	8[a]
Immunotherapy (anti-GD2 monoclonal antibody 3F8)	38	58
Radioimmunotherapy (anti-GD2 monoclonal antibody ^{131}I-3F8)	19	29[b]

[a] Five of 35 patients who underwent ABMT received TBI (14%)

[b] Nineteen of 38 patients who received immunotherapy received radioimmunotherapy (50%)

Table 18.2. Frequencies of late effects observed in neuroblastoma survivors followed in the Long-Term Follow-up Clinic at MSKCC (*n*=65)

Late effect	No. of patients	Percentage
Hearing loss	36	55
Ovarian failure	12	38[a]
Primary hypothyroidism	15	23
Musculoskeletal problems	10	15
Dental problems	8	12
Visual problems	8	12
Neurological deficits	7	11
Pulmonary dysfunction	7	11
Neurocognitive problems	6	9
Renal dysfunction	6	9
Gastrointestinal problems	6	9
Growth hormone deficiency	6	9
Second malignant neoplasm	4	6
Hepatitis C	4	6

[a] *n*=32 female patients

range, but speech frequencies can also be affected (Schell et al. 1989; Parsons et al. 1998). It is usually irreversible, but some patients experience partial recovery (Skinner et al. 1990). Risk factors for cisplatin-induced hearing loss include cumulative dose higher than 360 mg/m^2, young age at treatment, previous or concomitant cranial or head and neck irradiation, abnormal renal function, and use of other ototoxic drugs (e.g., aminoglycosides, loop diuretics) (Schell et al. 1989; Weatherly et al. 1991; Parsons et al. 1998). Hearing loss at a young age has a significant impact on the acquisition of speech and contributes to a lessened quality of life in survivors of advanced neuroblastoma (Barr et al. 2000). Early audiological interventions, such as hearing aids and speech and language therapy, are therefore mandatory to minimize the impact of the hearing loss. The use of chemoprotective agents, such as amifostine for platinum-induced ototoxicity, warrants further investigation (Cronin et al. 2000; Fulda et al. 2001).

In our cohort, 55% (36 of 65) of survivors have hearing loss: 10 patients (16% of the cohort) experience losses at high frequencies (500–2000 Hz) and 26 patients (40% of the cohort) at speech frequencies (500–2000 Hz). These results are in accordance with other studies showing that young age at treatment and high doses of platinum compounds are major risk factors for the development of hearing loss.

18.3.2 Endocrine

18.3.2.1 Thyroid Function

Primary hypothyroidism is a common late effect observed in cancer survivors who received head and neck radiation (Kaplan et al. 1983; Halperin et al. 1999). The occurrence of thyroid dysfunction is related, primarily, to the dose of radiotherapy administered but is also influenced by the age and gender of the patient and the time elapsed since the end of treatment (Sklar et al. 2000).

A higher incidence of clinically significant hypothyroidism is observed above radiation doses of 2000 cGy (Kaplan et al. 1983; Constine et al. 1984).

Current radiotherapy doses used for local control in high-risk neuroblastoma patients with thoracic or cervical tumors are often in this range (Halperin et al. 1999; Kushner et al. 2001). Patients who received total-body irradiation (TBI) are also at risk for hypothyroidism (Ogilvy-Stuart et al. 1992). The radiation-related risk persists more than 25 years after treatment (Hancock et al. 1991; Sklar et al. 2000). The addition of chemotherapy to radiation therapy does not seem to increase the risk of hypothyroidism (Van Santen et al. 2003).

Many cases of subclinical primary hypothyroidism have been described in neuroblastoma patients following the administration of ^{131}I-metaiodobenzylguanidine (^{131} I-MIBG; Garaventa et al. 1991; Picco et al. 1993; Picco et al. 1995; Van Santen et al. 2002). The reported incidence is 50–80% despite thyroid protection with high doses of potassium iodide before, during, and after the ^{131}I-MIBG (Picco et al. 1995; Van Santen et al. 2002). Optimal prophylaxis against the thyroidal damage induced by radio-iodinated substances is still unknown (Van Santen et al. 2002).

In our cohort, 23% of the patients developed primary hypothyroidism. Of these patients, 66% received ^{131}I-3F8 antibody (despite protection with potassium iodide and thyroid hormone suppression) and 33% received chest/mantle external-beam radiation therapy.

18.3.2.2 Reproductive Endocrine Function

Ovarian Dysfunction

Both chemotherapy and radiation therapy can induce ovarian dysfunction, which can be either transient or permanent. In the pre-pubertal state, ovaries are more resistant to chemotherapy-induced damage than in the post-pubertal individual (Rivkees and Crawford 1988; Halperin et al. 1999). Among all the chemotherapeutic agents, alkylating agents, including cyclophosphamide, ifosfamide, busulfan, BCNU, and CCNU, have most consistently caused ovarian damage. High doses of these agents are very toxic even to young ovaries (Thibaud et al. 1998; Sklar 1999). Patients who have undergone allogenic or autologous bone marrow transplant with high-dose alkylator therapy (e.g., busulfan, melphalan, or thiotepa) are at particularly high risk of developing ovarian failure (Thibaud et al. 1998; Sklar 1999). Furthermore, even if female patients recover ovarian function after treatment is completed, a significant proportion of these patients are at risk of experiencing premature menopause in the future (Byrne et al. 1992).

Radiation-induced ovarian failure is also common in female cancer survivors. As with chemotherapy, pre-pubertal ovaries seem to be more resistant to damage from irradiation than post-pubertal ovaries. Radiation doses above 1000–2000 cGy can, however, cause irreversible ovarian damage in young girls (Stillman et al. 1981; Wallace et al. 1989a); therefore, young females who receive abdominal, pelvic, or spinal irradiation for tumors such as neuroblastoma have a high risk of ovarian failure (Shalet et al. 1976; Stillman et al. 1981; Wallace et al. 1989a; Wallace et al. 1989b). Moreover, we can extrapolate that the concomitant use of intensive chemotherapy in neuroblastoma definitely increases the risk of ovarian failure and premature menopause. Patients who received TBI are also at significant risk of developing irreversible ovarian failure (Sklar 1995a). The use of more conformal radiation techniques, shielding of the ovaries, or oophoropexy are strategies used to lessen the occurrence of this complication (Halperin et al. 1999). Female patients who receive abdominal irradiation are also at increased risk for spontaneous abortion, preterm labor, and the delivery of low-birth-weight infants once they reach childbearing age (Li et al. 1987).

In our cohort, 12 of 32 patients (38%) developed ovarian dysfunction, which was transient in 3 of the patients. All 12 patients had received cyclophosphamide and 75% had also been treated with abdominal irradiation.

Testicular Dysfunction

Male germ cells are very vulnerable to both radiation and chemotherapy (Aubier et al. 1989; Halperin et al. 1999). Alkylating agents (cyclophosphamide, nitrosoureas) are very toxic to the germinal epithelium (the sperm-producing cells). This effect is more frequent and more severe at higher doses (Aubier et al.

include age less than 3 years, high-dose chemotherapy with autologous bone marrow transplantation, and cranial radiation (Phipps et al. 2000). The impact of TBI on the neurocognitive impairment remains controversial (Simms et al. 1988; Kramer et al. 1992; Phipps et al. 1995; Phipps et al. 2000). Notteghem et al. (2003) recently reviewed the neuropsychological outcomes of 46 high-risk neuroblastoma patients with a mean follow-up of 9.1 years. Survivors of neuroblastoma had an overall performance and skills in the normal range; however, patients who were younger than 3 years when they received the treatment had more visuospatial difficulties and a worse visual memory. Furthermore, hearing loss due to cisplatin was associated with defects in verbal performance (Notteghem et al. 2003).

A recent CCSS study evaluated the educational achievement of a large cohort of childhood cancer survivors. Compared with normal siblings, neuroblastoma survivors were significantly more likely to use special education services because of lower tests scores, and were significantly less likely to complete high school (odds ratio 1.7); however, when the neuroblastoma survivors received special education services, risk estimates approximated those of the sibling population. In the same study, age at diagnosis under 6 years and cranial radiation were associated independently with the use of special education services among all the survivors (Mitby et al. 2003). In contrast, another study reported a similar educational achievement between survivors of neuroblastoma and siblings (Kelaghan et al. 1988).

18.3.9 Subsequent Malignant Neoplasms

Second malignancy is an unfortunate consequence of childhood cancer treatment. The cumulative estimated incidence of subsequent malignant neoplasms (SMNs) 20 years after a diagnosis of childhood cancer is 3.2% (Neglia et al. 2001). For neuroblastoma survivors, the relative risk of developing an SMN has been reported as 6.59 when compared with the general population, with a cumulative incidence at 20 years of 1.87% (Neglia et al. 2001). This latter estimate is derived from a historical cohort that includes a large number of survivors treated for low/intermediate-risk disease and may not reflect the true risk for patients who are treated with more intensive contemporary regimens.

The most common secondary malignancies reported after neuroblastoma are myelodysplasia/leukemia, thyroid neoplasm, soft tissue sarcomas, and osteosarcomas (Shah et al. 1983; Meadows et al. 1985; de Vathaire et al. 1989; Tucker et al. 1991; Kushner et al. 1998; Tabone et al. 1999; Schiavetti et al. 2001; Acharya et al. 2003; Garaventa et al. 2003; Le Deley et al. 2003; Weiss et al. 2003). Treatment-related myelodysplasia/leukemia has been well described. The most common chemotherapeutic agents associated with this complication are topoisomerase-II inhibitors (etoposide, doxorubicin) and alkylating agents. The two classes of drugs are associated with specific and different cytogenetic abnormalities (Kushner et al. 1998; Le Deley et al. 2003). Among neuroblastoma survivors treated at MSKCC, Kushner et al. (1998) found a 3-year cumulative incidence of secondary myelodysplasia/leukemia of 7%; therefore, current intensive treatment for high-risk neuroblastoma is associated with a significant risk for treatment-related acute myeloid leukemia and warrants that these patients be monitored closely.

Secondary thyroid neoplasms are also common in neuroblastoma survivors due to chest and spinal irradiation at a young age (Tucker et al. 1991; Le Deley et al. 2003).

Recently, two studies reported on the risk of SMN (leukemia and solid tumors) with the administration of ^{131}I-MIBG (Garaventa et al. 2003; Weiss et al. 2003). In one of these studies, the cumulative risk of developing a second cancer was 20% within 15 years of receiving ^{131}I-MIBG (Garaventa et al. 2003).

18.4 Health-Related Quality of Life

Beyond survival and long-term late effects, health-related quality of life (HRQOL) is increasingly being appreciated as an important outcome measure for evaluating treatment effects in clinical research (Spilker 1996; Staquet 1998; Drotar 1998; Joyce 1999). Health-related quality of life is a subjective term, but it reflects the understanding that health is not only the absence of disease, but also a complex function of psychological, social, physical, and functional well-being. The very few HRQOL studies conducted on childhood cancer survivors to date have usually been limited to proxy reports from clinicians or parents, without considering the child's own perspective on his or her functioning and well-being. Practically no published HRQOL-related studies are specific to neuroblastoma survivors. One exception was a study of health status conducted by Barr and colleagues (2000) using health utility indexes. They sent questionnaires to parents of children who survived either Wilms' tumor (n=52) or advanced neuroblastoma (n=26), and compared scores related to health attributes and functional capacity. Children surviving high-risk neuroblastoma had a greater overall burden of morbidity, and a significantly higher likelihood of sensory deficits, specifically in speech and hearing, than did children surviving Wilms' tumor. In one measure representing constructs for memory and problem-solving skills, both groups showed indications of cognitive morbidity (Barr 2000). Psychological adjustment and psychosocial functioning among long-term neuroblastoma survivors has yet to be addressed in the clinical literature, although a cross-sectional study on HRQOL and family impact from the cancer experience is currently being conducted through the Children's Oncology Group. This study compares outcomes across neuroblastoma treatment regimens. Results from that study should be available soon.

18.5 Conclusion

Late effects of treatment are common among neuroblastoma survivors, mostly in high-risk patients. These complications are important and must be identified and treated early in order to minimize the impact on quality of life of the survivors. The new treatment paradigms for low- and intermediate-risk patients will probably result in a decrease in treatment-related morbidity. However, for high-risk patients, the intensification of therapy for these patients treated at a very young age can have severe late effects; therefore, close follow-up of these patients after completion of the therapy is strongly recommended. More specifically, ovarian function of female patients should be followed closely. All high-risk patients treated with platinum compounds should be screened for hearing loss, and early audiological interventions, such as hearing aids and speech and language therapy, should be implemented as needed. In addition, neurocognitive development should be monitored with serial psychometric testing and patients should be screened for subsequent malignant neoplasms. Because long-term survivors of high-risk neuroblastoma can have complex medical problems with multi-organ dysfunction, these children are optimally cared for by physicians familiar with the late effects of intensive chemotherapy and radiation. New therapeutic strategies for high-risk neuroblastoma that will lead to higher rates of survival as well as enhanced quality of life are desperately needed.

References

Acharya S, Sarafoglou K, LaQuaglia M et al. (2003) Thyroid neoplasms after therapeutic radiation for malignancies during childhood or adolescence. Cancer 97:2397–2403

Aubier F, Flamant F, Brauner R et al. (1989) Male gonadal function after chemotherapy for solid tumors in childhood. J Clin Oncol 7:304–309

Azizkhan RG, Shaw A, Chandler JG (1985) Surgical complications of neuroblastoma resection. Surgery 97:514–517

Barr RD, Chalmers D, De Pauw S et al. (2000) Health-related quality of life in survivors of Wilms' tumor and advanced neuroblastoma: a cross-sectional study. J Clin Oncol 18: 3280–3287

Brodeur GM (2003) Neuroblastoma: biological insights into a clinical enigma. Nat Rev Cancer 3:203–216

Brodeur GM, Maris JM (2002) Neuroblastoma. In: Pizzo PA, Poplack DG (eds) Principles and practice of pediatric oncology, 4th edn. Lippincott, Williams and Wilkins, Philadelphia, pp 895–937

Byrne J, Fears TR, Gail MH et al. (1992) Early menopause in long-term survivors of cancer during adolescence. Am J Obstet Gynecol 166:788–793

Cheung NKV, Kushner BH, Cheung IY et al. (1998) Anti-G_{D2} antibody treatment of minimal residual stage 4 neuroblastoma diagnosed at more than 1 year of age. J Clin Oncol 16:3053–3060

Cheung NKV, Kushner BH, LaQuaglia M et al. (2001) N7: a novel multi-modality therapy of high risk neuroblastoma (NB) in children diagnosed over 1 year of age. Med Pediatr Oncol 36:227–230

Constine LS, Donaldson SS, McDougall IR et al. (1984) Thyroid dysfunction after radiotherapy in children with Hodgkin's disease. Cancer 53:878–883
Cronin S, Uberti JP, Ayash LJ et al. (2000) Use of amifostine as a chemoprotectant during high-dose chemotherapy in autologous peripheral blood stem cell transplantation. Bone Marrow Transplant 26:1247–1249
Cruccetti A, Kiely EM, Spitz L et al. (2000) Pelvic neuroblastoma: low mortality and high morbidity. J Pediatr Surg 35:724–728
De Bernardi B, Pianco C, Pistamiglio P et al. (2001) Neuroblastoma with symptomatic spinal cord compression at diagnosis: treatment and results with 76 cases. J Clin Oncol 19:183–190
De Vathaire F, François P, Hill C et al. (1989) Role of radiotherapy and chemotherapy in the risk of second malignant neoplasms after cancer in childhood. Br J Cancer 59: 792–796
Drotar D (ed) Measuring health-related quality of life in children and adolescents: implications for research and practice. Lawrence Erlbaum Associates, Publishers, Mahwah, New Jersey
Estilo CL, Huryn JM, Kraus DH et al. (2003) Effects of therapy on dentofacial development in long-term survivors of head and neck rhabdomyosarcoma: the Memorial Sloan-Kettering Cancer Center Experience. J Pediatr Hematol Oncol 25:215–222
Fulda S, Fichtner I, Hero B et al. (2001) Preclinical and clinical aspects on the use of amifostine as chemoprotection in neuroblastoma patients. Med Pediatr Oncol 36:199–202
Garaventa A, Guerra P, Arrighini A et al. (1991) Treatment of advanced neuroblastoma with ^{131}I-meta-iodobenzylguanidine. Cancer 67:922–928
Garaventa A, Gambina C, Villavecchia G et al. (2003) Second malignancies in children with neuroblastoma after combined treatment with ^{131}I-metaiodobenzylguanidine. Cancer 97:1332–1338
Goren MP (2003) Cisplatin nephrotoxicity affects magnesium and calcium metabolism. Med Pediatr Oncol 41:186–189
Gupta M, Steinherz PG, Cheung NK et al. (2003) Late cardiotoxicity after bolus versus infusion anthracycline therapy for childhood cancers. Med Pediatr Oncol 40:343–347
Halperin EC, Constine LS, Tarbell NJ (1999) Late effects of cancer treatment. In: Halperin EC, Constine LS, Tarbell NJ, Kun LE (eds) Pediatric radiation oncology, 3rd edn. Lippincott, Williams and Wilkins, Philadelphia, pp 457–537
Hancock SL, Cox RS, McDougall IR (1991) Thyroid diseases after treatment of Hodgkin's disease. N Engl J Med 325:599–605
Hölttä P, Alaluusua S, Saarinen-Pihkala UM et al. (2002) Long-term adverse effects on dentition in children with poor-risk neuroblastoma treated with high-dose chemotherapy and autologous stem cell transplantation with or without total body irradiation. Bone Marrow Transplant 29:121–127
Hoover M, Bowman LC, Crawford SE et al. (1999) Long-term outcome of patients with intraspinal neuroblastoma. Med Pediatr Oncol 32:353–359
Hovi L, Saarinen-Pihkala UM, Vettenranta K et al. (1999) Growth in children with poor-risk neuroblastoma after regimens with or without total body irradiation in preparation for autologous bone marrow transplantation. Bone Marrow Transplant 24:1131–1136
Joyce CRB, O'Boyle CA, McGee H (1999) Individual quality of life: approaches to conceptualisation and assessment. Harwood, The Netherlands
Kajanti M (1983) Neuroblastoma in 88 children: clinical features, prognostic factors, results and late effects of therapy. Ann Clin Res 15 (Suppl 39):1–68
Kaplan MM, Garnick MB, Gelber R et al. (1983) Risk factors for thyroid abnormalities after neck irradiation for childhood cancer. Am J Med 74:272–280
Kaste SC, Hopking KP, Bowman LC et al. (1998) Dental abnormalities in children treated for neuroblastoma. Med Pediatr Oncol 30:22–27
Katzenstein HM, Kent PM, London WB et al. (2001) Treatment and outcome of 83 children with intraspinal neuroblastoma: the Pediatric Oncology Group experience. J Clin Oncol 19:1047–1055
Kelaghan J, Myers MH, Mulvihill JJ et al. (1988) Educational achievement of long-term survivors of childhood and adolescent cancer. Med Pediatr Oncol 16:320–326
Koyle MA, Hatch DA, Furness PD III et al. (2001) Long-term urological complications in survivors younger than 15 months of advanced stage abdominal neuroblastoma. J Urol 166: 1455–1458
Kramer JH, Crittenden MR, Halberg FE et al. (1992) A prospective study of cognitive functioning following low-dose cranial radiation for bone marrow transplantation. Pediatrics 90:447–450
Kushner BH, LaQuaglia MP, Bonilla MA et al. (1994) Highly effective induction therapy for stage 4 neuroblastoma in children over 1 year of age. J Clin Oncol 12:2607–2613
Kushner BH, Cheung NKV, LaQuaglia MP et al. (1996a) Survival from locally invasive or widespread neuroblastoma without cytotoxic therapy. J Clin Oncol 14:373–381
Kushner BH, Cheung NK, LaQuaglia MP et al. (1996b) International neuroblastoma staging system stage 1 neuroblastoma: a prospective study and literature review. J Clin Oncol 14:2174–2180
Kushner BH, Cheung NK, Kramer K et al. (1998) Neuroblastoma and treatment-related myelodysplasia/leukemia: the Memorial Sloan-Kettering experience and a literature review. J Clin Oncol 16:3880–3889
Kushner BH, Wolden S, LaQuaglia MP et al. (2001) Hyperfractionated low-dose radiotherapy for high-risk neuroblastoma after intensive chemotherapy and surgery. J Clin Oncol 19:2821–2828

Le Deley MC, Leblanc T, Shamsaldin A et al. (2003) Risk of secondary leukemia after a solid tumor in childhood according to the dose of epipodophyllotoxins and anthracyclines: a case-control study by the Société Française d'Oncologie Pédiatrique. J Clin Oncol 21:1074–1081

Li FP, Gimbrere K, Gelber RD et al. (1987) Outcome of pregnancy in survivors of Wilms' tumor. J Am Med Assoc 257:216–219

Lipshultz SE, Colan SD, Gelber RD et al. (1991) Late cardiac effects of doxorubicin therapy for acute lymphoblastic leukemia in childhood. N Engl J Med 324:808–815

Lipshultz SE, Lipsitz SR, Mone SM et al. (1995) Female sex and drug dose as risk factors for late cardiotoxic effects of doxorubicin therapy for childhood cancer. N Engl J Med 332:1738–1743

Loebstein R, Koren G (1998) Ifosfamide-induced nephrotoxicity in children: critical review of predictive risk factors. Pediatrics 101:E8

Mäkipernaa A, Heino M, Laitinen LA et al. (1989) Lung function following treatment of malignant tumors with surgery, radiotherapy, or cyclophosphamide in childhood: a follow-up study after 11 to 27 years. Cancer 63:625–630

Matthay KK, Sather HN, Seeger RC et al. (1989) Excellent outcome of stage II neuroblastoma is independent of residual disease and radiation therapy. J Clin Oncol 7:236–244

Matthay KK, Perez C, Seeger RC et al. (1998) Successful treatment of stage III neuroblastoma based on prospective biologic staging: a Children's Cancer Group Study. J Clin Oncol 16:1256–1264

Matthay KK, Villablanca JG, Seeger RC et al. (1999) Treatment of high-risk neuroblastoma with intensive chemotherapy, radiotherapy, autologous bone marrow transplantation, and 13-cis-retinoic acid. N Engl J Med 341:1165–1173

Mayfield JK, Riseborough EJ, Jaffe N et al. (1981) Spinal deformity in children treated for neuroblastoma: the effect of radiation and other forms of treatment. J Bone Joint Surg 63:183–193

Meadows AT, D'Angio GJ, Evans AE et al. (1975) Oncogenesis and other late effects of cancer treatment in children. Radiology 114:175–180

Meadows AT, Baum E, Fossati-Bellani F et al. (1985) Second malignant neoplasms in children: an update from the Late Effects Study Group. J Clin Oncol 3:532–538

Mertens AC, Yasui Y, Liu Y et al. (2002) Pulmonary complications in survivors of childhood and adolescent cancer: a report from the Childhood Cancer Survivor Study. Cancer 95:2431–2441

Mitby PA, Robison LL, Whitton JA et al. (2003) Utilization of special education services and educational attainment among long-term survivors of childhood cancer: a report from the Childhood Cancer Survivor Study. Cancer 97:1115–1126

Neglia JP, Friedman DL, Yasui Y et al. (2001) Second malignant neoplasms in five-year survivors of childhood cancer: Childhood Cancer Survivor Study. J Nat Cancer Inst 93:618–629

Nenadov Beck M, Meresse V, Hartmann O et al. (1995) Long-term pulmonary sequelae after autologous bone marrow transplantation in children without total body irradiation. Bone Marrow Transplant 16:771–775

Nève V, Foot ABM, Michon J et al. (1999) Longitudinal clinical and functional pulmonary follow-up after megatherapy, fractionated total body irradiation, and autologous bone marrow transplantation for metastatic neuroblastoma. Med Pediatr Oncol 32:170–176

Nitschke R, Smith EI, Shochat S et al. (1988) Localized neuroblastoma treated by surgery: a Pediatric Oncology Group Study. J Clin Oncol 6:1271–1279

Notteghem P, Soler C, Dellatolas G et al. (2003) Neuropsychological outcome in long-term survivors of a childhood extracranial solid tumor who have undergone autologous bone marrow transplantation. Bone Marrow Transplant 31:599–606

Ogilvy-Stuart AL, Clark DJ, Wallace WHB et al. (1992) Endocrine deficit after fractionated total body irradiation. Arch Dis Child 67:1107–1110

Olshan JS, Willi SM, Gruccio D et al. (1993) Growth hormone function and treatment following bone marrow transplant for neuroblastoma. Bone Marrow Transplant 12:381–385

Parsons SK, Neault MW, Lehmann LE et al. (1998) Severe ototoxicity following carboplatin-containing conditioning regimen for autologous marrow transplantation for neuroblastoma. Bone Marrow Transplant 22:669–674

Pastore G, Antonelli R, Fine W et al. (1982) Late effects of treatment of cancer in infancy. Med Pediatr Oncol 10:369–375

Pastore G, Zurlo MG, Acquaviva A et al. (1987) Health status of young children with cancer following discontinuation of therapy. Med Pediatr Oncol 15:1–6

Paulino AC, Mayr NA, Simon JH et al. (2002) Locoregional control in infants with neuroblastoma: role of radiation therapy and late toxicity. Int J Radiat Oncol Biol Phys 52:1025–1031

Perez CA, Matthay K, Atkinson JB et al. (2000) Biologic variables in the outcome of stages I and II neuroblastoma treated with surgery as primary therapy: a Children's Cancer Group Study. J Clin Oncol 18:18–26

Phipps S, Brenner M, Heslop H et al. (1995) Psychological effects of bone marrow transplantation on children and adolescents: preliminary report of a longitudinal study. Bone Marrow Transplant 15:829–835

Phipps S, Dunavant M, Srivastava DK et al. (2000) Cognitive and academic functioning in survivors of pediatric bone marrow transplantation. J Clin Oncol 18:1004–1011

Picco P, Garaventa A, Claudiani F et al. (1993) Primary hypothyroidism and ^{131}I-MIBG therapy in neuroblastoma [letter]. Lancet 342:57

Picco P, Garaventa A, Claudiani F et al. (1995) Primary hypothyroidism as a consequence of ^{131}I-metaiodobenzylguanidine treatment for children with neuroblastoma. Cancer 76:1662–1664

Piel J, Meyer D, Perlia CP et al. (1974) Effects of Cis-diamminedichloroplatinum (NSC-119875) on hearing function in man. Cancer Chemother Rep 58:871–875

Plantaz D, Rubie H, Michon J et al. (1996) The treatment of neuroblastoma with intraspinal extension with chemotherapy followed by surgical removal of residual disease: a prospective study of 42 patients – results of the NBL 90 Study of the French Society of Pediatric Oncology. Cancer 78:311–319

Schell MJ, McHaney VA, Green AA et al. (1989) Hearing loss in children and young adults receiving cisplatin with or without prior cranial irradiation. J Clin Oncol 7:754–760

Schiavetti A, Varrasso G, Maurizi P et al. (2001) Two secondary leukemias among 15 children given oral etoposide. Med Pediatr Oncol 37:148–149

Shah NR, Miller DR, Steinherz PG et al. (1983) Acute monoblastic leukemia as a second malignant neoplasm in metastatic neuroblastoma. Am J Pediatr Hematol Oncol 5:309–313

Shalet SM, Beardwell CG, Morris Jones PH et al. (1976) Ovarian failure following abdominal irradiation in childhood. Br J Cancer 33:655–658

Simms S, Kazak AE, Gannon T et al. (1988) Neuropsychological outcome of children undergoing bone marrow transplantation. Bone Marrow Transplant 22:181–184

Simon T, Hero B, Dupuis W et al. (2002) The incidence of hearing impairment after successful treatment of neuroblastoma. Klin Padiatr 214:149–152 [in German]

Skinner R (2003) Chronic ifosfamide nephrotoxicity in children. Med Pediatr Oncol 41:190–197

Skinner R, Pearson ADJ, Amineddine HA et al. (1990) Ototoxicity of cisplatinum in children and adolescents. Br J Cancer 61:927–931

Sklar C (1995a) Growth and endocrine disturbances after bone marrow transplantation in childhood. Acta Paediatr (Suppl) 411:57–62

Sklar CA (1995b) Growth following therapy for childhood cancer. Cancer Invest 13:511–516

Sklar C (1999) Reproductive physiology and treatment-related loss of sex hormone production. Med Pediatr Oncol 33:2–8

Sklar C, Whitton J, Mertens A et al. (2000) Abnormalities of the thyroid in survivors of Hodgkin's disease (HD): data from the Childhood Cancer Survivor Study. J Clin Endocrinol Metab 85:3227–3232

Sonis AL, Tarbell N, Valachovic RW et al. (1990) Dentofacial development in long-term survivors of acute lymphoblastic leukemia: a comparison of three treatment modalities. Cancer 66:2645–2652

Spilker B (ed) (1996) Quality of life and pharmacoeconomics in clinical trials, 2nd edn. Lippincott-Raven, Philadelphia

Staquet MJ, Hays RD, Fayers PM (1998) Quality of life assessment in clinical trials: methods and practice. Oxford University Press, New York

Steinherz LJ, Steinherz PG, Tan CTC et al. (1991) Cardiac toxicity 4 to 20 years after completing anthracycline therapy. J Am Med Assoc 266:1672–1677

Steinherz LJ, Steinherz PG, Tan C (1995) Cardiac failure and dysrhythmias 6–19 years after anthracycline therapy: a series of 15 patients. Med Pediatr Oncol 24:352–361

Stillman RJ, Shinfeld JS, Schiff I et al. (1981) Ovarian failure in long-term survivors of childhood malignancy. Am J Obstet Gynecol 139:62–66

Tabone MD, Terrier P, Pacquement H et al. (1999) Outcome of radiation-related osteosarcoma after treatment of childhood and adolescent cancer: a study of 23 cases. J Clin Oncol 17:2789–2795

Thibaud E, Rodriguez-Macias K, Trivin C et al. (1998) Ovarian function after bone marrow transplantation during childhood. Bone Marrow Transplant 21:287–290

Tucker MA, Morris Jones PH, Boice JD Jr et al. (1991) Therapeutic radiation at a young age is linked to secondary thyroid cancer. Cancer Res 51:2885–2888

Van Santen HM, de Kraker J, van Eck BLF et al. (2002) High incidence of thyroid dysfunction despite prophylaxis with potassium iodide during ^{131}I-metaiodobenzylguanidine treatment in children with neuroblastoma. Cancer 94:2081–2089

Van Santen HM, Vulsma T, Dijkgraaf MG et al. (2003) No damaging effect of chemotherapy in addition to radiotherapy on the thyroid axis in young adult survivors of childhood cancer. J Clin Endocrinol Metab 88:3657–3663

Wallace WH, Shalet SM, Crowne EC et al. (1989a) Ovarian failure following abdominal irradiation in childhood: natural history and prognosis. Clin Oncol (R Coll Radiol) 1:75–79

Wallace WH, Shalet SM, Hendry JH et al. (1989b) Ovarian failure following abdominal irradiation in childhood: the radiosensitivity of the human ovocyte. Br J Radiol 62:995–998

Weatherly RA, Owens JJ, Catlin FI et al. (1991) Cis-platinum ototoxicity in children. Laryngoscope 101:917–923

Weiss B, Vora A, Huberty J et al. (2003) Secondary myelodysplatic syndrome and leukemia following ^{131}I-metaiodobenzylguanidine therapy for relapsed neuroblastoma. J Pediatr Hematol Oncol 25:543–547

Willi SM, Cooke K, Goldwein J et al. (1992) Growth in children after bone marrow transplantation for advanced neuroblastoma compared with growth after transplantation for leukemia or aplastic anemia. J Pediatr 120:726–732

Perspectives and Future Directions

Nai-Kong V. Cheung, Susan L. Cohn

Contents

A hallmark of neuroblastoma (NB) is heterogeneity, with a wide spectrum of clinical behavior which varies according to age at diagnosis, the stage of disease, and tumor biology (Brodeur 2003). This heterogeneity is most evident in the numerous transformation-linked genetic changes identified in cell lines and tumors. Some of these aberrations are predictive of treatment response and outcome (see Chap. 4). Nevertheless, it is increasingly clear that despite such tissue heterogeneity, the clinical biology of NB is generally predictable. By and large, patients with stage-4S and local–regional tumors are curable with minimal or no therapy, whereas children with distant metastatic disease pose an enormous clinical challenge. Only small subsets of patients have elusive risk identities at diagnosis. Modern treatments stratifying patients according to both clinical and biological factors are now the standard (see Chap. 7). At the present time, because of disparities in classification and treatment approaches, it remains difficult to compare the results of clinical trials conducted in different regions of the world; however, efforts are currently underway to develop an International NB Risk Group (INRG) System.

All of the current risk grouping systems utilize age at diagnosis (≤vs >1 year), INSS stage, and tumor *MYCN* status. The COG Risk Classification System also includes tumor histology and ploidy, whereas other cooperative groups have incorporated the pattern of metastatic disease, tumor resectability, and the presence or absence of threatening symptoms (see Chaps. 7 and 11). As currently defined, each of the risk-classification systems has limitations. Small subsets of patients classified as low- or intermediate risk at diagnosis have acted clinically as aggressive disease, whereas other children, currently classified as high risk, have favorable outcomes and may not require the dose-intensive therapeutic approach presently prescribed. Some genetic abnormalities and molecular markers not utilized in the current classification schemas may help refine the definition of risk groups (see Chap. 4–5), and prospective studies investigating their clinical significance are ongoing. In addition, new techniques, such as comprehensive gene expression profiling, are being utilized to molecularly classify NB tumors (see Chap. 9). These studies are likely to lead to a refinement of the current risk-group classification systems and an improvement in risk-group based treatment strategies.

Although substantial progress has been made in the treatment approach toward patients with low- and intermediate-risk NB, the cure rate for metastatic NB in children remains unsatisfactory. As described in Chap. 11, most low-risk patients are successfully treated with surgery alone, and some infants do not require any treatment because their tumors have a high frequency of spontaneous regression (Chap. 2). Even for infants with stage 4 NB, >90% long-term survival is typical if the tumor *MCYN* oncogene is not amplified. Similarly, among patients with intermediate-risk tumors, >90% survival is expected following moderate-dose chemotherapy and surgery. In contrast, outcome remains poor for children older than 1 year with metastatic NB, with or without *MYCN* amplification, and during the past decade there has been only a modest improvement in cure. This small gain is due to intensification of induction chemotherapy, megatherapy consolidation, biological/immunological therapy and improved supportive care. Several clinical trials, including the large prospective randomized CCG-3891 study which demonstrated superior outcome for patients randomized to myeloablative therapy and bone marrow transplant vs chemotherapy during consolidation (Matthay et al. 1999), support the hypothesis that dose intensification is an important component to achieve successful treatment of metastatic NB (Cheung and Heller 1991). Whether intensification is most beneficial during induction or during consolidation remains controversial. Although promising results have also been observed in recent pilot studies testing tandem cycles of high-dose therapy plus stem-cell rescue (Grupp et al. 2000; Kletzel et al. 2002) (Chap. 11), further dose escalation is likely to be unacceptable. In addition, despite achieving complete clinical remission, the majority of children with high-risk disease will relapse due to drug-resistant residual disease. Eradication of refractory microscopic disease remains the most significant challenge in the treatment of metastatic NB. The paradigm of "more is better" should be questioned and additional high-risk trials testing biological and targeted agents need to be designed (Chap. 11).

Recently, the differentiation agent 13-cis retinoic acid was shown to be clinically effective when administered in the setting of minimal residual disease in the randomized CCG 3891 clinical trial (Matthay et al. 1999) (reviewed in Chap. 15). This seminal study demonstrated that a biological agent was capable of impacting outcome in high-risk NB. The COG is currently conducting a randomized prospective study comparing the efficacy of anti-GD2 ch14.18 antibody plus cytokines and 13-cis retinoic acid vs 13-cis retinoic acid alone in the setting of minimal residual disease. Clinical trials have also been developed in Europe to test immunotherapy in high-risk NB, and a single-arm study investigating the efficacy of the anti-GD2 antibody 3F8 plus GM-CSF, is ongoing at Memorial Sloan-Kettering Cancer Center. Additional phase-I and phase-II studies are testing other targeted therapies (see Chap. 12). As outlined in Chaps. 14–17, preliminary studies suggest that several immunotherapeutic molecules, new retinoids, anti-angiogenic agents, and other experimental therapeutics have activity against refractory disease.

As reviewed in Chap. 18, a variety of acute and late complications from NB and its treatment may occur; these include late effects of chemotherapy, radiation therapy, and surgery. High-risk patients are at greatest risk because of the intensive multi-modality treatment strategies that are currently utilized. Reliable identification of the subset of patients currently classified as high risk who do not require intensive therapy would significantly decrease long-term morbidity and treatment-related mortality for these very young patients. For example, data from both the POG and CCG indicate that toddlers 12–18 months of age with favorable biology stage-4 tumors may not require the current intensive high-risk treatment regimen to be cured (Schmidt et al. 2003; George et al. 2003); however, ultimate improvements in survival and reductions of late effects may require more targeted therapies. Research aimed at discovering new genes and pathways critical to NB tumorigenesis and drug resistance should be prioritized. It is hoped that these biologically based treatment approaches will prove to be more effective and less toxic than the current regimens.

We have learned important lessons from NB. The clinical biology of stage-4S and local-regional NB, when combined with the findings of the screening study (Chap. 2), have challenged accepted oncological principles. If clinical progression from local regional small NB to metastatic disease does not generally occur, adjuvant cytotoxic therapy is probably not necessary for the majority of these patients. On the other hand, despite general sensitivity of NB to chemotherapy, curing minimal residual metastasis remains difficult. Research focused on its measurement, control, or eradication should be emphasized. Most important of all, with the growing list of promising therapies, efforts devoted to their timely and effective integration into an overall curative strategy should have high priority.

References

Brodeur GM (2003) Neuroblastoma: biological insights into a clinical enigma. Nat Rev Cancer 3:203–216

Cheung NK, Heller G (1991) Chemotherapy dose intensity correlates strongly with response, median survival, and median progression-free survival in metastatic neuroblastoma. J Clin Oncol 9:1050–1058

George RE, London WB, Maris JM, Cohn SL, Diller L, Brodeur GM, Castleberry RP, Look AT. Hyperdiploidy plus Non-amplified *MYCN* Confers a Favorable Prognostic Group in Children 12 to 18 Month of Age with Disseminated Neuroblastoma: A Pediatric Oncology Group Study. J Clin Oncol (in press)

Grupp SA, Stern JW, Bunin N, Nancarrow C, Ross AA, Mogul M, Adams R, Grier HE, Gorlin JB, Shamberger R, Marcus K, Neuberg D, Weinstein HJ, Diller L (2000) Tandem high-dose therapy in rapid sequence for children with high-risk neuroblastoma. J Clin Oncol 18:2567–2575

Kletzel M, Katzenstein HM, Haut PR, Yu AL, Morgan E, Reynolds M, Geissler G, Marymount MH, Liu D, Kalapurakal JA, Shore RM, Bardo DM, Schmoldt J, Rademaker AW, Cohn SL (2002) Treatment of high-risk neuroblastoma with triple-tandem high-dose therapy and stem-cell rescue: results of the Chicago Pilot II Study. J Clin Oncol 20:2284–2292

Matthay KK, Villablanca JG, Seeger RC, Stram DO, Harris RE, Ramsay NK, Swift P, Shimada H, Black CT, Brodeur GM, Gerbing RB, Reynolds CP (1999) Treatment of high-risk neuroblastoma with intensive chemotherapy, radiotherapy, autologous bone marrow transplantation, and 13-*cis*-retinoic acid. N Engl J Med 341:1165–1173

Schmidt ML, Lal A, Seeger RC, Maris JM, Shimada H, O'Leary M, Gerbing RB, Matthay KK. Favorable prognosis for patients ages 12–18 month with stage 4 MYCN-nonamplified neuroblastoma. J Clin Oncol (in press)

Subject Index

S

T

U

V

W

X

Y

Z